Spinal Cord Injury

SPINAL CORD INJURY

ANDERS HOLTZ, MD, PHD
Department of Neurosurgery
Uppsala University Hospital
Uppsala, Sweden

RICHARD LEVI, MD, PHD
Department of Rehabilitation Medicine
Umeå University Hospital
Umeå, Sweden

New York   Oxford
OXFORD UNIVERSITY PRESS

2010

OXFORD
UNIVERSITY PRESS

Oxford University Press, Inc., publishes works that further
Oxford University's objective of excellence
in research, scholarship, and education.

Oxford   New York
Auckland   Cape Town   Dar es Salaam   Hong Kong   Karachi
Kuala Lumpur   Madrid   Melbourne   Mexico City   Nairobi
New Delhi   Shanghai   Taipei   Toronto

With offices in
Argentina   Austria   Brazil   Chile   Czech Republic   France   Greece
Guatemala   Hungary   Italy   Japan   Poland   Portugal   Singapore
South Korea   Switzerland   Thailand   Turkey   Ukraine   Vietnam

Published by Oxford University Press, Inc.
198 Madison Avenue, New York, New York 10016

www.oup.com

Oxford is a registered trademark of Oxford University Press

Library of Congress Cataloging-in-Publication Data

Holtz, Anders.
[Ryggmärgsskador. English]
Spinal cord injury / Anders Holtz, Richard Levi.
p.   ;   cm.
Translated from Swedish.
Includes bibliographical references and index.
ISBN-13: 978-0-19-537276-2 (alk. paper)
ISBN-10: 0-19-537276-X (alk. paper)
1. Spinal cord—Wounds and injuries.   I. Levi, Richard.   II. Title.
[DNLM: 1. Spinal Cord Injuries—therapy.   2. Spinal Cord Injuries—rehabilitation. WL 400 H758s 2010a]
RD594.3.H6513 2010
617.4'82044—dc22

                                                                2009011161

9   8   7   6   5   4   3   2   1

Printed in the United States of America
on acid-free paper

Preface

In your hands you are holding a translation of the first Swedish textbook on spinal cord injury (SCI), a volume that illuminates this topic from the time of injury through long-term rehabilitation. We had two reasons for writing. First, because we felt a need to document our experiences from the past two decades, during which time we were involved in caring for this group of patients, and second, to help fill a void that has existed in the literature up until now.

The theme of this book could justifiably be considered either extremely narrow or extremely broad. Narrow, because spinal cord lesions—irrespective of cause—are uncommon, much more so than lesions in adjacent structures, such as the brain or spinal column. Broad, since SCI often have far-reaching effects on the function of all body organ systems. And also broad because the care of SCI involves not only a large number of medical specialties, but to a large degree also the allied medical professions, as well as psychosocial and socioeconomic interventions.

Typically, SCI necessitates a dramatic readjustment in lifestyle. From having been free to engage in all activities associated with normal living, post injury even simple routine tasks now become a challenge. In addition to more or less extensive paralysis and sensory deficits below the level of lesion, patients often experience significant impairments involving urination, bowel movements, and sexual function. These deficits, often combined with problems such as pain, spasticity, and pressure ulcers, become a heavy burden for both the individual with the SCI and for family and friends. Preventive measures and treatment of problems resulting from the injury therefore comprise a natural theme for this book.

Definitive treatment—one that can restore neurologic deficits and return the patient to the same level of function that existed prior to the accident—does not yet exist. However, knowledge about the acute mechanisms of injury, emergent treatment at the scene of the accident and in the hospital, and long-term rehabilitation has increased significantly over the past few decades. This is also reflected in encouraging advances in injury prevention, a decrease in acute mortality, an increase in the number of incomplete (partial) versus complete injuries, and improvements in both prevention and treatment of secondary and tertiary complications, as well as more successful rehabilitation to an active lifestyle. Now it has become fully realistic for a person with a SCI to achieve a high degree of autonomy, have a family and a job, drive a car, actively pursue leisure activities, and enjoy a good quality of life for many decades after the time of the injury.

The purpose of this book is to present an overview of the fields of knowledge that are of central importance to the care of patients with SCI. This interdisciplinary approach equates to what is sometimes referred to as "spinal cord medicine." However, readers in many languages have been relegated to individual subsections of diverse texts in fields such as neurology, neurosurgery, orthopedics, rehabilitation medicine, internal medicine, general surgery, and urology. The focus of this book is on our areas of specialization: neurology, neurosurgery, and rehabilitation medicine. Those with special interests may supplement their reading with specialized literature primarily in urology, plastic surgery, hand surgery, andrology, gynecology, algology, psychiatry, and, of course, the crucial areas for rehabilitation outcome represented by the allied medical professions of physical therapy, occupational therapy, behavioral sciences, and the like. Largely for this reason, and in order to facilitate further study, we have provided a fairly comprehensive bibliography and reference section.

We hope that a broad readership with a variety of backgrounds will find this book to be useful and that as a whole, it will serve as an introduction to the care of this challenging patient group.

ACKNOWLEDGMENTS

In addition to acknowledgments to colleagues at the end of specific chapters, we would like to thank Kerstin Sund and Elisabeth Gustafsson for help with the content and Lena Lyons for creating the beautiful illustrations. Anders Holtz would like to thank his entire family, from Adam to Britt Maria, for everything from photos to moral support. Richard Levi would like to extend his warmest thanks to Prof. Åke Seiger; Mr. Göran Lagerström and Dr. Claes Hultling; as well as to his family for their continual encouragement and support.

Uppsala and Umeå, April 2010
Anders Holtz
Richard Levi
anders.holtz@akademiska.se
richard.levi@rehabmed.umu.se

Contents

SPINAL CORD INJURY

1 | History

Our historical knowledge of spinal cord injury (SCI) originates in ancient Egyptian society (Third Dynasty, 3000–2500 years BC). During this relatively peaceful era, great resources were dedicated to construction work, and most of all to the creation of the pyramids. It was possible, for the first time, to describe a variety of injuries seen within a relatively large population exposed to a high incidence of trauma. In 1862, the Egyptologist Edwin Smith purchased documents from this period describing different injuries to the human body. These documents are regarded as one of the world's most valuable treasures of medical history. The documents, later named the *Edwin Smith Papyrus*, contain 48 cases of trauma including six cases of spine and/or SCI. The case reports do not differentiate between injuries to the spinal column and the spinal cord. Imhotep, an Egyptian official and architect responsible for the step pyramid of Sakkara and a practicing surgeon, probably wrote the papyrus. The documents are dated to approximately 2500 BC and clearly illustrate biomechanics, clinical evaluation and diagnosis, treatment, and prognosis following different injuries ranging in severity from mild distortions without neurological impairment to fractures leading to complete SCI. In the classical case report number 33 "Instructions concerning a crushed vertebra in his neck" (here illustrated with a modern magnetic resonance imaging [MRI] sequence in Fig. 12.16), a complete SCI caused by a fracture in the cervical region is described. A vertebral body has been crushed against an adjacent one as a result of the flexed position of the head at the moment of injury.

The clinical status includes paralysis of both arms and legs (tetraplegia), loss of sensation below the level of injury, and loss of control of the urinary bladder. The patient also showed persistent involuntary painful erection (priapism)

and ejaculation. The case report is concluded with a declaration of the treatment strategy of that time—"an ailment not to be treated." The Egyptians refrained from surgical interventions but relieved urinary retention by using bronze catheters.

The next known reference to traumatic SCI is dated to the time of the Trojan War (circa 1100 BC). Three immortal brothers, Zeus, Poseidon, and Hades, ruled the sky and the living, the seas, and the nether world, respectively. In the epic tale of the Odyssey, the youngest of Odysseus' companions, Elpenor, fell from the palace roof, broke his neck, and his soul went down to Hades.

Seven hundred years later, Hippocrates (circa 460–377 BC), the "father of medicine," analyzed the relationship between vertebral injuries and paralysis. He observed that if damage to the spinal cord only occurred on one side, a subsequent paralysis always was located on the same side as the damage. Until the time of Hippocrates, Aesculapius, the sun-god Apollo's son, was considered in the Greek mythology to be the god of medical healing, and the ancients believed that all such healing flowed from him. With his observations and practical application of basic medical knowledge, however, Hippocrates succeeded in separating medicine from mythology. Because of his efforts, medicine became a worldly and rational endeavor. He is the main author of the book *Corpus Hippocraticum*, which summarizes the medical knowledge of that time, and in it he describes for the first time the clinical condition of chronic paralysis.

Hippocrates presents the difficulties, such as constipation, painful urination, pressure sores, and leg swelling, associated with the aftermath of traumatic SCI. He advocated a diet consisting of four to nine pints of milk combined with honey and a special mild white wine from Mendez in Egypt to mitigate these problems.

On Hippocrates advice, pressure sores were treated with exposure to the air in combination with the direct application of wine, juice, vinegar, and oils, as well as aluminum salt and lead. He recommended that the bandages be changed every third day to avoid infections.

The ancient Greeks frequently used spinal manipulations to manually reduce malformations. Hippocrates introduced two devices, the Hippocratic ladder and the Hippocratic board for this purpose (Fig. 1.1). The patient was placed in a prone position and was stretched from the shoulder area upward, and from the hips

downwards A medical orderly then either sat or stood on the deformity until reduction; alternatively, a wooden board was placed crosswise over the injured area to achieve a similar compression.

Only few fragments of written documentation remain regarding SCI from the Greco-Roman era. Aulus Cornelius Celsus, working during the 1st century BC, built upon the medical tradition of Hippocrates. He became aware of the importance of the spinal cord itself, and he was probably the first to document rapid death as a consequence of a cervical SCI. Celsus introduced the closing of small open pressure sores with female hair as suture material. Within the field of medicine, the Greco-Roman era was

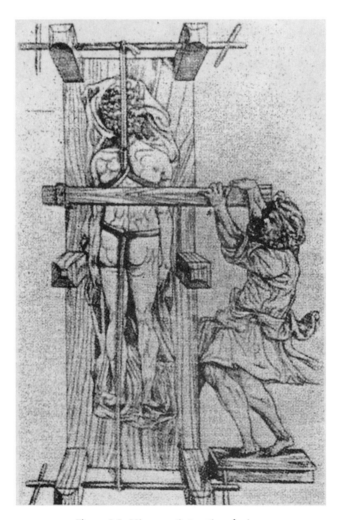

Figure 1.1 Hippocratic traction device.

represented by two prominent figures, Galen and Paul of Aegina.

The Greek Galen (129–199 AD), physician-in-ordinary to the Emperor Marcus Aurelius and also called the "second Hippocrates," was the first to report on the effect of experimental incisions of the spinal cord. Galen noted that a longitudinal incision to the spinal cord did not result in any symptoms but a transverse incision at the level of the second and third cervical vertebrae results in loss of motion and sensory functions below the level of the incision. He also described the number of vertebrae comprising the different parts of the spinal column and introduced the terms *scoliosis*, *lordosis*, and *kyphosis*.

The famous surgeon Paul (625–690), from the Greek island of Aegina, described the importance of clinical examination. He concluded that a fracture of the vertebra should be suspected if the physician was unable to palpate the spinous process belonging to the damaged vertebra. He proposed, on these occasions, the following treatment: "Make an incision of the skin externally and extract it (the fractured bone) and unite the wound with sutures." This is the first time that the removal of vertebral arches (i.e., a laminectomy) is described as a treatment for spinal fractures, and Paul of Aegina is considered the originator of this procedure.

Documents from India dated to the second and third century mention immobilization as a treatment option for fractures in the lumbar region. The *Sushruta Samhita*, a Sanskrit text on surgery, describes patients being laid on a table to which they were bound with ropes to correct spinal deformities. Hindu descriptions of treating spinal deformities with axial traction precede Hippocrates by a millennium.

Medical science during the medieval period was hampered by superstition and intellectual stagnation. Western medicine during this period is regarded as primitive, and was predominantly practiced by monks. The most important medical reference during this period, *The Canon of Medicine*, was written by the Persian astronomer and physician Avicenna (Ibn Seena).

Leonardo da Vinci (1452–1519) was the first to describe the physiological curvatures of the spine, and he also suggested the importance of the neck muscles in contributing to the stability of the cervical spine. His dissections of the spine formed the basis for highly detailed drawings of the joints, vertebrae, muscles, and tendons.

After nearly a thousand years of medical stagnation, in 1543, during the Renaissance, the Flemish anatomist and physician Andreas Vesalius published one of the greatest medical books ever written (Fig. 1.2). This treatise of seven volumes entitled *De Humani Corporis Fabrica* (The Fabric of the Human Body), contains for the first time drawings in which the human nervous system is correctly illustrated. The illustrator Johann Stephan van Calcar produced all the drawings for Vesalius' work. Because, until that time, the anatomical conception of the human body as presented by Galen had been based on studies done on monkeys, not humans, the work of Vesalius constitutes the first textbook to present human anatomy in a detailed and correct fashion.

The German surgeon Fabricius Hildanus in 1646 described a method to reduce dislocations in the cervical region. A clamp was inserted through the spinous processes in the neck, after which traction was applied. This closed reduction was supplemented by open reduction if necessary.

A very special event from a surgical point of view, happened, during the battle of Amenenburg in 1762. The surgeon Andre Louis successfully removed a bullet lodged in the lumbar spine, and the patient not only survived, but also regained functional movement in the lower extremities.

During the 19th century, two famous persons died following SCI. The first, Lord Nelson (Fig. 1.3), flaunting his characteristic and highly visible scarf, was shot in the thoracic spine during the battle of Trafalgar in 1805. He became paralyzed and died shortly after. Lord Nelson survived long enough to describe his paralysis to the ship's surgeon, Dr. Beatty, as follows: "That all power of motion and feeling below my chest are gone and you very well know that I can live but a shorter time." Doctor Beatty replied: "My Lord, unhappily for our country, nothing can be done to you."

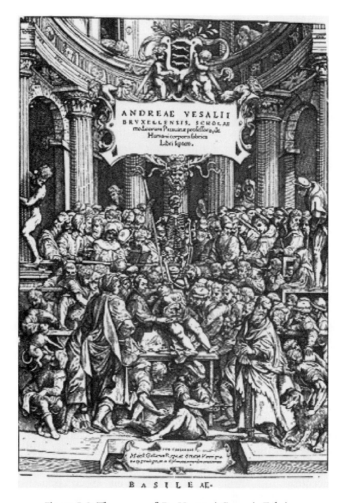

Figure 1.2 The cover of *De Humani Corporis Fabrica*.

The second celebrity, James Abram Garfield, the 20th president of the United States, became victim of an attempted assassination by a crazed gunman in Washington D.C., in 1881. One bullet lodged itself somewhere inside the President's body and was later found during autopsy a few inches from the spinal canal. The famous scientist and inventor Alexander Graham Bell devised a metal detector specifically for the purpose of finding the bullet, but the metal bed frame on which Garfield was lying made the instrument malfunction and the bullet was not found. The president died a few months later as a result of internal bleeding and infection, the latter probably caused by insertion of unsterilized instruments into the wound.

In 1814, the English surgeon Henry Cline performed a laminectomy at the thoracic level. The patient, who suffered a fracture and a SCI, died nine days later. This resulted in a quite nihilistic attitude toward this type of surgical intervention, as is illustrated by the following quotation from 1824: "Laying a patient upon his belly and by incisions laying bare bones and exposing the spinal marrow itself, exceeds all beliefs." However, a successful laminectomy performed following trauma was reported soon thereafter in 1829, by the American surgeon Gilpin Smith. The operation resulted in improved sensibility and the progressive neurological deterioration seen before surgery was reduced. Charles Bell introduced the clinically important concepts of spastic and

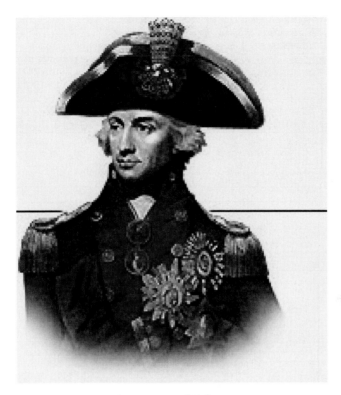

Figure 1.3 Lord Nelson.

flaccid paralysis in 1824, and he also described the concept of spinal shock.

During World War I, mortality following SCI was as high as 80% within the first two weeks following injury. Given these poor prognostic figures, a nihilistic attitude toward treatment persisted during the 1920s and 1930s, until the modern era of rehabilitation began in 1943. In that year, the Stoke Mandeville National Spinal Injuries Centre was opened in England by neurosurgeon Sir Ludwig Guttmann. A similar pioneering work was conducted by Bors in the USA. The well-structured and comprehensive rehabilitation at the center did not only help patients survive but also to readapt to society. The Stoke Mandeville Centre was, and is still, a model for many other rehabilitation units around the world. The implementation of the treatment model developed by Guttmann, together with concurrent progress within other fields of medicine, has prolonged the survival time for this group of patients by approximately 2000% since 1940.

Modern care of the SCI patient requires knowledge within a variety of medical fields such as rehabilitation, urology, intensive care, algology, orthopedics, neurosurgery, fertility, and pharmacology, and also an interest in research and development. At present, the goal of healing the injured spinal cord is still out of reach. There exist, however, many therapeutic measures to offer the SCI patient as to improve his health and quality of life. Within the field of SCI, the main focus of research is currently directed toward neuroprotection and, especially, regeneration. Another ongoing challenge within the area of rehabilitation is to offer treatments in order to ensure a long, healthy, and fulfilling life.

Suggested Reading

Lifshutz J, Colohan A. A brief history of therapy for traumatic SCI. *Neurosurg Focus* 2004;16(1):1–8.

Sonntag VKH. History of spinal disorders. In: Menezes AH, Sonntag VKH, eds., *Principles of Spinal Surgery*. New York: McGraw-Hill, 1996:3–23.

Wilkins RH. Neurosurgical classic: XVII Edwin Smith Surgical Papyrus. *Neurosurgery* 1964; March:240–244.

Wiltse LL. The history of spinal disorders. In: Frymoyer JW, ed., *The Adult Spine: Principles and Practice*. New York: Raven Press, 1991:3–42.

Internet

Fabulous historical overviews, entitled "History of Spinal Surgery" were presented in the digital edition of *Neurosurgical Focus* in January 2004. One excellent manuscript illustrates the history of SCI (see Lifshutz and Colohan, above). www.thejns.org Search for Lifshutz J, Colohan A. A brief history of therapy for traumatic SCI. *Neurosurg Focus* 2004;16(1):1–8. The manuscript is for free.

2 Epidemiology

Trauma to the vertebral column and spinal cord may result in a broad spectrum of injuries. Such injuries span the spectrum from simple soft-tissue injuries, via isolated vertebral fractures, to the most serious form of injury—a transection of the spinal cord. Few patient groups are as meticulously classified as those with SCI, and an abundance of epidemiological data are recounted in the medical literature. The majority of statistics referred to in this chapter is taken from the National SCI Database, which was established in 1973 and captures data from 15% of the SCI population in the United States. Table 2.1 summarizes the most pertinent facts.

INCIDENCE AND PREVALENCE

The incidence i.e., the annual rate of acute traumatic SCI varies in industrialized countries between about 10 and 50 cases per million inhabitants. In the United States, the incidence is estimated at about 40 cases per million; thus, every year about 12,000 persons sustain an acute traumatic SCI. The prevalence (i.e., the number of persons presently living with such injuries) is estimated at 850 per 100,000 inhabitants in the United States.

AGE

Over 50% of all spinal injuries occur in persons between the ages of 16 and 30. The mean age is just over 33 years. Advancing age is accompanied by increasing spinal column stiffness (particularly in certain spinal disorders such as ankylosing spondylitis), degenerative encroachment of the spinal canal and foramina, and osteoporosis of the spinal column. Under these circumstances even low-energy trauma may result in a serious SCI.

GENDER DISTRIBUTION

Approximately 80% of all traumatic SCI patients are men. This gender distribution reflects the fact that certain high-risk behaviors are more common among men (especially young men).

EXTENT OF NEUROLOGICAL INJURY

Residual Function Below the Level of Injury

Almost 50% of all traumatic SCI results in complete loss of function below the level of injury. This equates to an American Spinal Injury Association Impairment Scale (AIS) grade A injury; grades B, C, and D are associated with incomplete impairment below the level of injury. Each of these grades corresponds to progressively less severe impairment. Interestingly, the proportion of patients with complete SCI has dropped from 70% in 1969 to 44% in 2004. This may be the result of safer cars, better care at, and transport from, the scene of the injury to the hospital, and improved care focusing on the special problems seen in patients with acute SCI.

Level of injury

About 55% of all traumatic injuries to the spine affect the cervical spine. The remaining lesions involve the thoracic spine, the thoracolumbar transition (T11–T12 to L1–L2), and the lumbar spine and sacrum (L2–S5), with 15% of injuries occurring at each level. Injuries to the thoracic spine more frequently result in complete SCI than do injuries at other levels. Among patients who are immediately judged to have a clinically complete injury, the prognosis for some return of neurological function is better the higher the level of SCI.

TABLE 2.1 Epidemiological data relating to traumatic SCI in a European country (Sweden).

Incidence	10–15
Prevalence	5,000
Age	
Mean age at injury	31 years
Age at injury <30 years	50–70%
Age at injury >50 years	25%
Gender	
male: female	4:1
Completeness of lesion	
Complete	45%
(AIS A)	
Incomplete	
AIS B	15%
AIS C	10%
AIS D	30%
Level of lesion	
Cervical spine	55%
Thoracic spine	15%
Thoracolumbar spine	15%
Lower lumbar spine and sacrum	15%
Ratio of paraplegia to tetraplegia	3:2
Most common level of injury	
Cervical	C5
Thoracic	Th12
Most common etiology	
Motor vehicle accidents	40–50%
Relationship to moderate/severe head injury	
SCI: head injury	1:30
Remaining life expectancy (injured at 20 years of age)	
High tetraplegic	33 years
Low tetraplegic	39 years
Paraplegic	44 years

The occurrence of SCI is further subdivided by the AIS as:

- Tetraplegia (complete) 20%
- Tetraparesis (incomplete) 30%
- Paraplegia (complete) 30%
- Paraparesis (incomplete) 20%

Paresis refers to incomplete injury, which means that some degree of residual neurological function is present below the level of injury. *Plegia* and *Paralysis* refer to complete injury. *Tetra* indicates neurological involvement of both arms and legs, whereas *para* indicates that only the lower extremities are involved. The most common level of neurological injury in the cervical spine is C5. Among paraplegics, T12 is the most common level of neurological injury.

ETIOLOGY

Motor vehicle accidents are by far the most common cause of acute SCI (44%). Accidents related to acts of violence (24%), falls (22%), sports (8%), and other factors (2%) are other common causes. In Europe, falls are more commonly the cause of SCI, and in some countries falls have become the dominant cause. Additionally, the presence of acts of violence varies considerably between regions and over time.

Relationship to Head Injuries

According to the U.S. Centers for Disease Control (CDC), for each case of traumatic SCI there occurs about 30 cases of moderate (Glasgow Coma Scale [GCS] 9–13) to severe (GCS 3–8) traumatic brain injury.

In about 20% of cases, other severe injuries, such as brain and thoracic injuries, also occur among SCI patients. Only one-fifth of acutely injured SCI patients have an isolated spinal cord lesion.

SOCIOECONOMIC DATA

In addition to the personal tragedy associated with SCI for the patient and family, society is also burdened by massive costs resulting from these injuries and their sequelae. The cost of medical care for the first year for a patient with high tetraplegia is estimated at $800,000; for a patient with low tetraplegia it is estimated at over $500,000; and for a patient with paraplegia at $300,000. If a person sustains a SCI at the age of 25, lifetime medical costs are estimated at over $3.3 million in the case of high tetraplegia, $1.8 million for low tetraplegia, and $1.1 million for paraplegia. About half of all acutely injured patients are single at the time of injury. The marriage rate is about 60% lower and the divorce rate is about 2.5 times higher than in the noninjured population.

MORTALITY AND LIFE EXPECTANCY

The immediate or early mortality for this patient group is probably relatively high and largely dependent on other injuries such as head injury, multiple trauma, and/or respiratory arrest in cases of high tetraplegia. However, mortality during subsequent hospital care is only 3% during the acute phase. In the past, death over the long term was mainly due to renal failure. Advances in urinary tract management have led to a significant reduction in renal failure as cause of death. Instead, deaths today are predominantly due to cardiovascular diseases, pneumonia, pulmonary emboli, and septicemia.

The remaining life expectancy of individuals injured at age 20 has been calculated to:

- 33 years with high tetraplegia
- 39 years with low tetraplegia
- 44 years with paraplegia

High tetraplegia usually refers to a neurological level of injury at C5 or higher (see Chapter 8). The prognosis for long-term survival is particularly unfavorable among ventilator-dependent patients.

Suggested Reading

DeVivo MJ, Vogel LC. Epidemiology of spinal cord injury in children and adolescence. *J Spinal Cord Med* 2004;27(Suppl 1):S4–S10.

Divanoglou A, Levi R. Incidence of traumatic spinal cord injury in Thessaloniki, Greece and Stockholm, Sweden: a prospective population-based study. *Spinal Cord* April 2009. Epub ahead of print.

Furlan JC, Krassioukov AV, Fehlings MG. The effects of gender on clinical and neurological outcomes after acute cervical spinal cord injury. *J Neurotrauma* 2005;22(3):368–381.

Garrison A, Clifford K, Gleason SF, et al. Alcohol use associated with cervical spinal cord injury. *J Spinal Cord Med* 2004;27(2):111–115.

Kirshblum S, Millis S, McKinley W, Tulsky D. Late neurological recovery after spinal cord injury. *Arch Phys Med Rehab* 2004;85(11):1818–1825.

Kraus JF, Silberman TA, McArthur DL. Epidemiology of spinal cord injury. In: Menezes AH, Sonntag VKH, eds., *Principles of Spinal Surgery*. New York: McGraw-Hill, 1996:41–58.

Krause JS, Zhai Y, Saunders LL, Carter RE. Risk of mortality after spinal cord injury: an 8-year prospective study. *Arch Phys Med Rehabil* 2009; 90(10):1708–1715.

Levi R. The Stockholm spinal cord injury study: medical, economical and psycho-social outcomes in a prevalence population (doctoral dissertation). Stockholm: Karolinska Institutet, 1996.

National Spinal Cord Injury Data Base. *Arch Phys Med Rehab* 1999;80(11):1363.

Tator C. Epidemiology and general characteristics of the spinal cord-injured patient. In: Tator CH, Benzel CH, eds., *Contemporary Management of Spinal Cord Injury: From Impact to Rehabilitation*. Park Ridge, IL: American Association of Neurological Surgeons, 2000:72–73.

3   Anatomy and Physiology

A brief review of the spinal cord anatomy and physiology is presented in this chapter. The spinal cord transmits sensory information to the brain and also plays a crucial part in the regulation of motor and autonomic function. Knowledge of some basic anatomy and physiology, will make it easier to understand the clinical conditions presented later in this book. We have deliberately omitted description of vertebral column anatomy here; the anatomy of the spinal column and adjacent supporting structures will be illustrated in Chapters 10–15, in association with the presentation of fracture classifications.

GROSS ANATOMY

The human spinal cord is cylindrical in appearance and has a diameter of approximately 1 cm. It is slightly flattened anteriorly as well as posteriorly. The spinal cord originates from the caudal part of the medulla oblongata. It leaves the skull through the foramen magnum and extends down into the vertebral canal (Fig. 3.1A,B,C). Caudally, in adults, it ends approximately at the disk level between the first and second lumbar vertebrae (L1 and L2), and its length ranges between 42 and 45 cm. The spinal cord is divided, in the craniocaudal direction, into the pars cervicalis, pars thoracica, pars lumbalis, and pars sacralis. The pars cervicalis, for example, corresponds to that part of the spinal cord from which eight pairs of cervical spinal nerves emanate. The spinal cord contains two thicker regions – intumescentia cervicalis and lumbalis. The cervical enlargement (intumescentia cervicalis) is located between the fifth cervical (C5) and the first thoracic (T1) vertebrae. The spinal nerves originating from the intumescentia cervicalis comprise the brachial plexus that innervates the upper limbs. The

lumbar enlargement (intumescentia lumbosacralis) gives rise to nervous structures forming the lumbar (L1–L5) and sacral (SI–S3) plexus, which innervate the lower limbs.

The terminal end of the spinal cord becomes narrower in shape and is denoted the *conus medullaris*. It contains the sacral segments responsible for sensory information from the lower part of the abdomen and genitals, for regulation of motor sphincter functions and for parasympathetic innervation of the bladder wall and distal part of the bowel (Fig. 3.1C; see same figure in the Color Plate section).

The caudal extension of the conus medullaris is called the *filum terminale*. It is enclosed in the pia mater and extends down to the coccyx. The filum terminale is finally attached, together with the dural sac extension (coccygeal ligament), to the coccygeal periosteum. The spinal cord is localized centrally in the spinal canal by result of this attachment. Nerve roots originating from the lumbar and sacral level surround the filum terminale. The bundles of nerves resembles a horse's tail, and this structure is thus called the *cauda equina*. Horizontal extensions of the pia mater are attached through the arachnoid to the dural sac on each side of the spinal cord between the dorsal and ventral roots. These structures, the *ligamenta denticulata*, are located between the foramen magnum and the vertebral level of T 12 to L1 and prevent the spinal cord from undesired movements.

The spinal cord contains 31 pairs of spinal nerves (8 cervical, 12 thoracic, 5 lumbar, 5 sacral and 1 coccygeal; Fig. 3.1A) and their corresponding 31 segments. Each pair of nerve roots exits the spinal canal through the intervertebral foramina. The first seven pairs of cervical nerve roots exit through the intervertebral foramina above the correspondingly numbered vertebra.

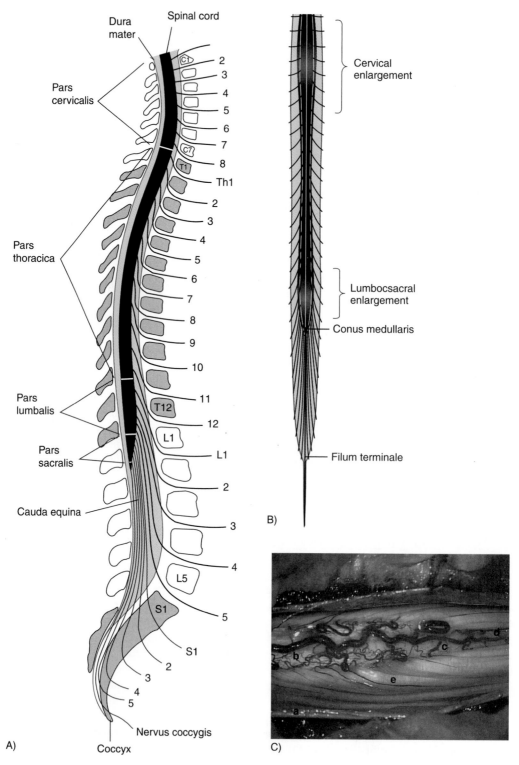

Figure 3.1 Spinal cord topography. A: Side view. B: Front view C: Exposed spinal cord. *a*, dural sac; *b*, spinal cord; *c*, conus medullaris; *d*, filum terminale; *e*, dorsal nerve root. See also Color Plate Fig. 3.1C.

However, the eighth pair of cervical nerve roots leave the spinal canal between the C7 and T1 vertebra due to the existence of only seven cervical vertebrae. The thoracic, lumbar, sacral and coccygeal nerve roots then exit through intervertebral foramina located below the correspondingly numbered vertebra. The third thoracic pair of nerve roots, as an example, extends through the intervertebral foramina between the third and fourth vertebral bodies.

The lengths of the spinal column and spinal cord are equal in the first trimester of fetal development. Connections are established during that period between the peripheral structures such as skeletal muscle fibers and spinal nerves, the latter extending through the intervertebral foramina almost horizontally. The vertebral column then grows caudally during the second and third trimester of development. The spinal cord, however, does not extend to the same degree. Consequently, each part of the spinal cord is located more cranial to its corresponding vertebra. The length of each nerve root located in the spinal canal increases the more caudally the pair of nerve root exits the spinal canal as a result of this discrepancy in growth. The shortest intraspinally located pair of nerve roots are thus located within the cervical spine and the longest at the sacral level.

The relation between vertebral spinous processes and corresponding spinal cord segments can be estimated as follows. As rule of thumb, add one to the number of the spinous processes of C2–C5 to obtain the corresponding segment of the spinal cord. Correspondingly, add two between the spinous processes of C6–T6, and finally add three in the interval between T7–T10. The spinous process of the fifth thoracic vertebra is, for example, located at the level of the seventh thoracic segment of the spinal cord.

The spinous processes of T11–T12 are located at the level of the fifth lumbar spinal cord segment and the spinous process of LI is located at the level of the fifth sacral spinal cord segment. This discrepancy between the numbering of vertebrae and spinal cord segments has important clinical implications. For example, patients exhibiting deteriorated sensory function from the T9 segment (dermatome)

and below usually suffer from fractures located at the level of the T6 vertebra.

The Spinal Cord Meninges

Three layers of coverings (i.e., spinal meninges; Fig. 3.2A,B) surround the spinal cord. The outermost of these, the *dura mater*, consists of elastic connective tissue and forms a sheath around the spinal cord. The spinal dura is single-layered and lacks the periosteal layer of the cranial dura. It is therefore separated from the inner surface of the bone forming the spinal canal, leaving a potential space between the dura and the bony surface, the *epidural space*. This space contains mainly fatty tissue and venous plexuses. The spinal dura extends cranially to the level of foramen magnum and joins the inner meningeal layer of the cranial dura. Caudally, approximately at the level of the second sacral vertebra, the dural sac becomes narrower, in order to cover the filum terminale, and is finally attached to the coccygeal periosteum.

The *arachnoid membrane,* the middle covering, is attached to the inner surface of the dural sac. Normally, there is no space between these two coverings, and the arachnoid membrane follows the dural sac caudally to the level of S2, where the cauda equina is finally enclosed. The innermost layer, the *pia mater,* covers spinal cord. The pia mater continues caudally as the filum terminale and attaches with dural sac to the coccygeal periosteum, thereby preventing unnecessary movement of the spinal cord.

The subarachnoid space, i.e., that space between the arachnoid membrane and pia mater, contains cerebrospinal fluid (CSF). The lumbar cistern, i.e., that area of the spinal canal containing the most CSF, is located between the second lumbar and second sacral vertebral bodies (Fig. 3.3). This enlargement of the subarachnoid space is routinely accessed for sampling of CSF. Lumbar puncture ("spinal tap") is performed with low risk despite the proximity of multiple nerve roots in the cistern. These nerve roots, bathed in the CSF, slide away from the contact of the needle and are not injured during the procedure.

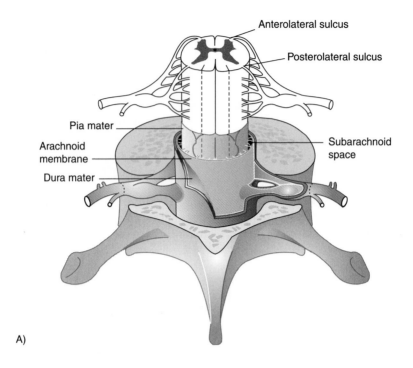

A)

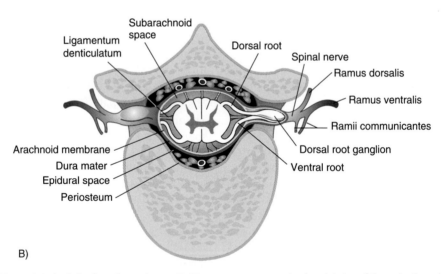

B)

Figure 3.2 A: Spinal cord meninges. B: Nerve root anatomy in the vicinity of the spinal cord.

NEUROANATOMICAL OVERVIEW

Each spinal nerve contains a dorsal root transmitting sensory information and a ventral root regulating the activity of the skeletal muscles. Spinal nerves are connected to their corresponding body segment during the early stage of development in order to innervate appropriate muscle groups (myotomes) and sensory areas (dermatomes). Sensory (afferent) information from, for example, pain, temperature, and touch receptors, is transmitted from the body to the spinal cord via the *dorsal roots* (Figs. 3.1C, 3.2B, 3.4, and 3.5). The dorsal roots enter the

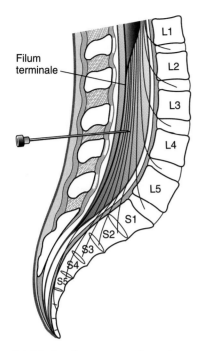

Filum
terminale

Figure 3.3 The lumbar cistern and its relation to the cauda equina and filum terminale.

spinal cord through the *posterolateral sulcus,* located in the posterior area of the spinal cord. The cell bodies belonging to the afferent nerve fibers are located in the dorsal root (spinal) ganglia.

The *ventral roots* transmit motor (efferent) signals from the spinal cord to skeletal muscles and leave the spinal cord through the *anterolateral sulcus*. The dorsal and ventral roots merge just distally to the spinal ganglion, at the level of the intervertebral foramina, to create a spinal nerve. Each spinal nerve represents a body segment and thus contains sensory as well motor nerve fibres (Fig. 3.2A,B). Each spinal nerve root divides into a ventral and dorsal branch (ramus ventralis and ramus dorsalis), both of which incorporate sensory and motor nerve fibers, shortly after they exit the intervertebral foramina.

A transverse section of the spinal cord shows central butterfly- or H-shaped gray matter surrounded by peripherally located white matter (Figs. 3.4 and 3.5). The gray matter consists mainly of nerve cell bodies giving rise to ascending and descending pathways, local neurons (interneurons), and glial cells (supportive cells). The surrounding white matter contains ascending and descending myelinated and unmyelinated axons and glial cells. The white appearance is caused by the presence of myelin, which is mainly composed of lipids. The gray matter acts as the "computer" of the spinal cord, while the white matter provides the gray matter with a network of connecting "cables."

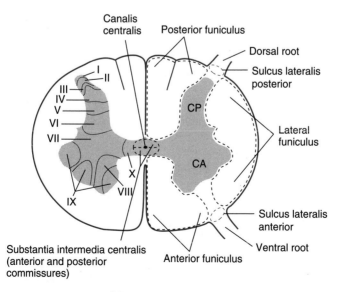

Figure 3.4 Neuroanatomic organization of the spinal cord. *CP*, cornu posterior; *CA*, cornu anterior. Roman numerals indicate the cytoarchitectonic map according to Rexed.

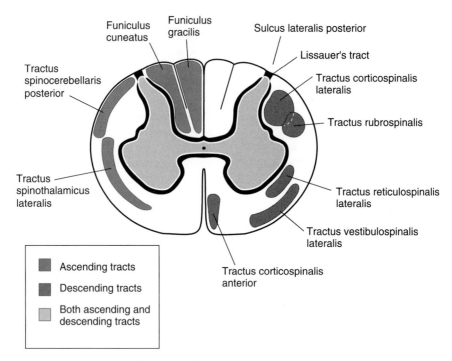

Figure 3.5 Cross-sectional illustration showing the distribution of the spinal cord pathways.

Gray Substance (Substantia Grisea)

Both halves of the gray matter are connected at the midline by a structure called the *substantia intermedia centralis* (Fig. 3.4). The anterior and posterior part of the substantia intermedia centralis is also called the anterior and posterior commissure, respectively. The central canal (canalis centralis) is located in the center of the gray substance and serves as a CSF pathway between the fourth ventricle in the brainstem and the ventriculus terminalis, which constitutes the ventricular system termination in the conus medullaris. The H-shaped gray matter is further divided, on the left as well as the right side, into anterior and posterior horns, the cornu anterior and posterior, respectively. The entire gray substance is also divided into ten laminae named after the Swedish neuroanatomist, Bror Rexed. The Rexed laminae I–VI constitute the posterior horn, while the laminae VII–X are located in the anterior horns and substantia intermedia centralis.

Nerve cells mediating sensory (afferent) information are, as previously mentioned, located in the posterior horns. Neurons, with their cell bodies located in the dorsal root ganglia, transmit impulses to neurons in the posterior horns via *synapses*. The sensory information is thereafter either conveyed cranially to centers in the brain or into the local spinal cord circuitry. The anterior horn contains mainly motor neurons innervating skeletal muscles and interneurons. Lateral horns (not illustrated) are found in the thoracic and upper two lumbar segments of the spinal cord only. They contain preganglionic sympathetic neurons which belong to the autonomic nervous system. The axons of the lateral horns exit the spinal cord through the ventral roots together with the axons of the motor neurons.

White Substance (Substantia Alba)

White matter is composed of, as previously mentioned, bundles of ascending and descending myelinated and unmyelinated axons (fasciculi or tracts) running in a craniocaudal direction. A bundle containing two or more tracts is called a *funiculus*. The white matter contains three funiculi on each side of the midline, the anterior, lateral, and posterior funiculi (Figs. 3.4 and 3.5). The posterior funiculi from C1 to T6 are subdivided into a medial (fasciculus gracilis) and lateral part (fasciculus cuneatus). Axons coursing within the gray matter of one segment constitute the basis for the segmental reflex arc. Bundles running just outside the gray matter form intersegmental (propriospinal) tracts that interconnect spinal cord segments. Finally, there are neurons connecting both the segmental and intersegmental tracts, with centers mainly located in the brain.

SPINAL CORD PATHWAYS

Ascending Tracts

Posterior Funiculi

The posterior funiculi are often referred to as the dorsal (posterior) columns (Figs 3.5 and 3.6). The heavily myelinated axons located in the posterior columns are responsible for conscious proprioception: kinesthesia (sense of position and movement) and discriminative touch (ability to separate two points and to localize touch stimuli). Injuries to the dorsal columns lead to reduced or lost ability for vibratory sense, stereognosis (the capacity to identify the form and shape of various objects), two-point tactile discrimination, touch, and weight perception ipsilaterally caudally to the level of injury. The sensory fibers entering the spinal cord below the sixth thoracic segment form the *fasciculus gracilis*, whereas those entering above that level form the *fasciculus cuneatus*. The vast majority of the sacral and cervical nerve cell axons are located medially and laterally in these pathways, respectively.

Complete damage to the dorsal columns results in loss of position and movement ability, and this sensory loss leads to clumsy, poorly coordinated movements. This condition is referred to as *dorsal column ataxia* or *sensory ataxia*.

Posterior Spinocerebellar Tracts

The posterior spinocerebellar tracts are uncrossed pathways that convey proprioceptive information—sensory signals from receptors in joints, tendons, and muscles—to the cerebellum. Most of the impulses reach the spinal cord through the dorsal roots and fasciculus

gracilis after which they synapse, one or two segments cranially, in nucleus dorsalis located in Rexed lamina VII. Corresponding information above the level of C8 is transmitted via the fasciculus cuneatus to the medulla oblongata. The proprioceptive information is integrated with impulses from mechanoreceptors of the inner ear by the cerebellum, providing a basis for maintenance of body balance and position.

The Anterolateral System

The anterolateral systems, which includes the lateral spinothalamic tracts, constitutes one of the most important clinical pathways in the spinal cord (Figs. 3.5 and 3.7). This pathway transmits pain and temperature impulses from the skin, joint capsules, and skeletal muscle to the thalamus. Cell bodies of the peripheral sensory

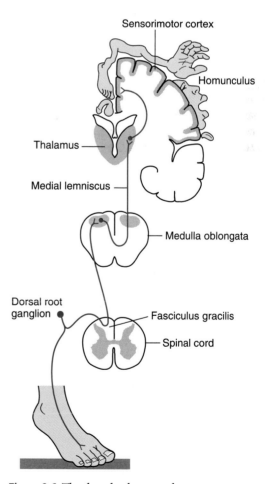

Figure 3.6 The dorsal column pathway.

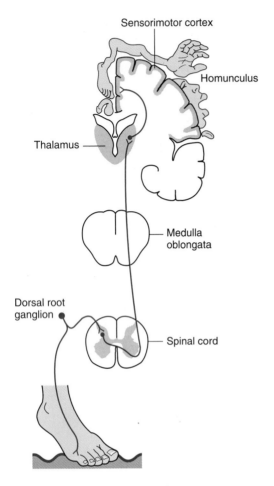

Figure 3.7 The lateral spinothalamic tract.

neurons are located in the dorsal root ganglia. Impulses from these primary sensory neurons synapse in Rexed lamina I–V in the posterior horn and are further transmitted by secondary sensory neurons to the thalamus before reaching cerebral cortex.

These secondary neurons cross the midline through the anterior white commissure one or two segments above their entrance into the spinal cord, forming the lateral *spinothalamic tract*. The spinothalamic tract is located in the anterior part of the lateral funiculus, and the ascending fibers show a somatotopic organization. Fibers originating from the sacral and lumbar parts are located dorsolaterally, whereas those arising from the cervical part are located ventromedially; that is, inversely compared to the organization of the dorsal column.

Lesions located in the lateral funiculus will produce a diminished or lost sensation of pain and temperature on the contralateral side of the lesion, starting one or two segments below the lesion. A similar loss of function is observed following damage to the primary sensory neurons, although these patients lose sensation of pain and temperature in one ipsilateral segment at the level of injury. This distinction is of importance in determining if pain originates from the spinal cord or from a peripheral nerve lesion.

Lesions to the anterior commissure result in a bilateral segmental loss of pain and temperature sensation corresponding to the level of injury. This pattern of symptoms is seen following the formation of intramedullary cavities involving the anterior commissure in the central area of the spinal cord, a condition denoted *syringomyelia*. The remaining sensory qualities are unimpaired, producing a condition known as *dissociated sensory loss*. The Brown-Séquard syndrome, caused by a hemisection of the spinal cord (see Fig. 5.3) presents partly with an ipsilateral loss of pain and temperature sensation as a result of a lesion to the anterior commissure and partly with loss of these qualities on the opposite side of the body starting one or two segments below the level of injury, since the spinothalamic tract crosses the midline.

The anterolateral system also contains neurons transmitting information from superficial touch receptors. These neurons synapse in Rexed laminae III–V (Fig. 3.4), and secondary sensory neuron axons cross the midline through the white commissure in several segments. Light touch sensation is also mediated through other pathways, such as the dorsal columns. Lesions located exclusively in the anterolateral tracts do not, therefore, result in a loss of sensation for light touch, whereas the ability to feel itch, tickle, and sensual touch will disappear since these sensation qualities are solely transmitted by the anterolateral tract.

Descending Tracts

Corticospinal Tracts

The corticospinal tract originates from the cerebral cortex and is considered the most important descending pathway. The axons pass laterally to the diencephalon, through the brainstem, and terminate within the spinal cord. The corticospinal tract consists mainly of nerve cells that influence spinal cord motor neurons. The overall function is consequently to mediate voluntary movements in skeletal muscles. Between 80% and 90% of the nerve fibers cross to the contralateral side at the transition between the medulla oblongata and spinal cord (the pyramidal decussation), and the lateral corticospinal tract is formed (Figs. 3.5 and 3.8). The somatotopic organization established in the cortex persists, and cervical fibers are located medially and are followed in a lateral direction by the thoracic, lumbar, and sacral nerve fibers. The lateral corticospinal tract influences spinal cord motor neurons innervating the upper and lower limbs, and mediates skill and precision in

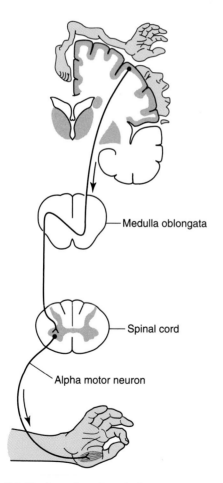

Figure 3.8 The lateral corticospinal tract.

Medulla oblongata

Spinal cord

Alpha motor neuron

movement. This tract is considered particularly important in regulating the precise movements of the fingers. About 10–20% of the nerve fibers of the corticospinal tract remain uncrossed as they descend to the spinal cord, and these fibers form the anterior corticospinal tracts. This pathway contributes to the innervation of muscle located in the neck and trunk. It contains consequently both uncrossed nerve fibers as well as nerve fibers crossing the midline segmentally in the spinal cord before they synapse with contralaterally located neurons.

The neurons forming the corticospinal tracts are called *upper motor neurons*. The α-motor neurons located in the anterior horn of the spinal cord and their axons innervating the skeletal muscles are the *lower motor neurons*. Acute lesions affecting the upper motor neurons result initially in a complete block of the nervous activity below the lesion, since stimulation of the segmental reflex activity ceases. These patients present with a flaccid paralysis of muscles, muscular hypotonia and, also, a loss of bowel and urinary bladder reflexes (*spinal shock*) as conduction activity is lost. If, the lesion is located above T6, symptoms such as bradycardia and hypotension will also appear. This circulatory condition is called *neurogenic shock*. The segmental reflex activity returns within a few days or weeks following the acute motor neuron lesion, due to activation of previously "silent" synapses and sprouting activity of surviving axons finding new possibilities for synaptic connections. Symptoms such as spasticity, hyperactive bowel and bladder, tendon reflex activity, and presence of the Babinski sign indicate returning nervous activity. However, a partial or complete inability to perform voluntary motor activity often remains also after the spinal shock has resolved.

Extrapyramidal Tracts

The extrapyramidal tracts refer to the pathways and nuclei that, in addition to the pyramidal tracts, mediate voluntary movements. The *tractus rubrospinalis* consists of axons that cross the midbrain in midline. They originate from neurons located in the nucleus ruber and travel through the spinal cord in the lateral funiculus. The function of this tract is, according to the standard view, connected to the lateral corticospinal tract and associated with mediation of voluntary movements. The *lateral vestibulospinal tract* is an uncrossed tract originating from neurons located in the lateral vestibular nucleus situated in the borderland between the medulla oblongata and the pons. It regulates extensor muscle tonus, in order to maintain the upright position. The more devastating lesions to the lateral spinothalamic tract often camouflage the

consequence of injuries to this tract. The *medial vestibulospinal tract* cooperates with the labyrinths of the inner ear to control head position. The *reticulospinal tracts* contain neurons originating from the formatio reticularis located in the brainstem at the level of the pons and medulla oblongata. The pathways are uncrossed and descend down to the anterior and lateral funiculi of the spinal cord. It has been demonstrated in animal studies that this pathway modulates voluntary muscle movements, muscle tone, reflex activity, and breathing capacity.

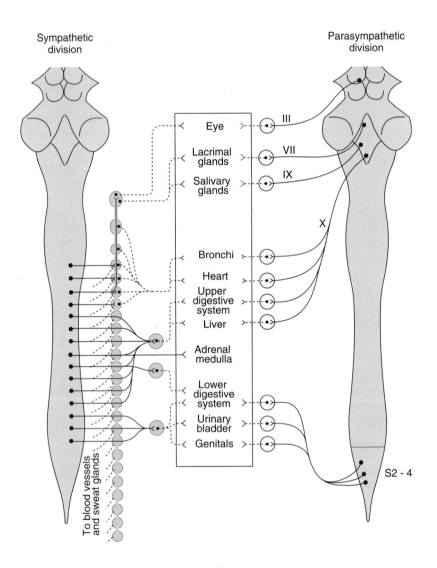

Figure 3.9 The autonomic nervous system.

Autonomic Nervous System

The autonomic nervous system regulates automatic and involuntary functions that maintain the internal environment of the body (Fig. 3.9). Blood pressure, respiration, heart rate and contractile force, reproductive hormone levels, renal function, and body temperature are some examples of the functions regulated by the autonomic nervous system. The autonomic pathways originate in the hypothalamus, where different regulating centers are located. The autonomic nervous system is divided into the sympathetic and parasympathetic nervous system. The descending tracts are mainly located in the lateral funiculi and end in the preganglionic sympathetic and parasympathetic neurons located in the brainstem and at the levels of T1–L2 and S2–S4, respectively. The sympathetic nerve fibers join the sympathetic chain located bilaterally on the anterior part of the vertebral body, while the parasympathetic fibers descend to the lower part of the urinary tract and bowel. A lesion occurring above or at the level of T1 results in *Horner syndrome*, due to damage of the sympathetic innervation to the eye. The consequence of an injury to the descending autonomic pathways innervating the preganglionic parasympathetic neurons above the level of S2 is a loss of normal bowel and bladder function, as well as impotence.

BLOOD SUPPLY OF THE SPINAL CORD

Arterial Blood Supply

Vessels from the intracranial part of both vertebral arteries (Figs. 3.10 and 3.11) supply the spinal cord. Multiple segmentally arranged branches, the radicular arteries, originating in part from the cervical part of the vertebral arteries and in part from the posterior intercostal arteries (Fig. 3.12) also provide arterial blood flow to the spinal cord.

Anterior Spinal Artery

One anterior and two posterior branches arise from each vertebral artery. The anterior branches unite and form the anterior spinal artery (Figs. 3.10 and 3.11). The anterior two-

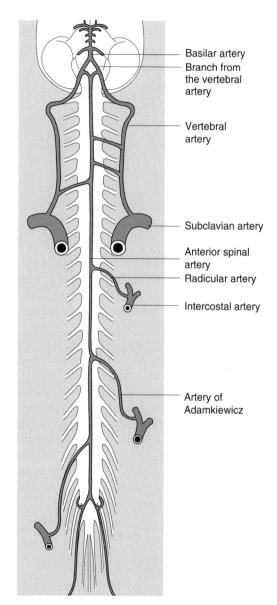

Basilar artery

Branch from the vertebral artery

Vertebral artery

Subclavian artery

Anterior spinal artery

Radicular artery

Intercostal artery

Artery of Adamkiewicz

Figure 3.10 The longitudinal arterial supply of the spinal cord.

thirds of every spinal cord segment is supplied by the anterior spinal artery. Damage to these vessels result in the anterior cord syndrome characterized by dissociated sensory loss. It includes bilateral loss of pain and temperature sensations (lesions of both the lateral spinothalamic tracts) and preserved deep sensations (kinesthesia and discriminative touch) since the posterior funiculi is spared (see also Chapter 5).

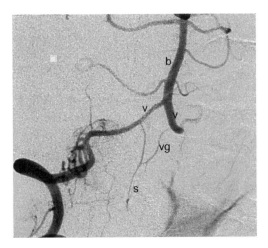

Figure 3.11 Angiography illustrating the merging of vertebral arteries (*v*) forming the basilar artery (*b*). Each vertebral artery contributes one branch (*vg*) that unites and forms the anterior spinal artery (*s*).

Posterior Spinal Artery

The posterior spinal arteries arise from the vertebral arteries as those run on the surface of the medulla oblongata. The posterior spinal arteries descend on the posterior surface of the spinal cord slightly medial to the posterior roots (Fig. 3.12). They supply the posterior one-third of the spinal cord. Anastomotic arteries, the *vasocorona arteries*, located between the anterior and posterior circulation, supply the peripheral part of the lateral funiculi (Fig. 3.12).

Radicular Arteries

Segmental vessels, the spinal rami of the intercostals arteries, join the nerve roots as they pass through the intervertebral foramina, after which they bifurcate into an anterior and posterior radicular artery (Fig. 3.13). The radicular arteries merge with the anterior and posterior circulation, respectively, creating a circumferential arterial supply to the spinal cord. One of the anterior radicular arteries in the lumbar region, the artery of Adamkiewicz, has a larger diameter compared to the other. This vessel is typically located on the left side and enters the spinal cord in its lower thoracic or upper lumbar part. The artery of Adamkiewicz is vital for the circulation of the anterior two-thirds of the spinal cord, including the lumbosacral enlargement. Damage to the artery of Adamkiewicz leads to infarction of the spinal cord and usually a subsequent paraplegia. The largest distance between two major contributing radicular vessels is seen in the thoracic part of the spinal cord. The interval between T1 and T4 and the L1 segment are consequently particularly vulnerable levels. Occlusion of only one of the radicular arteries in this sensitive area may

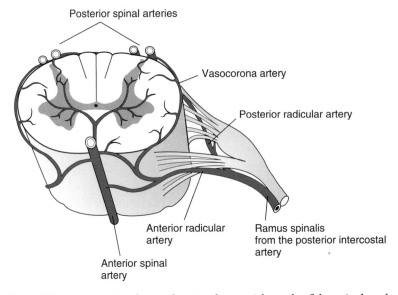

Figure 3.12 Cross-sectional view showing the arterial supply of the spinal cord.

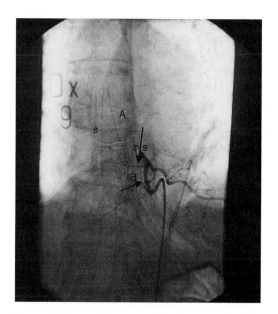

Figure 3.13 Spinal angiography depicting a segmental intercostal artery (*ia*). The ramus spinalis artery (*rs*) exits the intercostal artery and passes through the intervertebral foramen (vertical arrow.) The radicular artery of Adamkiewicz (*A*) continues into the anterior spinal artery (*s*).

result in an infarction and severe clinical symptoms.

Spinal Cord Veins

The spinal cord veins exhibit a pattern similar to that of the spinal arteries. Six veins drain the spinal cord. Three are located anteriorly and three posteriorly. They communicate with each other and are drained by anterior and posterior radicular veins. These vessels empty into the anterior and posterior epidural venous plexus, respectively, after which the plexuses pass cranially in the spinal canal and through the foramen magnum. The venous blood is finally emptied into the veins and dural sinuses of the skull. The epidural venous plexuses also communicate with external plexuses located on the surface of the vertebral bodies. The spinal cord veins lack valves, which increases the risk of dissemination of tumor cells and microorganisms as valves normally present a mechanical obstacle to such dissemination.

SPINAL CORD REFLEXES

Physiologically, signals from the brain, spinal cord, and peripheral nerves interplay. The spinal cord may metaphorically be considered a "cable" connecting the brain with the rest of the body in this interplay. However, it should also be considered as a "satellite" of the brain since an abundance of activities are initiated and modulated without the influence of the brain. The spinal cord reflexes and some activities related to the ability to walk could be given as illustrations of these spinal cord initiated and mediated activities. The spinal reflexes are partly autonomic, related to smooth muscle and partly somatic, related to the striated skeletal musculature. A brief overview of the somatic spinal cord reflexes will be given in this chapter, while the autonomic reflexes will be described later in chapters presenting various organ systems. Knowledge of the intrinsic activity of the spinal cord is of importance in understanding spasticity and other motor disturbances following lesions to the spinal cord, and for the rationale behind the development of certain treatment strategies.

The Stretch Reflex

Muscle fiber stretching stimulates muscle spindles, and reflexogenic contractions are initiated as a result of this stimulation. The afferent nerve impulses are directly relayed to the α-neurons of the spinal cord. The α-neurons discharge, resulting in contraction of the activated muscle. This is an example of a *monosynaptic reflex* (Fig. 3.14).

The sensitivity of muscle spindles is regulated by the γ-motor neurons located in the anterior horn of the spinal cord. Increased γ-motor neuron activity results in increased contraction of certain muscle fibers, the *intrafusal muscle fibers*, in the muscle spindles. The muscle spindle sensitivity to stretching of the muscle increases following the contraction of intrafusal muscle fibers.

A simultaneous contraction of the antagonist to the activated muscle will be prevented by impulses emanating from the activated muscle, which activates inhibitory interneurons located in the spinal cord. This mechanism is called *reciprocal inhibition*.

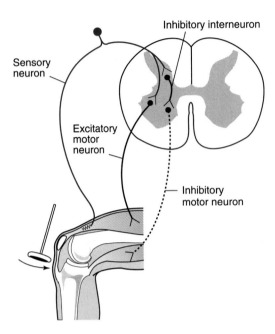

Inhibitory interneuron

Sensory neuron

Excitatory motor neuron

Inhibitory motor neuron

Figure 3.14 Monosynaptic stretch reflex.

The activity of the α-motor neurons is also regulated through collateral nerve fibers. This additional regulation of the α-motor neurons is mediated by inhibitory interneurons, the so called *Renshaw cells*. This mechanism is denoted *recurrent inhibition*, and it blocks an extensive discharge frequency from the α-motor neurons.

Muscle fibers also contain so-called *Golgi tendon organs*, which are located at the insertion of skeletal muscle fibers into their corresponding tendons. The Golgi tendon organs record muscle tension and are thus activated during muscle contractions. This stimulation initiates afferent impulses that inhibit contraction of the muscle (autogenic inhibition or Golgi inhibition) and stimulate antagonist muscles spindles.

Flexor Reflex

The flexor reflex (Fig. 3.15) is initiated by nociceptive stimuli, as, for instance, when you tread on a nail.

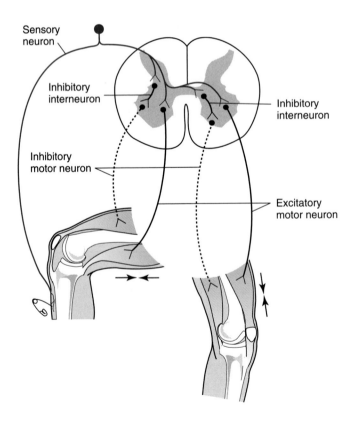

Sensory neuron

Inhibitory interneuron

Inhibitory motor neuron

Inhibitory interneuron

Excitatory motor neuron

Figure 3.15 Flexor reflex.

Afferent impulses, initiated by pain receptors, synapse via interneurons to ipsilaterally located flexor muscles, after which the flexor muscles contract. A simultaneous contraction of the extensor muscles located ipsilaterally is inhibited. Impulses also reach the contralateral side of the spinal cord, resulting in an opposite pattern of muscle activity. The extensor muscles thus contract while flexor muscle activity is inhibited.

A connection exists between the afferent limb of the flexor reflex and normal walking pattern. So-called "central pattern generators" have been found, causing an oscillating activity between the flexion and extension neurons.

ACKNOWLEDGMENTS

The authors would like to express their gratitude to Professor Håkan Aldskogius, Department of Neuroscience, Neuroanatomy, University of Uppsala. His knowledge and enthusiasm has strongly contributed to this chapter.

Suggested Reading

Er U, Fraser K, Lanzino G. The anterior spinal artery origin: a microanatomical study. *Spinal Cord* 2008; 46(1):45–49. Epub 2007 April 3.

Felten D, Jozefowicz RF, eds. *Netter's Atlas of Human Neuroscience*. ISBN 1–929007–16–7.

Goshgarian HG. Anatomy and function of the spinal cord. In: VW Lin, ed., *Spinal Cord Medicine. Principles and Practice*. New York: Demos Medical Publishing, 1996:15–34.

Özgen S, Pait TG, Caglar YS. The V2 segment of the vertebral artery and its branches. *J Neurosurg Spine* 2004;1(3):299–305.

Sobotta J. In: Putz R, Pabst R, eds., *Atlas of Human Anatomy*. Elsevier Science, 2008. ISBN 9780702033230.

Watson C. *Basic Human Neuroanatomy: An Introductory Atlas*. New York: Little Brown, 1995.

4

Pathophysiology

Injuries to the spinal cord typically occur following severe trauma, such as that caused by vehicular accidents or falls. Extraspinal injuries and complications are often seen in several organ systems both acutely, as well as in later stages. This chapter addresses the posttraumatic events that occur locally in the spinal cord.

Our knowledge about the complex pathophysiological processes that are seen following trauma to the spinal cord has increased during the last decades, although crucial pieces of the puzzle are still missing. A close cooperation between basic scientists and scientifically active clinicians has been established to map and better understand the various mechanisms that are activated following an injury to the spinal cord. However, most of our knowledge regarding these processes has been obtained from experimental animal studies (Table 4.1).

ANIMAL EXPERIMENTAL MODELS

Trauma to the spinal cord activates a variety of mechanisms, each of which might influence spinal cord function and viability. The acute, millisecond instance when the spinal cord is compressed by a fractured vertebral body, for example, is often followed by a sustained compression caused by extruded disk material, fractured bone, or hematoma. It has therefore been difficult to establish an "ultimate SCI model" mimicking all such components. Rather, several complementary models have been developed, each of which represents to a varying degree the true events in the pathophysiology of SCI.

The most commonly used method is the weight-drop technique, introduced by Allen in 1911, causing a contusion to the cord (Table 4.1). This kinetic model reflects the initial damage caused by a blow to the cord in the clinical setting. The device used in the experimental situation consists of a cylinder, placed perpendicularly to the spinal cord, and a plastic impounder that rests on the intact dura mater. A weight is then dropped from a predetermined height, resulting in a kinetic impact to the spinal cord. The intensity of the injury is described in terms of gram–centimeter–force (GCF).

By contrast, static models, in which the spinal cord is compressed but not impacted, represent yet another component of the real-life injury mechanism. Here, the load is sustained for up to several minutes by a steady compression, thus reflecting an aspect of "true" trauma different from the very transient and abrupt kinetic impact caused by the weight-drop technique. The compression model mimics a clinical situation in which sustained compression is caused by, for example, bony fragments, extruded disk material or epidural hematoma (Fig. 4.1).

MORPHOLOGICAL DEFINITIONS

The morphological damage to the spinal cord following trauma can, according to Hulsebosch, be classified into four morphological characteristics (see Table 4.1).

1. **Cord maceration** results in extensive morphological changes affecting the entire cross-section of the spinal cord. All structures are more or less damaged (destroyed/crushed).

2. **Laceration injury** (e.g., gunshot or knife wound) typically results in a sharp transection of the spinal cord.

3. **Contusion injury** is characterized by a central hemorrhage mainly located in the

gray matter of the spinal cord. This causes a conduction block in the initial phase, even if the surround-ing white matter is not severely damaged. The hemorrhage is absorbed over time and replaced in the chronic stage either by a cavity or by a widening of the central canal.

4. **Solid cord injury** is characterized by the absence of a central focus of damage. Changes are instead observed in patches across the entire cross-section of the spinal cord.

The first two categories are characterized by damage to the surface of the spinal cord. Here, a substantial amount of connective tissue will be seen growing into the spinal cord during posttraumatic healing. The remaining two types of injuries are characterized by an intact surface and minimal connective tissue penetration into the spinal cord. In reality, however, the spinal cord is not usually subjected to a singular type of injury, and this is reflected clinically by a very mixed variety of symptoms and signs.

The type(s) of injury is of great importance in the management of the SCI patient. The amount of immediately and irreversible injured tissue is high when cord maceration and laceration dominate the injury pattern. Neurological function is then irrevocably lost, and no currently extant treatment can improve or restore that function.

The contusion injury is the most common morphologic type of injury (Fig. 4.2A–C). This type of injury does not result in immediate irreversible tissue damage, since the amount of lacerated and macerated nervous tissue is relatively low. Instead, this injury is progressive in nature. The initial (primary), mechanically induced damage to the nervous and other tissues initiates a cascade of secondary tissue destructive reactions. This progressive nature of tissue destruction provides the prerequisite window of opportunity for treatment, which aims at preventing the effects of the secondary injury mechanisms. Contusion injury models are the most frequently used animal models, and the results from such experiments constitute the basis of our knowledge about the course of events following trauma to the spinal cord.

Characteristic morphological changes occur in the spinal cord over time following trauma. The extent of these changes is related to the type and severity of trauma. Small petechial bleeding formed by seeping through the injured endothelium of the blood vessels, is observed within 5–15 minutes of injury (Fig. 4.2A). Mechanical trauma is also responsible for centrally located hemorrhage into the gray matter. Damage to the endothelium of the blood vessels, axon destruction, and accumulation of inflammatory mediators as a result of reduced spinal cord blood flow, thus *ischemia*, is seen as early as 4 hours after injury. These ischemic changes are visualized in areas that initially show signs of hemorrhagic necrosis (cell death) and that develop, in the late stage, into cavities. These morphological changes result in loss of impulse propagation and consequently loss of neurological function below the level of lesion.

PRIMARY SPINAL CORD INJURY

The pathophysiological events following a lesion to the spinal cord are customarily divided into primary and secondary, followed by a chronic stage (Table 4.2). The primary injury mechanism corresponds to the acute mechanical damage, whereas subsequent secondary injury mechanisms consist of a cascade of vascular, biochemical, and cellular processes, initiated by the primary injury. The duration of the acute period varies according to the literature from minutes to days.

Primary injury to the spinal cord is caused by the initial mechanical impact in combination with sustained pressure caused by bony fragments, blood, and disk material. Vertebral body dislocations and/or severe ligamentous injuries may initiate similar compression mechanisms even in the absence of concomittant fractures. The mechanical damage to the spinal cord caused by the primary injury is considered irreversible. No presently known treatment can restore disrupted axons and injuries to the blood vessels. The acute primary injury is thus characterized by an immediate mechanical injury, which typically causes a centrally located bleed in the gray matter, affecting both the nervous tissue and vascular structures. This sudden

TABLE 4.1 Animal experimental models of SCI

Model	Performance	Mimicking	Morphological definitions
Contusion injury			
Weight-drop technique	Different weigths are dropped from a predetermined height on the exposed dura sac (gram-centimeter-force (GCF).	Initial millisecond impact to the spinal cord	3 Contusion injury
Compression injury			
Extradural-balloon technique	A balloon located between the dura sac and vertebral arch is rapidly inflated with liquid.	Sustained compression caused by bone, blood and/or disk material	1 + 3 Cord maceration + contusion injury
Blocking-weight technique (Fig. 4.1)	A predetermined weight is gradually applied on the exposed dura.		
Crush injury			
Extradural clip compression	Modified aneurysm clips exerting various closing forces are applied extradurally around the exposed spinal cord	Initial millisecond impact to the spinal cord	1 Cord maceration
Miscellanous			
Transection	The spinal cord is transected with a scalpel	Laceration injury following knife wound and/or gunshot	2 Laceration injury
Aortic occlusion	The aorta is closed below the renal artery	Ischemia	4 Solid cord injury

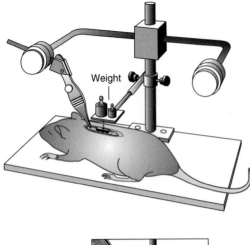

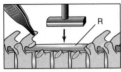

Figure 4.1 Static compression injury model. R = exposed dural sac.

mechanical damage results in tissue necrosis in contused areas; this damage seems to adversely affect the gray matter earlier in the injury process than the white matter. A ring of preserved white matter surrounding the necrotic gray tissue thus remain in the post-acute period.

The injured nerve cells, during the first minutes following trauma, initiate increased firing of action potentials before impulse conduction ceases. An intracellular increase of sodium and calcium and an extracellular increase of potassium to toxic levels are examples of ionic derangements observed. These early changes consequently result in a failure of normal impulse transmission.

SECONDARY SPINAL CORD INJURY

The secondary injury mechanisms begin within minutes to days following injury. These mechanisms include a variety of processes that, taken individually or together, lead to cellular damage and, ultimately, to cell death (see Table 4.2). Vascular and biochemical changes, inflammation, edema, and apoptosis are examples of key mechanisms occurring in the period after acute mechanical damage.

VASCULAR MECHANISMS

A transient increase in systemic arterial blood pressure, followed by hypotension, is seen in immediate connection to the injury. These cardiovascular alterations are caused by the response of the sympathetic nervous system. The sustained hypotension, together with the damage to the spinal cord itself, results in a decrease in spinal cord blood flow. It has been proposed that this reduction in spinal cord blood flow is the major contributing factor behind most of the dynamic secondary injury mechanisms. The term *hypoperfusion* describes a situation with impaired or reduced spinal cord blood flow without reaching the critical threshold to result in damage to the spinal cord tissue. *Ischemia* occurs if the reduction of spinal cord blood flow is severe enough and the duration of the reduction persists long enough so that tissue injury appears. Various secondary injury mechanisms are triggered as a consequence of ischemia, and those contribute to an ongoing destruction (autodestruction) of spinal cord tissue.

Changes in spinal cord blood flow may affect initially undamaged tissues of the gray and white matter in various ways. Local minor bleeding and reduced spinal cord blood flow can be observed in the gray matter after only 5 minutes. A correlation exists between the degree of spinal cord blood flow reduction and the severity of spinal cord tissue damage. It has been shown in animal experiments that spinal cord blood perfusion remains reduced for at least 24 hours following the initial insult. The blood flow in the white matter is simultaneously reduced after 5 minutes, but, conversely to that in gray matter, resumes relatively quickly, sometimes within 15 minutes of initial insult, if permitted by the condition of the tissue. Vascular changes, such as damaged microcirculation and reduced or eliminated autoregulation, are responsible for reduced spinal cord blood flow, subsequent ischemia, and ultimate cell death.

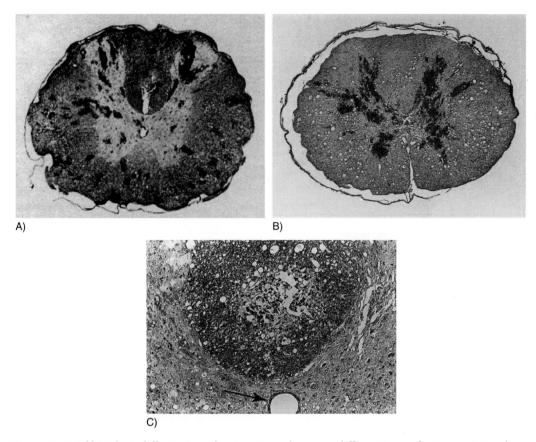

Figure 4.2 Axial histological illustrations showing tissue changes at different times after injury. A: One hour post-injury. Observe the small petechial bleedings mainly located in the gray matter. B: Twenty-four hours post-injury. Extensive bleeding is seen in the gray matter. Blister-like vacuoles are seen within the white matter. C: Nine days after injury. A necrotic area is seen in the posterior column region. The central canal is indicated with an arrow.

Damage to the microcirculation is caused by vasospasm, mediated by excitatory amino acids, accumulation of blood cells that occlude the vessels (thrombosis), and edema in the endothelial cells, forming the walls of the tiny capillaries.

Circulatory autoregulation is an important function which is altered by tissue injury. It comprises processes which help maintain homeostasis in the body. Vital organs, such as the brain and spinal cord, are normally guaranteed a fairly constant blood flow within a range of systolic blood pressure of 50 to 160 mm Hg, regardless of the degree of blood supply to other less-vital organ systems. By contrast, spinal cord blood flow in injured areas becomes virtually totally dependent on systemic blood pressure when autoregulatory ability is lost. Since systemic hypotension will develop if the SCI is severe enough, a loss of autoregulation therefore results in significantly reduced perfusion of damaged areas. It has been shown in animal experimental models that autoregulation remains intact during the first 60–90 minutes following an injury to the spinal cord, after which time a gradual loss occurs. This happens in conjunction with a simultaneous reduction of spinal cord blood flow and the development of ischemia. Logically, counteracting the hypotension, for example by elevating systemic blood pressure, should compensate for the loss of autoregulation. Hypothetically, this would improve

TABLE 4.2 Pathophysiological mechanisms

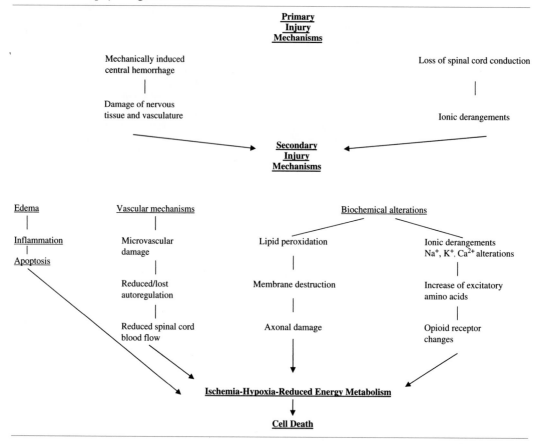

spinal cord blood flow and reduce the cascade of secondary injury processes. This is a very important aspect in the emergency treatment of this group of patients.

BIOCHEMICAL CHANGES

It is widely accepted that biochemical alterations play an important role in the aftermath of SCI. Here we briefly present certain events that have been the focus of research during the past few decades (for review see Table 4.2).

Axonal Damage Caused by Free Oxygen Radicals

Free oxygen radicals (Fig. 4.3) are naturally occurring byproducts that occur after various biochemical reactions. These radicals are characterized by the presence of unpaired or single

Superoxide dismutase (SOD; cofactored with Cu/ZN or Mn)

$$2 \cdot O_2^- + 2H^+ \rightarrow H_2O_2 + O_2$$

Catalase

$$2H_2O_2 \rightarrow 2H_2O + O_2$$

Figure 4.3 The endogenous defense mechanisms that lead to the formation of free oxygen radicals.

electrons (O_2^-) in the outer electron shell. The formation of these molecules occur during the normal metabolism of oxygen, and takes part in the oxidation of polydesaturated fatty acids in the lipid-containing cell membranes (lipid peroxidation) of the central nervous system (CNS). The free oxygen radical superoxide (O_2^-) is normally formed during mitochondrial metabolism and is later detoxified to hydrogen peroxide (H_2O_2) by the enzyme superoxide dismutase. The H_2O_2 is eventually converted by the enzyme catalase to water (H_2O) and oxygen (O_2). The protective effect of these enzymes on these reactive (toxic) free oxygen radicals may, metaphorically, be compared to that of a sponge which absorbs liberated free oxygen radicals and converts them to H_2O and O_2.

Changes in the oxidative mechanisms are seen following injury to the spinal cord. Iron (Fe^{2+}) is, for instance, released from hemoglobin, and the extremely powerful hydroxyl radical ($\cdot OH$) is formed instead of H_2O_2 (Fig. 4.4). The hydroxyl radicals initiate an accelerated lipid peroxidation, a process somewhat similar to the growth of a snowball rolling downhill. This process begins only a few minutes after trauma. It results in the breakdown of the polydesaturated fatty acids in the lipid-containing cell membranes and

---

Fentons reaction

$$Fe^{2+} + H_2O_2 \quad Fe^{3+} + \cdot OH + OH^-$$

Haber-Weiss reaction catalysed by iron ions

$$\cdot O_2^- + H_2O_2 \rightarrow \cdot OH + HO^- + O_2$$

Figure 4.4 The two most common mechanisms behind the formation of hydroxyl radicals (OH).

ultimately to cell death. This pathological lipid peroxidation is probably mediated by excitatory amino acids and by a simultaneous increase in the intracellular calcium level.

Ionic Mechanisms

The neurons of the spinal cord contain voltage-regulating membranes responsible for neuronal impulse transmission (Fig. 4.5). The levels of mainly extracellular sodium and chloride and intracellular potassium determine the membrane potential. This membrane potential results from an energy consuming transportation of ions across the cell membrane and the permeability of the membrane to these ions. The voltage of an inactive cell remains close to a resting potential, with excess of negative charge contained inside the cell. The cell triggers an action potential when the membrane of an excitable cell becomes depolarized beyond a threshold; that is, an impulse is transmitted. The availability of energy, in the form of adenosine diphosphate (ADP), is reduced when spinal cord blood flow is decreased following damage to the axons. The ionic equilibrium is lost, and the membrane potential (depolarization) is reduced. Sodium enters the intracellular space and remains there permanently.

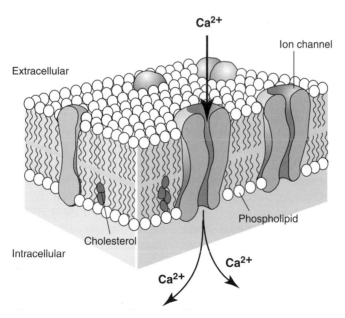

Figure 4.5 Ca^+ ion influx following damage to the cellular membranes.

This influx of sodium results in a corresponding influx of calcium, which further accelerates nerve cell breakdown. The increase of intracellular calcium is related to cell death, although the precise mechanism is unknown. Possibly, increased intracellular calcium influences enzymes, such as phospholipases and phosphatases, to promote the breakdown of the cell membrane. These breakdowns results in the liberation of free fatty acids, which are converted to, among other substances, prostaglandins. The presence of prostaglandins further increases the constriction of the blood vessels (vasospasm), which in its turn also contributes to final cell death.

Excitatory Amino Acids

Glutamate and other excitatory amino acids accumulate in the extracellular space within 15 minutes following injury. The concentration of these amino acids reaches toxic levels, with concentrations about six to eight times above normal values. The precise destructive mechanism of the excitatory amino acids is still unknown. However, calcium and the excitatory amino acids pass into dendrites and cell bodies when sodium channels are opened at the time of injury. Various receptors are affected by the released glutamates, resulting in an additional influx of calcium and other positive ions. Accumulation of calcium in the intracellular space is probably the most likely mechanism behind the neurotoxic action of the excitatory amino acids.

Opioid Receptors

Opioids are synthetic as well as endogenous (i.e., originating from within the body) chemical compounds resembling morphine. The endogenous opioids, including peptides, are associated with injuries within the CNS. An increase in endogenous opioids has been demonstrated in the damaged spinal cord following animal experimental trauma. It has also been experimentally shown that the microcirculation is affected by peptide activity, resulting in a decrease of spinal cord blood flow, and also that the number of peptide receptors increases after injury. It has been possible to hamper this peptide-mediated reduction of spinal cord blood flow in experimental models. Introduction of receptor-binding opioid receptor antagonists has been shown to prevent peptides from attaching to the receptors and their effect on spinal cord blood flow is thus blocked. The postulated possible beneficial effect of opioid receptor antagonists resulted in a clinical trial using naloxone, although beneficial effects could not be confirmed by these clinical studies.

INFLAMMATION

The CNS is usually protected from inflammatory reactions due to the ability of the blood–brain barrier to keep immunologically active cells away from brain and spinal cord. An invasion of immunologically active cells to the damaged spinal cord is seen following the demolition of the blood–brain barrier and results in an initiation of the inflammatory response. Neutrophils, T-lymphocytes, and macrophages are cells participating in this inflammatory response. The invading T-lymphocytes release cytokines, proteins, and peptides with signalling properties that act like hormones and neurotransmitters. These cytokines are of great interest in research because of their cytotoxic effects. The cellular process of phagocytosis is the most important property of the macrophages, but these cells also release substances with cytotoxic properties. Inflammatory mediators are consequently responsible for an increase in spinal cord tissue damage, and many inflammatory mediators such as prostaglandins, serotonins, and leukotrienes contribute to this tissue destruction.

APOPTOSIS

An injured cell may die either through apoptosis or through cell necrosis, although mitochondria play an important role in either scenario. Apoptosis is a molecularly mediated cell death. It is often referred to as "programmed" cell death. Apoptosis is genetically programmed during embryonic development and results in a steady state or homeostasis between cell death and the development of new cells. Apoptotic cell death is, in contrast to cell necrosis, energy consuming. The mitochondrial envelopes are slightly opened if energy access in the damaged tissue is restricted to 60–70% of normal levels. Injurious molecules enter into the cells and initiate a chain reaction of molecular events. The enzyme caspase is one of these injurious molecules, promoting cutting and breaking down of other proteins. The final stage of apoptosis includes a caspase-dependent activation of enzymes, which cleaves DNA. The DNA of the cells is thus reduced to fragments, leading to cell death. Apoptosis is morphologically characterized by cell shrinkage, chromatin condensation, and chromosomal fragmentation. The macrophages absorb dead cells without initiating an inflammatory response. The cellular content is not transported to the extracellular space, and the disposal of cellular debris does not damage the organism. Apoptosis strikes the oligodendrocytes most frequently. Demyelinization occurs if oligodendrocytes die, since these cell provide myelin to the surviving axons (see also Chapter 34).

Necrosis, by contrast, is a less energy-dependent process. The mitochondria are activated if the energy access in the tissue is reduced to less than 30% of normal levels. The ionic pumps lose their function, and lysis of all cell structures begins. Cellular edema and damage to the mitochondria, disruption of the cellular membranes, and an inflammatory response morphologically characterize necrosis. This results in a release of intracellular contents to the extracellular surroundings and, finally, cell lysis.

EDEMA

Normally, intra- and extracellular fluid diffuses through the semipermeable endothelium in a balanced ebb and flow. However, the largest volume of fluid is accumulated in the intercellular space following trauma to the spinal cord. Signs of edema (an increased accumulation of fluid) occur shortly after injury, and this edema is mainly located in the border zone between gray and white matter. Damage to the endothelium constitutes the prerequisite for edema formation and results in fluid leakage into the extracellular space. Arachidonic acid and its metabolites mediate the progressive edema accumulation. Edema formation reaches its peak 2–3 days after injury and regresses at the end of the first posttraumatic week. Spinal cord edema often extends one to two levels above injury level and probably contributes to the neurological deterioration seen immediately following injury. Aggravation of edema formation occur with excessive administration of i.v. fluids in the acute stage (see Chapter 6). Excessive infusions of fluid constitute a threat to the function of the spinal cord in the first 2–3 days following injury. The accumulation of edema initiates, preserves, and prolongs most of the other secondary injury processes, and this eventually contributes to increased cell death in the early posttraumatic stage. The tissue destruction continues to progress both rostrally and caudally from the injury site during the final chronic stage. This chronic stage may persist for many years. Various receptors and ionic channels change their degree of activity, and macrophages as well as neutrophil polymorphs remove devitalized tissue. A continuing demyelinization of the white matter results in a progressive transmission failure of nervous impulses. The axons degenerate (*Wallerian degeneration*, i.e., breakdown of axons distal to the lesion), and the spinal cord shows signs of atrophy. Cavities, with or without fluid, develop. Adhesion of the spinal cord to adjacent structures (e.g., the spinal meninges) is seen in areas subjected to infiltration of connective tissue, as when there is damage to the outer surface of the spinal cord. The diameter of the central canal increases, and the continuing accumulation of cerebrospinal fluid results in the formation of cyst cavities in about 50% of spinal cord injured patients.

CONCLUSION

The pathophysiological events following an injury to the spinal cord can be divided into primary, secondary, and chronic phases. The primary injury comprises direct mechanical destruction of nervous tissue and vascular structures. The effects of the primary trauma are considered irreversible—no known treatments can repair these damages and improve neurological function. A transformation from primary to secondary injury mechanisms occurs gradually, during a period ranging from minutes to days after injury. A cascade of vascular mechanisms, biochemical alterations, inflammation, edema, and apoptosis contributes to an ongoing auto-destruction of the spinal cord tissue. The apoptosis progresses in both cranial and caudal direction during the chronic stage. This stage ranges from days to years. Receptors, ion channels, and other structures try to restore functions, and damaged spinal cord tissue is removed from the site of injury. The demyelinization of the white matter continues, leading to an atrophy of the spinal cord. Cyst formation located in previously injured areas of the spinal cord and/or a widening of the central canal appears (syringomyelia) during this chronic stage. The spinal cord is often tethered or attached to the dural sac (see Chapter 30). The primary injury cannot be treated, but only avoided by prevention. An adequate and acutely initiated intensive care and careful rehabilitation may, however, minimize the consequences of secondary injury mechanisms. Active rehabilitation and, in some selected cases, surgical treatment may relieve some of the negative consequences of SCI during the chronic stage.

ACKNOWLEDGMENTS

The authors wish to express their gratitude to assistent professor Anders Lewén, Department of Neuroscience, Neurosurgery, University of Uppsala, Sweden, for his valuable contribution and support in the creation of this chapter.

Suggested Reading

Agrawal SK, Fehlings MG. Mechanisms of secondary injury to spinal cord axons in vitro: role of Na$^+$, Na($^+$)-K($^+$)-ATPase, the Na($^+$)-H$^+$ exchanger, and the Na($^+$)-Ca2$^+$ exchanger. *J Neurosci* 1996;16(2): 545–552.

Agrawal SK, Theriault E, Fehlings MG. Role of group I metabotropic glutamate receptors in traumatic spinal cord white matter injury. *J Neurotrauma* 1998;15(11): 929–941.

Beattie MS, Hermann GE, Rogers RC, Bresnahan JC. Cell death in models of spinal cord injury. *Prog Brain Res* 2002;137:37–47. Review.

Bramlett HM, Dietrich WD. Progressive damage after brain and spinal cord injury: pathomechanisms and treatment strategies. *Prog Brain Res* 2007;161:125–141.

Carlson GD, Gorden C. Current developments in spinal cord injury research. *Spine J* 2002;2(2):116–128. Review.

Choo AM, Liu J, Dvorak M, et al. Secondary pathology following contusion, dislocation, and distraction spinal cord injuries. *Exp Neurol* 2008;212(2):490–506. Epub 2008 May 14.

Dumont RJ, Okonkwo DO, Verma S, et al. Acute spinal cord injury, part I: pathophysiologic mechanisms. *Clin Neuropharmacol* 2001; 24(5):254–264. Review.

Fehlings MG, Agrawal S. Role of sodium in the pathophysiology of secondary spinal cord injury. *Spine* 1995; 20(20):2187–2191.

Fehlings MMG, Sekhon LSH. Cellular, ionic, and biomolecular mechanisms of the injury process. In: Tator CH, Benzel CH, eds., *Contemporary Management of Spinal Cord Injury: From Impact to Rehabilitation.* Park Ridge, IL: American Association of Neurological Surgeons, 2000: 33–50.

Kim DH, Vaccaro AR, Henderson FC, Benzel EC. Molecular biology of cervical myelopathy and spinal cord injury: role of oligodendrocyte apoptosis. *Spine J* 2003; 3(6):510–519. Review.

Kwon BK, Tetzlaff W, Grauer JN, et al. Pathophysiology and pharmacologic treatment of acute spinal cord injury. *Spine J* 2004;4(4):451–464.

Park E, Velumian AA, Fehlings MG. The role of excitotoxicity in secondary mechanisms of spinal cord injury: a review with an emphasis on the implications for white matter degeneration. *J Neurotrauma* 2004; 21(6):754–774. Review.

Pouw MH, Hosman AJ, van Middendorp JJ, et al. Biomarkers in spinal cord injury. *Spinal Cord* 2009;47(7):519–25. Epub 2009 January 20. Review.

Sekhon LH, Fehlings MG. Epidemiology, demographics, and pathophysiology of acute spinal cord injury. *Spine* 2001;26(24 Suppl):S2–12. Review.

Swartz KR, Scheff NN, Roberts KN, Fee DB. Exacerbation of spinal cord injury due to static compression occurring early after onset. *J Neurosurg Spine* 2009;11 (5):570–574.

Tator CH. Experimental and clinical studies of the pathophysiology and management of acute spinal cord injury. *J Spinal Cord Med* 1996;19(4):206–214. Review.

Tator CH, Koyanagi I. Vascular mechanisms in the pathophysiology of human spinal cord injury. 1997. Available online at www.aans.org.

5

Clinical Examination

The spinal cord connects the brain with the rest of the body with respect to motor, sensory, and autonomic functions. In addition, the spinal cord contains several neural networks ("minibrains") that participate in both simple reflexes, as well as in more complex events (such as gait, bladder, bowel, and sexual functions).

The ascending and descending pathways run longitudinally along the periphery of the spinal cord. For example, axons to or from the lower extremities travel nearly the entire length of the spinal cord, and an injury anywhere along its length can result in motor and/or sensory deficit in the legs.

In addition, the spinal cord demonstrates a segmental arrangement, in which the spinal nerves exit from the "stem" of the spinal cord in an organized fashion, like the branches of a tree. This "stem" with its numerous transverse branches forms the anatomical basis for symptoms relating to spinal cord lesions. The patient will experience symptoms below a particular level on the body that corresponds to the injured spinal cord segment.

As a result, motor, sensory, and/or autonomic symptoms may occur. Such symptoms may be due to neural deficit (such as paralysis and sensory loss) or to neural irritation (such as pain and paresthesias). Sometimes, interruption of an inhibitory supraspinal influence on the spinal cord's intrinsic structure may lead to what is known as a *release phenomenon*, with increased muscular tension and increased deep tendon reflexes (spasticity).

A sudden injury, such as acute spinal cord compression, results in a constellation of symptoms somewhat different from that of a slowly progressive disorder. A complete injury that involves a transection of the spinal cord results in different symptoms than an incomplete injury that involves only a part of the cord cross-section. The spectrum of symptoms of incomplete injuries varies depending on whether the spinal cord is injured anteriorly, posteriorly, centrally, or laterally. Finally, symptoms will vary according to whether the injury is focal, multifocal, or diffuse.

Knowledge of spinal cord anatomy will allow the location and extent of injury to be deduced from the spectrum of symptoms. Such a "topographic" diagnosis (i.e., "Where?") is the first step in making the diagnosis. The second step is to ascertain the cause of injury (i.e., "What?").

History and physical exam remain the most important diagnostic tools. Of course, the clinical diagnosis typically must be confirmed or refuted through additional laboratory, radiologic, and/or neurophysiologic diagnostic methods. These methods are described in Chapter 8, as well as in conjunction with discussions of specific injuries.

HISTORY

The history in acute trauma cases focuses heavily on the circumstances surrounding the trauma and on the symptoms that indicate neurological involvement (see Chapter 7). Preexisting spinal disease involving the back, such as spinal stenosis or ankylosing spondylitis, increases the probability of neurological involvement in trauma cases.

History taking in cases of suspected nontraumatic spinal cord disease is appropriately initiated by discussing the patient's current complaints. Each symptom is noted and analyzed separately in regard to onset and progression. Common symptoms in cases of spinal cord disease include localized back pain, radiating or diffuse pain, impaired gait due to muscle weakness and/or sensory disturbance, stiffness, impaired fine motor function/clumsiness, sensory disturbance, increased urinary urgency and/or impaired bladder function, incontinence, and erectile dysfunction. The symptoms may involve one or both arms and legs, as well as the trunk. The distribution of sensorimotor symptoms may indicate either "para" (both legs) or "tetra" (both arms and both legs) involvement. In other words, the symptoms indicate a horizontal level—which is most common—or, in rare cases, a "hemi" involvement, or vertical level. Information about previous and current known disorders may provide important etiological clues. Examples of diseases that may affect the spinal cord include cancer, multiple sclerosis (MS), amyotrophic lateral sclerosis (ALS), herniated disk, rheumatoid arthritis, acquired immunodeficiency syndrome (AIDS), malnutrition, and arteriosclerosis. As regards past medical history, it is particularly important to inquire about previous back and tumor diseases. A prior history of meningitis, subarachnoid hemorrhage, back surgery, or myelography with intrathecal contrast injection may lead to scarring of the meninges, with subsequent spinal cord involvement. Social history should include questions about alcohol and drug abuse. Intravenous drug users comprise a risk group for spinal epidural abscess. The clinician should obtain the patient's family history of neurological disease, since several hereditary diseases may be associated with spinal cord involvement.

PHYSICAL EXAM

Generally, the focus of the neurological exam varies depending on the suspected area of injury as indicated by the history (e.g., the brain, spinal cord, nerve roots, peripheral nerves, or muscles), and depending on whether a unifocal, multifocal, or diffuse pathologic process is contemplated.

The neuro exam for suspected spinal cord involvement should include sensation, motor function, deep tendon reflexes (DTRs), and muscle tone of the arms, legs, and trunk. Higher functions such as cognition, speech, and memory, of course, reflect brain rather than spinal function and are therefore of

secondary importance in lesions that are limited to the spinal cord. However, a screening examination of these functions should generally be carried out. With respect to the cranial nerves, high cervical spinal cord lesions may sometimes impair function of the accessory and trigeminal nerves, as well as the sympathetic innervation to the eye and face (Horner syndrome). Please refer to neurology textbooks for a description of a general neuro exam.

A complete neurological examination is time consuming; that which may be considered a reasonably comprehensive physical examination varies according to circumstances. Time is of the essence when examining patients in emergency situations and, understandably, the neuro exam in such instances must therefore be more cursive. In emergency situations, *repeated* examinations (to detect changes, such as worsening paralysis or deteriorating level of consciousness) are given priority over a single highly detailed examination.

In the case of acute trauma to the spine it is of fundamental importance to verify whether neurological signs are present. If so, the *level of neurological injury* must be identified (the most caudal level of the spinal cord with normal function) and *the degree of neurological involvement* must be assessed (whether all sensory function and voluntary motor function is absent below the level of injury—a *complete* injury; or if any sensory and/or voluntary motor function remains—an *incomplete* injury). In traumatic SCI, we use a standardized method of examination based on the American Spinal Injury Association (ASIA) classification system (see Chapter 2). The minimum emergency examination also includes an assessment of the stability of the vertebral column, and every suspected case of spinal trauma should be treated as if the vertebral column were unstable until proven otherwise. Additional radiologic examinations are carried out in regular order on such occasions, typically including plain x-ray, magnetic resonance imaging (MRI) and/or computed tomography (CT); see also Chapter 6.

For rapidly progressing nontraumatic cases involving the spine, the clinician must consider several possible etiologies (e.g., herniated disk, abscess, infarction, hemorrhage, or myelitis), necessitating a thorough analysis of the history. Here, too, the neurological examination should primarily focus on establishing whether neurological involvement is present and if so, the probable level of injury should be ascertained. In cases of para- or tetraparesis, spinal cord compression must be either ruled out or treated emergently.

For slowly progressing nontraumatic cases involving the spine, the differential diagnoses are even more numerous, and the clinician must carry out a comprehensive review of the history and physical examination. Here, the time element is not as critical as in emergency situations, and workup can often be done electively on an outpatient basis (see also Chapter 19).

SEGMENTAL AND LONG-TRACT SYMPTOMS

For a more comprehensive review, please refer to Chapter 3, including its illustrations. In cases of *focal* (circumscribed) spinal cord lesions, regardless of etiology, we expect to find a segmental, roughly horizontal level on the body, with normal function cranial to this level, and impaired or absent function caudal to this level. The segmental level is a reflection of the skin innervation (*dermatome*) and muscle innervation (*myotome*). Knowledge about the body's segmental innervation is required to correctly diagnose levels.

Establishing the *sensory level* is an important component of the neurological examination in cases of suspected spinal cord involvement. The sensory examination should include at least the modalities light touch and pain.

In the myotomes innervated from the injured spinal cord segment(s), signs of what is known as a *lower motor neuron injury* may be demonstrated. This is caused by injury to the segmental α-motor neurons in the anterior horns of the spinal cord. When these lower motor neurons are injured, a paralysis occurs characterized by *muscular hypotonia* (flaccid paresis), *pronounced atrophy, decreased or absent deep tendon reflexes,* and *fasciculations* (involuntary contractions in individual muscle fiber bundles). Clinically manifest paresis due to injury of the α-motor

neurons does not occur until at least 50% of the motor neuron pool has been destroyed.

As the segmental α-motor neurons are injured, the descending motor tracts passing through the area of injury along the longitudinal axis of the spinal cord are typically also injured. These are known as the *upper motor neurons*. The α-motor neurons in the spinal cord below the level of injury thus lose their supraspinal connection, and the muscles innervated by intact α-motor neurons are therefore also affected by paresis, although this type of paresis is instead characterized by *muscular hypertonia* (spastic paresis), *only a slight degree of atrophy, increased deep tendon reflexes,* and *absence of fasciculations.* Clinically manifest paresis typically does not occur until at least 50% of the upper motor neurons have ceased functioning, and total paralysis does not occur until more than 90% of the neurons cease to function.

It is easy to be confused by the fact that lower motor neuron paresis can be present *above* upper motor neuron paresis. Also note that in the case of acute injuries, also paresis related to upper motor neuron damage will at first be flaccid, with decreased or absent reflexes. This transient condition is known as *spinal shock* and is described in greater detail later.

A spectrum of symptoms with segmental flaccid paresis at the level of injury and spastic paresis below the level of injury thus typify focal spinal cord lesions. Such lesions may be seen with trauma, transverse myelitis, spinal cord tumors, spinal epidural abscess, and cervical spinal stenosis. However, symptoms may be more complex in cases of diffuse or multifocal spinal cord involvement along the longitudinal and/or transverse axes, and a definite level of injury may then be lacking or difficult to define.

SENSORY FUNCTION

Assessment of sensory function requires patient cooperation. Granted, expressions such as grimacing and other nonverbal behavioral pain reactions may indicate that the patient perceives a painful stimulus but, to a large extent, testing sensory function is reliant upon the patient's ability to adequately report his perceptions. In the case of sensory deficit, stimulation may also elicit reflex motor responses, such as a flexor reflex. It is not unusual that a patient may very well experience pain in an area of the body completely devoid of sensation. On the trunk of the body, sensory testing is the primary method of establishing the neurological lesion level. It is also important to underscore that sensation includes not just one, but several distinct modalities (pain, temperature, light touch, deep pressure, vibration), and that sensory loss may very well be selective for one modality or another. A more detailed discussion is found in the next sections.

Light Touch

Light touch, including *two-point discrimination* (the ability to distinguish between two simultaneous, closely spaced sensory stimuli as separate), is mediated in part through the dorsal columns and in part via the ventral spinothalamic fasciculus on the contralateral side. Since the impulses travel through the spinal cord in not one, but two anatomically distinct pathways, a total loss of light touch sensation below the neurological level generally implies a total or near-total transverse lesion.

Dorsal Columns

Proprioception provides information about joint position and movements. Conscious proprioception is initially transmitted through the dorsal columns of the spinal cord to reach conscious awareness at the cortical level. Unconscious proprioception is transmitted through the dorsal and ventral spinocerebellar tracts to the cerebellum. Impaired proprioception is an important sign of dorsal column lesions. Generally, we begin testing in the most distal parts of the extremity. The examiner fixes the distal interphalangeal joint of the finger or toe (usually the thumb or large toe) from the sides with one hand, and then flexes or extends the distal phalanx by gripping the sides of the finger/toe between the thumb and index finger of the examiner's other hand. Patients should be able to perceive a couple of millimeters of movement. In the case of a distal deficit, proprioception should also be tested in more proximal joints. Proprioception is

not lost until about 75% of the dorsal column axons are nonfunctional.

Vibration stimuli are also mainly mediated through the dorsal columns. Testing vibration is of great value in cases where polyneuropathy is suspected (diffuse disease of the peripheral nerves), in which impairment of vibration sense is often one of the earliest signs. A vibrating tuning fork is first placed on top of the patient's large toe. If the patient does not sense vibration here, the tuning fork is serially applied more proximally and cranially to the medial malleolus, proximal tibia, anterior superior iliac spine, the costal arch, and finally the clavicle.

Pathology affecting the dorsal columns may lead to *sensory ataxia,* in which impaired sensory feedback in regard to position of the extremities leads to clumsy, imprecise movements. In addition, paresthesias often occur, and are probably due to spontaneous impulses arising from within the injured axons. Common descriptions include "pins and needles," perception of vibration, sensation of a tightly drawn band, and/or hypersensitivity to touch (hyperesthesia) below the level of injury. One distinct type of paresthesia elicited from the dorsal column is known as the *L'hermitte's sign,* which involves an unpleasant sensation—similar to electrical shocks—shooting down the back when the neck is flexed.

Pain and Temperature

Pain is mediated via several spinal pathways, the most important of which is the lateral spinothalamic tract. An injury to this pathway system causes decreased sensitivity to pain and temperature stimuli from the contralateral side of the body starting one or two dermatomes below the level of the lesion. Lesions of the pain pathways may also result in irritative symptoms that manifest as a perception of pain below the level of lesion. Such pain may be described as dull or more distinctly as burning or lancinating. When testing sensitivity to pain, the patient should be instructed to indicate the presence or absence of pain when pricked with a pin. Even when sensitivity to pain is absent, the patient may still have intact sensation to touch, and may thus experience being pricked. Therefore asking patients whether they "feel the pinprick" is not enough; it is necessary to specifically ask whether *pain* is present.

Temperature, like pain, is mediated via the lateral spinothalamic tract. When lesions are centrally located in the spinal cord (such as syringomyelia), the fibers that cross over and convey pain and temperature are those mainly affected. Clinically, this manifests as loss of sensation for these modalities within a band-shaped area reflecting the affected spinal cord segments. In the case of complete spinal cord lesions, temperature sensitivity is lost below the level of injury. A change in perception of temperature sensitivity may be an early sign of a lesion in the spinothalamic tract. The patient may note an absence of sensitivity to heat and/or cold within the affected area of skin, for example while showering or bathing. Since neural impulses for pain and temperature travel in the same pathways, it is usually sufficient to test only sensitivity to pain. If nevertheless temperature sensitivity is being tested, it is convenient to do this by touching the patient's skin with a metal tuning fork. The patient should be able to discern variations in skin temperature of just a few degrees in either a hot or cold direction.

Particular care should be exercised when the patient uses the descriptor "numb." This may denote a sensation of heaviness in a partially paralyzed extremity (even in the *absence* of any sensory loss!), paresthesias (indicating irritation), or a de facto sensory deficit or complete absence of sensation.

Patients may often detect discrete sensory disturbances even when the examiner is unable to discover any pathology during the examination. In particular, this applies to irritative symptoms such as pain and paresthesias.

MOTOR FUNCTION

Motor function testing has the advantage over sensory testing in that examiners can directly use their own senses to verify the findings. However, patients may intentionally choose not to fully exert themselves (or perhaps not even try to volitionally activate the muscle at all). In addition, pain may inhibit patients from fully

activating their muscles, and a "true" paresis may not actually be present. The concept of "normal" strength varies greatly among different people. The normal strength of a 20-year-old male body-builder is of course extremely exceeding that of an 80-year-old woman. A helpful suggestion is thus to use the patient as his own point of reference, by comparing strength on the left and right sides and between arms and legs. It furthermore should be remembered that not all motor function is voluntary. During voluntary activation, a spastic muscle may react with a superimposed involuntary contraction, which may distort the assessment of volitional strength. Motor function testing in cases of suspected spinal cord lesions focuses on the extremities, as it is difficult or impossible to evaluate segmental motor function in the trunk.

Muscle strength is conventionally assessed according to a 6-point scale, where $0 =$ total paralysis and $5 =$ normal function (see Chapter 8).

If the injury is at the level of the cervical spine, the paralysis will encompass both arms and legs (i.e., *tetraplegia*). If the level of injury is below the cervical spine, the paralysis will encompass the legs and possibly the trunk, (i.e., *paraplegia*). Even if these concepts are used in everyday clinical practice to describe both complete and incomplete injuries, it is more accurate to speak of tetra- or para*paresis* in cases of incomplete loss of motor function (where a degree of voluntary motor function remains below the level of injury), and to reserve the terms tetra- or para*plegia* for total loss of motor function (where no voluntary motor function remains below the level of injury). The term *paralysis* is also used, and generally refers to cases of complete loss of function.

The clinical picture seen when motor pathways are affected varies, as mentioned earlier, depending on whether the upper or lower motor neurons are involved. In the case of early involvement of the upper motor neurons a subtle sensation of stiffness in the affected extremity is the first symptom, often combined with a tendency to stumble and problems negotiating stairs. Patients often drag or shuffle their feet in a characteristic manner. Muscular atrophy is slight in the case of upper motor neuron lesions. (Injuries to the lower motor neuron may result in loss of up to 80% of muscle volume, whereas lesions of the upper motor neurons entail no more than about a 20% loss of muscle volume). Muscle tone and deep tendon reflexes are increased. In general, upper motor neuron lesions first lead to impairment of distal fine motor function and subsequently to impairment of gross motor strength. Distal motor function can be tested by having patients "play the piano" with their fingers in the air, or by wiggling their toes. A subtle sign of upper motor neuron involvement is that such movements are carried out more slowly and clumsily.

Patients are often able to notice symptoms of discrete upper motor neuron injury earlier than the examiner can detect them. Conversely, in lower motor neuron injury, the examiner often notes findings in the physical exam before the patient subjectively experiences any symptoms.

Reflexes

Testing of *deep tendon reflexes* is a key part of the neurological examination. Increased deep tendon reflexes are signs of upper motor neuron damage, whereas weakened or absent reflexes suggest damage to the afferent or efferent fibers of the segmental reflex arc. The reflexes that are routinely tested include the biceps, brachioradial, triceps, patellar, and Achilles. There is considerable individual variation in regard to how easily reflexes can be elicited. The most important sign of pathology is a *discrepancy in reflex response* between different muscle groups in the same patient, rather than the overall briskness in reflex response per se.

In focal spinal cord lesions, normal deep tendon reflexes are typically noted above the level of injury, impaired or absent reflexes are found at the level of injury, and increased reflexes are elicited below the level of injury.

Unlike deep tendon reflexes, which are monosynaptic, the *abdominal reflexes* are polysynaptic. These latter reflexes are abolished by both upper and segmental lower motor neuron lesions. The abdominal reflexes are most easily examined by gently scratching the skin in the four quadrants of the abdomen surrounding the umbilicus and observing the resultant muscle contraction, which normally pulls the umbilicus toward the

area of stimulus. In older and/or overweight persons, abdominal reflexes are often difficult to demonstrate.

Babinski sign is a pathological reflex response expressed by dorsal extension of the big toe in response to a stimulus exerted along the lateral edge of the foot in a proximal to distal direction and then turning in toward the medial side of the forefoot, proximal to the base of the toes. This maneuver is often accompanied by a simultaneous fanning out or spreading of the other toes. The presence of the Babinski sign indicates upper motor neuron damage in the brain or spinal cord.

Muscle Tone and Spasticity

Muscle tone—the involuntary basal tension of a muscle—may be normal, decreased, or increased. *Decreased* muscle tone accompanies paralysis due to a lower motor neuron injury and is also seen in the acute phase following an upper motor neuron injury (i.e., during spinal shock). *Increased* muscle tone accompanies the post acute and chronic phases following an upper motor neuron injury. This is known as spasticity (spastic increase in muscle tone) and should be distinguished from other types of muscular hypertonia, especially *rigidity*, which characterizes conditions such as Parkinson's disease.

Spasticity in turn is a complex and multifaceted aspect of a phenomenon known as the *upper motor neuron syndrome*. SCI is often accompanied by pronounced and sometimes problematic spasticity.

An *acute* spinal cord lesion initially results in flaccid paralysis below the level of injury, with muscular hypotonia and loss of deep tendon and superficial reflexes. This is assumed to be the result of a conduction block of electrical transmission in the spinal cord. This transient phase is called *spinal shock*. After a period of time spanning days to weeks, muscle tone and reflexes below the level of injury return and become increased, likely due to activation of so-called *silent synapses* (i.e., previously inactive synapses in motor neurons linked to segmental reflex activity). In addition, afferent fibers in the dorsal root grow out and establish new synapses (*sprouting*). Taken together, these two mechanisms cause the paresis to convert from flaccid to spastic, with hypertonia and increased deep tendon reflexes.

In cases of a more *gradual* onset of the spinal cord lesion, these plastic mechanisms have time to offset the loss of descending stimuli. Spinal shock with transient muscular hypotonia thus will not occur. Instead, we will note a gradually increasing spasticity accompanying the paresis.

Spasticity among patients with SCI may vary in severity. An assessment of muscle tone is important in choosing appropriate therapy.

Muscular hypertonicity in SCI can manifest clinically at least in three different ways:

1. *Spasticity*: A rapid monosynaptic reaction. *Clonus* is a repetitive phenomenon of this type.
2. *Flexor spasms*: A contraction reflex in the lower extremities in which a Babinski sign comprises part of this reflex. Sustained flexor spasms may result in muscle contractures and joint subluxation, such as in the hip joint.
3. *Spastic rigidity*: A slow, polysynaptic, extensive reaction in which the increased muscular tone may persist over a long period of time.

Functional impairment caused by increased muscle tone may also be classified according to its severity. Thus, severity may vary from mild gait disturbances in patients with incomplete injury, to painful and disabling spastic rigidity. In the past, severe spasticity was treated surgically by cutting tendons, nerve roots, and muscles, but such methods are now rarely used. Other types of therapy include nerve blocks (botulinum toxin, phenol) and administration of oral medications (baclofen, benzodiazepines, clonidine, dantrolene). Baclofen is usually administered orally, but is associated with limiting side effects such as fatigue, headache, nausea, confusion, and respiratory depression. These side effects are dose dependent and most pronounced early in the course of treatment. The sedative properties of the drug limit the maximum daily dose, which is about 100–120 mg (see Chapter 30).

Muscle tone can be tested in many ways. When checking muscle tone in the lower extremities with the patient in a supine position, the examiner may place one arm under the patient's knees and begin by carefully "rolling" the patient's legs from side to side to help the patient relax. Next, the examiner may quickly lift the patient's legs by raising the arm under the patient's knees. If the lower leg stiffly follows along, the exam suggests an increase in muscle tone, because normally this maneuver only causes knee flexion and the patient's heel remains in contact with the examination table. For the upper extremities, the examiner may instead hold the patient's hand, as when shaking hands, and carry out a maneuver that results in gentle flexion and extension of the patient's elbow and wrist. Once the patient relaxes, the examiner adds a maneuver to rotate the forearm. If muscle tone is increased, a distinct "catch" (sudden increased resistance) is noted during passive supination of the patient's forearm.

In addition to an increase in *tonic reflexes*, which can be documented with assessment scales such as the Ashworth scale, spastic muscle contractions may also lead to involuntary movements, known as *spasms*. Spasm frequency can be documented with the Penn Spasm Frequency Score or similar instruments.

Briskness of the deep tendon reflexes, in which heightened reflexes indicate an increase in *phasic reflex activity*, can be clinically graded according to the following scale:

0 = absent reflex
+ = decreased reflex
++ = normal reflex
+++ = pathologically increased reflex

In spastic paresis, muscular hypertonia is strongest in those muscles that have best-preserved strength. In the arms, these muscles include the shoulder adductors, elbow flexors, wrist flexors, and finger flexors. In contrast, in the legs, the hip extensors, knee extensors, and plantar flexors dominate. However, the dominance of extensor muscles in the legs (*paraplegia-in-extension*) may convert into a dominance of flexors (*paraplegia-in-flexion*) in response to chronic nociceptive stimuli (e.g., as a result of pressure ulcers).

In addition to spasticity, the upper motor neuron syndrome also includes pathologically increased flexor reflexes in the lower extremities and impaired distal fine motor function and decreased gross muscle strength. Stimulation of the foot may elicit flexor reflexes, expressed as an involuntary dorsal extension of the big toe and simultaneous flexion of the ankle, knee, and hip joints. Other spasticity-related phenomena include spread (*irradiation*) of extensor reflexes in response to percussion, as well as repetitive flexor contractions (*clonus*) in response to a sustained extensor stimulus. The upper motor neuron syndrome is also accompanied by certain changes in the physical properties of the tissues that further increase resistance to movements. These changes include decreased elasticity, fibrosis, and contractures.

In summary, several factors interact to impede or preclude a particular movement in the setting of an upper motor neuron syndrome: agonist muscle paresis, antagonist co-contraction (simultaneous, and thereby movement-impeding contraction) and antagonist muscle spasticity, joint contractures, and physical changes in the antagonist muscles.

SPINAL CORD SYNDROMES

Depending on the extent of the cross-sectional injury to the spinal cord or cauda equina, the disruption in the connections between the brain and body below the level of injury will be either *complete* or *incomplete*. The consequences of incomplete injuries vary depending on whether they involve the anterior, posterior, central, or lateral portions of the spinal cord cross-section. Certain patterns of injury are sufficiently common to justify specific syndrome nomenclature. We briefly describe these syndromes here. Note that the syndrome designations in and of themselves only describe the *extent and/or location* of an injury within the spinal cord. They say nothing about the cause of injury, even though certain syndromes are typically associated with specific etiologies.

Total Cord Syndrome

Total cord syndrome (Fig. 5.1), or total transverse lesion, occurs when conductivity is interrupted in all ascending and descending pathways of the spinal cord, leading to loss of all sensation and all voluntary motor function below the level of the lesion. Bladder and bowel control is also lost. Sexual function is affected, with impairment of the ability to have an erection, ejaculate, and experience orgasm in men, and decreased vaginal lubrication and impaired ability to experience orgasm in women.

Anterior Cord Syndrome

Anterior cord syndrome occurs with injury to the anterior two-thirds of the spinal cord, encompassing the corticospinal tract, spinothalamic

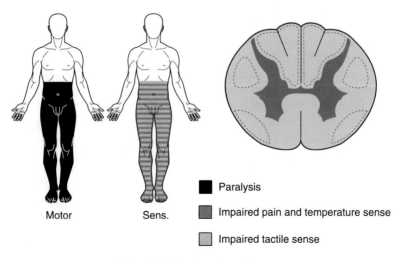

Motor   Sens.

■ Paralysis

▨ Impaired pain and temperature sense

▨ Impaired tactile sense

Figure 5.1 Total cord syndrome.

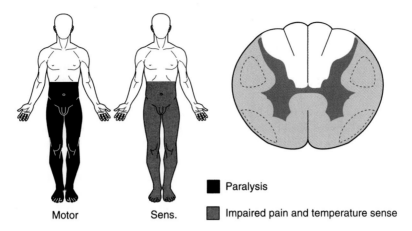

Paralysis

Impaired pain and temperature sense

Motor   Sens.

Figure 5.2 Anterior cord syndrome.

tract, and descending autonomic pathways to the sacral center for bladder control (Fig. 5.2). Clinically, this syndrome involves loss of voluntary motor function below the level of injury, but preserved function in the dorsal columns. In regard to activities of daily living (ADL), these patients are on a par with those who experience a total transverse lesion at the corresponding level, but incomplete lesions are associated with a better prognosis for return of function. Partially preserved sensory function also makes it easier for these patients to detect early signs of developing pressure ulcers.

Lateral Cord Syndrome (Brown-Séquard Syndrome)

Lateral cord syndrome, better known as *Brown-Séquard syndrome* (Fig. 5.3), occurs with hemitransection (right or left side) of the spinal cord with unilateral involvement of the dorsal columns, corticospinal tract, and spinothalamic tract. The syndrome encompasses a decrease in sensation to touch and paralysis on the ipsilateral side of the injury and loss of pain and temperature sensation on the contralateral side. Unilateral SCI usually does not affect bladder

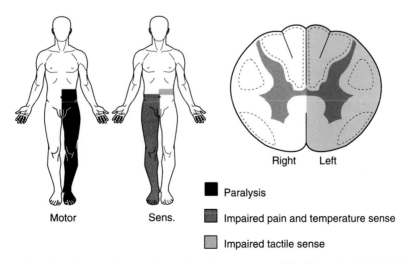

Right   Left

Paralysis

Impaired pain and temperature sense

Impaired tactile sense

Motor   Sens.

Figure 5.3 Lateral cord syndrome (Brown-Séquard syndrome), exemplified here by a left-sided injury to the spinal cord.

or bowel function. These patients typically have a better prognosis for both restoration of function and ADL.

Central Cord Syndrome

Central cord syndrome results from lesions of the central portion of the spinal cord cross-section (Fig. 5.4). Clinically, the syndrome is characterized by loss of pain and temperature sensation within one or more adjacent dermatomes (corresponding to the level[s] of the lesion) due to disruption of the crossing spinothalamic tracts. Should this central lesion expand, it may also come to involve the medial portions of the corticospinal tracts and/or the gray matter in the anterior horns, which would then cause paresis within the affected myotomes. Fibers in the

segmental reflex arcs are disrupted as they pass from the dorsal to the ventral spinal cord horns, which also causes loss of deep tendon reflexes within the affected segments.

The most common cause is traumatic injury to the cervical spinal cord, usually the result of hyperextension trauma in association with some degree of preexisting spinal stenosis. Patients with central cord syndrome due to a lesion of the cervical spinal cord will have more severe impairment of function in the arms than in the legs. Bladder, bowel, and sexual function, as well as gait, may be relatively well preserved.

Posterior Cord Syndrome

Posterior cord syndrome arises as a result of bilateral involvement of the dorsal columns (Fig. 5.5).

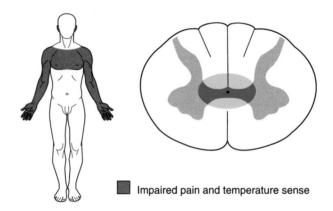

■ Impaired pain and temperature sense

Figure 5.4 Central cord syndrome.

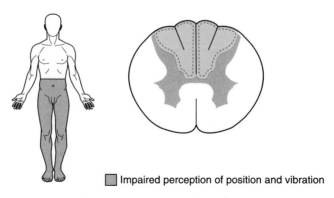

▨ Impaired perception of position and vibration

Figure 5.5 Posterior cord syndrome.

This syndrome is rare. Clinically, it is characterized by a loss of proprioception and vibration sense, with preserved motor function as well as preserved pain and temperature sensation.

Mixed Syndrome

In most traumatic cases, damage has a patchy distribution in the cross-section of the spinal cord, and the clinical picture fails to fit neatly into any of the syndromes just described (Fig. 5.6). In such cases, we refer to a *mixed syndrome.*

Pure Motor Spinal Cord Syndrome

A nontraumatic *pure motor spinal cord syndrome* may involve only the upper motor neurons, only the lower motor neurons, or a combination of upper and lower motor neurons (Fig. 5.7). An example of the latter can be seen in motor neuron disease, in which paralysis, spasticity, hyperreflexia, Babinski sign, pronounced muscle atrophy, and fasciculations may all occur simultaneously. In such cases, sensory function remains intact, as do bladder and bowel control.

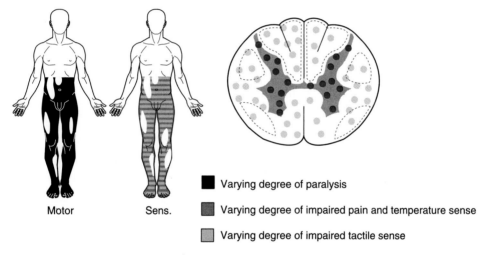

Motor   Sens.

■ Varying degree of paralysis

▨ Varying degree of impaired pain and temperature sense

▦ Varying degree of impaired tactile sense

Figure 5.6 Mixed syndrome.

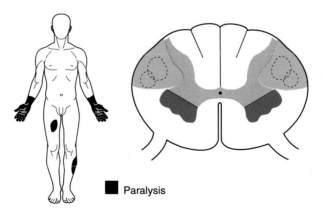

■ Paralysis

Figure 5.7 Pure motor spinal cord syndrome.

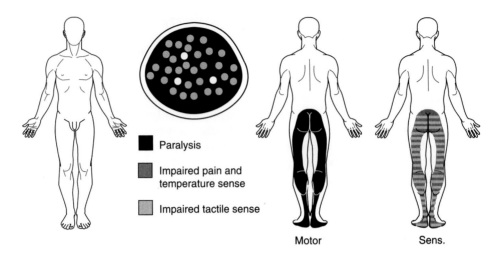

Figure 5.8 Cauda equina syndrome.

Cauda Equina Syndrome

In addition to these syndromes involving the spinal cord proper, we somewhat illogically also include *cauda equina syndrome* (Fig. 5.8). This syndrome does not entail injury to the spinal cord itself, but is caused by a loss of function in two or more of the 18 lumbosacral nerve roots that form the cauda equina. The deficit typically involves the perineal and gluteal areas, as well as the medial thighs. The motor deficit is characteristically of the lower motor neuron type.

Suggested Reading

McKinley W, Santos K, Meade M, Brooke K. Incidence and outcomes of spinal cord injury clinical syndromes. *J Spinal Cord Med* 2007;30(3):215–224.

Nielsen JB, Crone C, Hultborn H. The spinal pathophysiology of spasticity—from a basic science point of view. *Acta Physiol (Oxf)* 2007;189(2):171–180. Review.

6 Management at the Accident Scene

The management of the acutely spinal cord injured patients has, in addition to the fundamental life-saving goal, three main objectives: to minimize neurological deterioration, to mobilize the patient as soon as possible, and to implement an adequate rehabilitation. The early care of the injured patient starts immediately, at the site of accident. It has previously been shown that up to 25% of spinal cord injured patients suffer further neurological deterioration before arriving at the hospital. In some instances, this could be avoided.

Adequate management immediately after injury is vital and will optimize survival in the short term and the ultimate neurological outcome in the long term. The proportion of patients with complete lesions has diminished from 65% during the 1970s to approximately 45% in later studies. The number of patients with deteriorating neurological function during prehospital transfers has also been reduced.

Improved care at the site of the accident is one reason for this improved neurological outcome. The importance of secondary injury mechanisms has been clearly shown in animal experiments (see Chapter 4), and improved clinical outcomes likely reflect a reduction in secondary injury through proper management.

In cases of incomplete SCI, which results in subtotal loss of function below the level of injury, the prognosis is better and the consequences less devastating as compared to those associated with a complete lesion, which results in total loss of function below the level of injury. Since most traumas result in incomplete SCI, careful and adequate care at the site of the accident in combination with qualified medical management at the emergency hospital are vital prerequisites to reduce the impact of secondary injury and give the injured individual the best hope of regaining at least some neurological function.

MANAGEMENT AT THE ACCIDENT SCENE

Up to 60% of all patients with acute traumatic SCI prove to have injuries to other organ systems as well. Head trauma associated with unconsciousness, injuries to the chest and abdomen, and multiple fractures occur frequently (Table 6.1). Identification of trauma patients at risk is the first step in the evaluation and management at the site of an accident. The circumstances indicating an increased risk of SCI are described in Table 6.2. It is sometimes easy to overlook SCI, especially among patients with impaired consciousness. Therefore, it is a great advantage to establish a dialogue, at the site of the accident, with the injured patient. Tables 6.3 through 6.5 present those circumstances that may indicate that a person has suffered an SCI, but also and of equal importance, conditions indicating that an injury to the spine and/or spinal cord is very unlikely.

ADVANCED TRAUMA LIFE SUPPORT

The management of vital functions such as breathing and circulation, as well as controlling extensive blood loss (fractures, chest or abdominal hemorrhage) always has the highest priority. Most professionals treating patients at the site of accident use the Advanced Trauma Life Support (ATLS) guidelines developed and continuously revised (every fourth year) by the American College of Surgeons.

TABLE 6.1   The approximate frequency of injuries to other organ systems (operational definition within the brackets) among patients with acute SCI (given in per cent).

Head injury (coma >6 hours)	19%
Chest injury (requiring active treatment; e.g., Bülow drainage)	15%
Abdominal injury (requiring laparotomy)	2%
Multiple fractures including additional vertebral injuries	22%

TABLE 6.2   Circumstances indicating risk of injury to the spinal cord. Patients presenting with one or several of these symptoms should be treated as if suffering from SCI until proven contrarywise.

All high-energy trauma
Depressed/clouded consciousness
High speed traffic or motorcycle accidents
Falls >5 meters (>15 feet)
Severe facial injury
Severe pain at the site of the seat belt

TABLE 6.3   Circumstances, in awake patients, indicating an injury to the spinal cord. Patients presenting with one or several of these symptoms should be treated as if suffering from SCI until proven contrarywise.

Vertebral column pain
Reduced strength in arms and/or legs
Lack of movement in arms and/or legs
Numbness and loss of sensory function
Pain in arms ("burning hands" syndrome) and legs
Signs of urinary leakage and incontinence

TABLE 6.4   Circumstances, in unconscious patients, indicating an injury to the spinal cord. Patients presenting with one or several of these symptoms should be treated as if suffering from SCI until proven contrarywise.

Respiratory distress; paradoxical breathing
No response following pain stimulation below the level of injury
Loss of reflexes below the level of injury
Priapism
Hypotension in association with normal heart rate or bradycardia (indicates a high thoracic or cervical level lesion)

TABLE 6.5   Circumstances speaking against a lesion of cervical spine/spinal cord. Such lesions may be excluded if all criteria are present.

The patient is awake and shows no signs of disorientation
No signs of head injury
No signs of alcohol and drug intoxication
No pain from the cervical region
No signs of neurological deficits
No distracting pain that may divert the patient's attention from pain localized in the neck region

Five main tasks of pre-hospital management (i.e., at the scene of the accident) take precedence according to the ATLS guidelines:

- Evaluation
- Resuscitation
- Immobilization
- Extrication
- Transportation

These responsibilities are presented separately here, but are, of course, often performed simultaneously in view of the needs of each individual.

Evaluation

According to the ATLS guidelines, evaluation consists of a primary and secondary survey (examination and treatment). The ABCDEs during the primary and secondary surveys are to examine and treat the following body functions:

- *Airway.* Airway maintenance including administration of oxygen. The cervical spine must be protected if an injury to the cervical spine or spinal cord is suspected.
- *Breathing and ventilation.* The patient must be guaranteed adequate ventilation. Oro- or nasotracheal intubation if breathing capacity is inadequate.
- *Circulation with hemorrhage control.* Ensure adequate circulation by stopping ongoing external bleeding and initiating intravenous fluid therapy with balanced body-temperature saline solutions.
- *Disability.* Consciousness (according to Glasgow Coma Scale [GCS]) is assessed, as is the motor and sensory function in arms and legs.
- *Exposure/environmental control.* Evaluate the environment of the scene of accident. This includes measures to prevent hyper- and hypothermia, respectively. If needed, undress the patient completely.

The aim of this primary survey is to confirm that life-saving measures have been performed. The subsequent secondary survey consists of a more careful head to toe evaluation, to detect possible additional injuries. This evaluation includes a characterization of the approximate neurological level and completeness of the sensorimotor losses. The secondary survey does not start until the primary survey is finished, resuscitative measures are established, and the patient is showing stabilized and normalized vital functions. The secondary survey includes a brief but comprehensive patient evaluation that includes a history and physical examination of all body organs.

The patient should be asked about pain, numbness, and weakness. The presence of a burning pain in the hands (burning hand syndrome) indicates an injury to the cervical spinal cord. The aim of the initial neurological evaluation is to confirm or exclude the presence of any functional impairment in the arms and/or legs. The patient is asked to make a fist and to wiggle his feet. The sensory level is evaluated by assessment of sensation of pain and light touch. This will give a good indication regarding neurological status. Incontinence, urine retention, priapism, and reduced body temperature are other important signs of a SCI. The presence of unstable fractures is controlled for, in addition to the evaluation of sensory and motor losses. The patient should, during the examination of the back, be carefully log-rolled by multiple personnel, after which he is placed on a spine board (backboard) later used for transport.

Resuscitation

Aggressive resuscitation and treatment of life-threatening injuries is simultaneously performed with the primary survey. Resuscitation is focused on airway, breathing and circulation (the ABCs).

Airway

Airway control is of highest priority, and an open airway may be maintained by correct positioning of the mandible. This maneuver (using either the head tilt/chin lift or jaw thrust maneuvers) will release any obstruction of the posterior pharynx caused by the tongue. To perform the head tilt/chin lift maneuver, a backward pressure is applied to the patient's forehead using the palm of one hand. The fingers of the other hand are placed under the bony part of the chin. The chin is lifted forward while the jaw is supported, thus helping to tilt the head back.

The jaw thrust displaces the mandible forward and is done by grasping the angles of the mandible and lifting it in an upward motion. This method is preferred if an injury to the spinal cord is suspected, since it resembles the motion used for bag-valve mask ventilation. It also produces less flexion and extension movement of the cervical spine, which secondarily may reduce the effect of existing compression of the spinal cord by vertebral fragments.

Oropharyngeal airway insertion, suction of the airways, and/or removal of foreign bodies constitute the next step in airway management, in cases of inadequate oxygenation. Endotracheal intubation is required only if a free airway is still at risk. It is of greatest importance that cervical alignment and immobilization be maintained during these procedures, and it has been shown that neurological function does not deteriorate if an orotracheal insertion is performed correctly. It is thus vital that, during the intubation procedure, neutral position remains unchanged (see Immobilization).

Patients with a suspected SCI should receive supplemental oxygen during transport to the hospital. Oxygen can be given by nasal cannula or face mask if the patient is awake. The jaw thrust maneuver and insertion of an oropharyngeal tube may facilitate oxygenation if the patient is not fully awake and endotracheal intubation is not considered necessary.

Breathing

The patient must always be guaranteed adequate ventilation. Airway management is concentrated on breathing (ventilation) as soon as the airway is secured. The respiratory rate and pattern is observed, since ventilation is affected by paralysis of the diaphragm and respiratory accessory muscles following SCI. The ventilation may also be hampered following multitrauma by a flail chest (due to multiple rib fractures), and/or open pneumothorax.

The patient must be intubated if ventilation is impaired. This means logistically a return to "Airway" in order to secure the airway. Intubation is necessary if the patient is unconscious or suffers from impaired consciousness, has reduced ventilatory capacity, or if an obstruction of the airway is suspected. The ATLS guidelines point out that experience rather than technique decides whether orotracheal or nasopharyngeal intubation is to be performed. The latter requires, however, that the patient exhibit adequate spontaneous respiration.

According to ATLS guidelines, fractures to the skull base must be suspected if facial or other injuries above the level of the clavicle are diagnosed. If fractures to the skull base have not been excluded, nasopharyngeal intubation is consequently contraindicated, and orotracheal intubation is usually preferred if an injury to the spinal cord is suspected. The inflated orotracheal cuff serves two functions: It prevents reflow of gas during assisted ventilation, and it prevents aspiration of blood, gastric contents, and/or cerebrospinal fluid. The neck must be kept in a neutral position, and this is achieved by a second person stabilizing the neck during the intubation procedure. It is highly recommended that the anterior part of the rigid cervical collar be opened during the intubation maneuver, to facilitate opening the patient's mouth without hyperextending the neck. It has been shown that intubation while using hard cervical collar immobilization induced significant movement of the cervical spine, whereas intubation in neutral position did not produce a corresponding movement of the vertebrae.

Circulation

Control of the hemodynamics is the next important step in the management of the traumatized patient. The heart rate and blood pressure is measured repeatedly. Active bleeding is stopped, usually by direct local pressure, and intravenous lines are inserted. There is some controversy regarding the choice of the initially administered fluid. The standard procedure is to administer Ringer's lactate since hypovolemia, caused by excessive bleeding, is the most common cause of shock, and all patients in shock are considered to have a hemorrhagic shock until proven otherwise. The hypotension associated with shock may, however, among patients with cervical and high thoracic SCI (above the level of T4-T6) be caused by the SCI itself, a condition known as *neurogenic shock*. These high-level injuries to the spinal cord result in a loss of sympathetically induced regulation of peripheral vascular tone, thus an accumulation of blood in the extremities, and a reduced central venous return. This altered distribution of blood leads to a reduced cardiac preload and secondarily to a decreased cardiovascular function. Hypotension (usually a systolic

TABLE 6.6 Characteristics of neurogenic versus hemorrhagic shock.

	Neurogenic Shock	Hemorrhagic Shock
Hypotension	Yes	Yes
Pulse	Bradycardia	Tachycardia
Skin	Warm and dry	Cool and clammy
Mental status	Normal	Affected
Urine production	Normal	Low

blood pressure of approximately 70 mm Hg or lower) and bradycardia are the most obvious signs of reduced cardiovascular function. The latter symptom is seen as a consequence of reduced sympathetic outflow to the heart. Table 6.6 illustrates the major differences between these two causes of shock. A low pulse rate (bradycardia), usually below 60, together with hypotension should be considered a sign of neurogenic shock. Infusion with Ringer's lactate will be ineffective in raising low blood pressure in neurogenic shock, and heart failure may occur if excessive volumes are provided. Placing the patient in the Trendelenburg position is the easiest way of treating shock, regardless of origin. This maneuver decreases the pooling of blood in the lower extremities, and the return of blood from the periphery is facilitated.

Immobilization

The purpose of immobilization is to prevent unnecessary movements (e.g., distractions) of the spine, thus preventing further trauma to the spinal cord. It is recommended that all patients be immobilized at the scene of accident if a spinal column or cord injury is either suspected or verified. Immobilization is performed as soon as possible, with regard to the patient's general condition.

Traction using weights has been used as a immobilization device, but this method should not be used due to the risk of overdistraction of the cervical column in situations where severe disruption, mainly to the upper cervical region, may be present. Overdistraction may cause

secondary mechanical injury to the spinal cord and further deterioration of neurological symptoms. Up to 20% of spinal cord injured patients present with more than one fracture to the spinal column. The entire body must, therefore, be immobilized and secured in order to prevent unnecessary movement of the spinal column. Consequently, a rigid cervical collar, sandbags placed to each side of the head, and taping the forehead down to the board secures the neck while the rest of the body is fully immobilized using foam blocks and tape on a long spineboard.

Patient Found on the Ground

If a patient is found on the ground at the scene of an accident, neutral in-line immobilization of the neck should be effected as soon as possible. One person ("Person 1") carefully grasps the patient's head and moves it into a neutral in-line or "eyes-forward" position (Fig. 6.1). This maneuver must be done very gently and stopped if pain increases, ventilation is disturbed, and/or neurological symptoms increase. The neck should be immobilized in a non–in-line position if any of these symptoms occurs. A second person ("Person 2") applies a hard cervical collar once the neutral position is obtained (Fig. 6.2) while Person 1 maintains the eyes-forward position and prevents any movement of the cervical column. It is important that the hard cervical collar be sized correctly to avoid having the chin rest inside the collar support. The

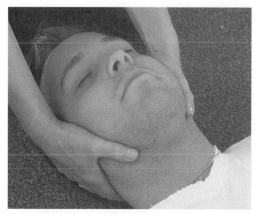

Figure 6.1 Neutral in-line or "eyes-forward" position.

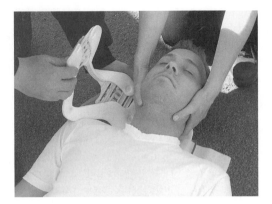

Figure 6.2 A hard cervical collar is applied.

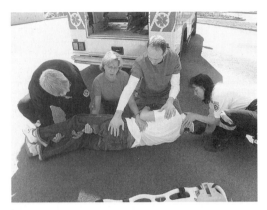

Figure 6.4 Log-rolling maneuvers second phase.

cervical collar should be applied before any other part of the body is moved.

Log-roll Maneuver and Placement on the Spine Board

The patient is rotated to one side using the log-roll maneuver with spine precautions in order to examine the spinal column (Figs. 6.3 and 6.4). The technique demands at least four individuals and aims to avoid movement in the spinal column during the rotation, thus making it possible to investigate the spine while it remains in a straight position. Person 1 is responsible for maintaining the neutral in-line position of the head and neck and coordinates the subsequent log-roll maneuver and placement of the patient on the spine board. The remaining three individuals simultaneously turn the chest, pelvis, and

extremities. Signs such as local tenderness, focal hematomas, and an increased distance between spinal processes (Fig. 6.4), indicate skeletal, muscle, and/or ligament injury. The patient is turned back to the supine position, using a reverse log-roll maneuver, after the examination is finished and is simultaneously placed on a spine board (backboard; Fig. 6.5).

The cervical collar alone does not completely immobilize the cervical spine. The head must be secured using adhesive tape or its equivalent after the patient's body has been placed on the spine board; this prevents rotational movement and achieves complete immobilization (Fig. 6.6).

The spine board is an excellent means of transportation for immobilized patients, but because of the risk of pressure ulcers (especially in the sacral region), patients should not be immobilized thus for more than 2 hours. Protective padding, such

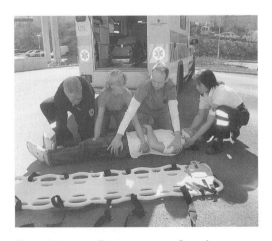

Figure 6.3 Log-rolling maneuver, first phase.

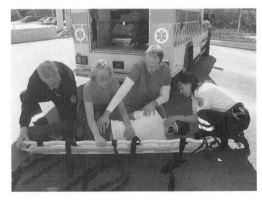

Figure 6.5 The patient is placed on the spine board.

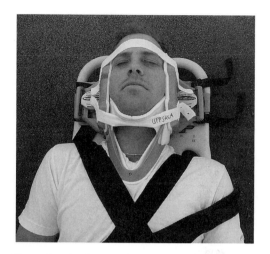

Figure 6.6 Final cervical spine immobilization.

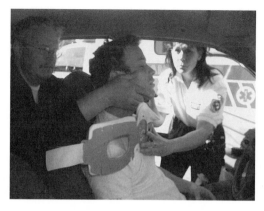

Figure 6.7 Cervical collar is placed on the patient while still in vehicle.

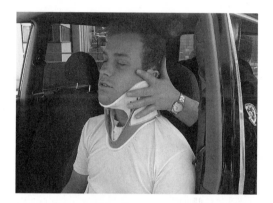

Figure 6.8 Immobilization following a motor vehicle accident.

as a gel mattress, may be used to minimize the risk of pressure sores.

Immobilization with a cervical collar and spineboard involves some risks; these are, however, offset by the risk of developing further neurological deterioration. Immobilization is uncomfortable, and often results in pain from the spinal column and jaw and/or headache. The risk of increased intracerebral pressure (venous return from the brain is compromised by the mechanical compression of the neck veins by the cervical collar) and aspiration must be accounted for and guarded against during prolonged immobilization.

Motor Vehicle Accident

Following a motor vehicle accident, the neck is secured using a similar program of immobilization used for a patient found on the ground, adapting the in-line immobilization as needed to the situation (Figs. 6.7 and 6.8).

Motorcycle Accident

In general, helmets need not be removed unless airway problems are detected, the helmet obscures extensive hemorrhage, or if it is too loose to secure an acceptable immobilization. If the helmet is removed, this is done by two individuals using a three-step procedure (Figs. 6.9–6.11).

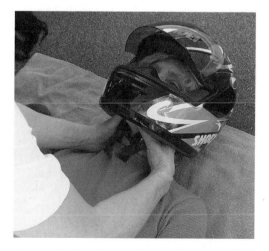

Figure 6.9 Helmet removal I. In helmet removal, the first rescuer places her hands on the mandible, which allows the neck to remain in a neutral position.

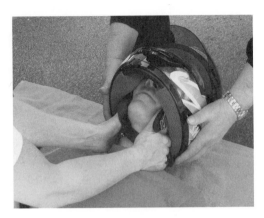

Figure 6.10 Helmet removal II. The second rescuer opens the chinstrap after which the first rescuer continues to stabilize the mandible and neck.

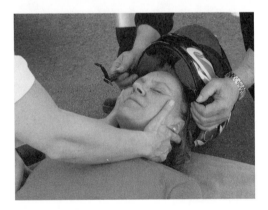

Figure 6.11 Helmet removal III. The second individual then removes the helmet and the helmet is initially expanded to uncover the ears. The first rescuer holds the head in neutral position while the second person finally applies the hard cervical collar.

Diving Accident

Individuals who sustain a diving accident should be treated as if an SCI is present until disproved. If the patient is found face down in the water, the immediate essential goal is to rotate him into a supine (face up) position. Person 1 places one arm on the injured patient's spine and his other arm under the patient's chest. He then backs away and simultaneously rotates the victim to a supine position. One hand is again placed beneath the chest, which enables the patient's head to rest on the

rescuer's upper arm. The other hand is used to stabilize the head and perform assisted ventilation if needed. A second provider delivers the backboard and slides it under the victim, after which the immobilization follows the steps previously described under "Patient Found on the Ground."

Extrication and Transportation

The final step in the ATLS guidelines involves the extrication of the patient from the scene of the accident and into an ambulance or helicopter. The overall goal is to remove the spinal cord injured patient from the scene of accident safely for transportation; that is, without aggravating his neurological status. Speed may be important, but the most important goal is to stabilize all vital organ systems before transporting the patient to an emergency unit.

A wide variety of literature covers all aspects of pre-hospital patient care and transport. The following suggested reading list reflects the forefront of research and best practices on this topic. Chapter 7, picks up where this chapter leaves off.

ACKNOWLEDGMENTS

The authors would like to express their gratitude to ATLS nurse Ragnhild Klum, Department of Anesthesiology, Akademiska Sjukhuset, Uppsala, Sweden, and to our colleague Staffan Pålsson, Department of Anesthesiology, Norrtälje Hospital, Sweden, for valuable contributions in the creation of this chapter.

Suggested Reading

American College of Surgeons Committee on Trauma. Advanced trauma life support for doctors. Student course manual 1997. ISBN-1-880696.

Ball PA, Chicoine RE, Gettinger A. Anesthesia and critical care management of spinal cord injury. In: Tator CH, Benzel CH, eds., *Contemporary Management of Spinal Cord Injury: From Impact to Rehabilitation.* Park Ridge, IL: American Association of Neurological Surgeons, 2000:99–108.

Bernhard M, Gries A, Kremer P, Böttiger BW. Spinal cord injury (SCI)—prehospital management. *Resuscitation* 2005;66(2):127–139. Review.

Crosby ET. Airway management in adults after cervical spine trauma. *Anesthesiology* 2006;104(6):1293–1318.

Dyson-Hudson TA, Stein AB. Acute management of traumatic cervical spinal cord injuries. *Mt Sinai J Med* 1999;66(3):170–178.

Fehlings MG, Louw D. Initial stabilization and medical management of acute spinal cord injury. *Am Fam Physician* 1996;54(1):155–162.

Hadley MN, ed. Cervical spine immobilization before admission to hospital. *Neurosurgery* 2002;50(3): S7–S17.

Hadley MN, ed. Transportation of patients with acute traumatic cervical spine injuries. *Neurosurgery* 2002; 50(3):S18–S20.

Rabinovici R, Ovadia P, Mathiak G, Abdullah F. Abdominal injuries associated with lumbar spine fractures in blunt trauma. *Injury* 1999;30(7): 471–474.

Rengacharry SS, Alton SM. Resuscitation and early medical management of the spinal cord injury patient. In: Tator CH, Benzel CH, eds., *Contemporary Management of Spinal Cord Injury: From Impact to Rehabilitation.* Park Ridge, IL: American Association of Neurological Surgeons, 2000:61–71.

Sheerin F. Spinal cord injury: acute care management. *J Bone Joint Surg Am* 2009;91(11):2568–2576.

Tator CH, Duncan EG, Edmonds VE, et al. Changes in epidemiology of acute spinal cord injury from 1947 to 1981. *Surg Neurol* 1994;40:207–215.

Tator CH, Duncan EG, Edmonds VE, et al. Neurological recovery, mortality and length of stay after acute spinal cord injury associated with changes in management. *Paraplegia* 1995; 33(5):254–262.

Whetstone W. Prehospital management of spinal cord injured patients. In: VW Lin, ed., *Spinal Cord Medicine: Principles and Practice.* New York: Demos Medical Publishing, 1996:107–111.

7   Management at the Hospital

Patients having sustained a SCI are treated according to similar general principles as individuals with multiple trauma. The focus of this chapter is, however, directed toward the specific aspects of treatment related to SCI, assuming that all facilities needed to optimize the treatment of this patient group are available at the receiving hospital. It is not possible to describe all treatment routines in detail, so only general principles are presented in this chapter.

Patients having sustained an acute, severe injury to the spinal cord, especially at the cervical level, may quite often exhibit hypotension, hypoxia, and pulmonary dysfunction. This may result in hemodynamic instability and insufficient ventilation even if circulation and breathing capacity is considered normal during the initial period following injury. A risk always exists for further neurological deterioration upon and immediately after arrival to the hospital. The incidence of neurological deterioration in such instances is not well surveyed; neurological deterioration was observed in 5% of patients after arrival to hospitals in the National Acute SCI Study (NASCIS II) published in 1990. This is an improved rate compared to those reported by previously performed retrospective studies.

NASCIS patients were treated at intensive care units during the acute stage following injury. Monitoring of ventilation and circulation parameters revealed hemodynamic instability, heart rhythm disturbances, and insufficient ventilation resulting in hypoxia. The identification and treatment of these complications is of crucial importance to minimize morbidity and mortality. Avoiding further neurological deterioration and optimizing the chances for recovery of neurological function is the goal of aggressive

intensive care treatment in the acute stage following SCI.

In 1984, Tator and coworkers presented the results of administering volume expanders (using crystalloid solutions, plasma, and whole blood) to avoid hypotension; the use of adequate ventilation, including endotracheal intubation and assisted ventilation if required; and routines to avoid sepsis and urological complications to reduce the consequences of secondary injury in SCI patients, versus a comparable group not receiving similar therapy. These measures resulted in a reduced mortality and morbidity, shorter in-hospital stays, and reduced overall costs. At the time, this study set the gold standard for the intensive care treatment of SCI patients.

The treatment protocol of the NASCIS II study (see Chapter 9) represents the introduction of modern intensive care, equal to that given to multi-trauma patients, also to this group of patients.

The necessity for rapid and active treatment of the SCI patient is based on the theory of primary and secondary injury mechanisms. Every patient, regardless of severity of neurological deficits, should be treated as if he had a potential of regaining function on a spinal cord and/or a spinal root level. Therefore, the goal of therapy is to preserve neurological function by preventing secondary injury mechanisms through the correction of hypoxia and/or hypotension, the treatment of associated injuries, and an ongoing monitoring of the neurological status. These goals are reached through active intensive care that focus on ventilation, circulation, pharmacological treatment, repeated neurological examinations, adequate radiological investigations and, if needed, surgical repair.

INTENSIVE CARE OF THE INJURED SPINAL CORD

There are six cornerstones to the treatment of the injured spinal cord: respiratory management, cardiovascular considerations, neurological examination, radiological evaluation, pharmacological treatment, and surgical decision-making.

Respiratory Management

Supporting ventilation is probably the most important therapeutic measures in treating the consequences following an injury to the spinal cord. An adequate supply of oxygen is not only necessary to guarantee the spinal cord sufficient oxygenation but also prevents additional organ failure.

Preservation of adequate oxygenation is likewise of utmost importance (Table 7.1). Respiratory insufficiency is common, especially among patients with high cervical lesions. Paralysis of diaphragm and respiratory accessory muscles result in insufficient breathing ability, and the patient exhibits a significantly reduced inspiratory capacity. This results in relative hypoxia, which may lead to impaired oxygen supply to the spinal cord. The resulting hypoxia accelerates and augments the destructive effects of secondary injury mechanisms.

Diaphragmatic function requires at least one functioning phrenic nerve. This nerve contains fibers from the third, fourth, and fifth cervical roots. Diaphragmatic breathing is thus impaired if a lesion occurs at C5 or above, resulting in hypoxia. The degree of impairment is correlated with the extent of lesion at those levels. The intercostal muscles are also affected if an injury occurs at the cervical level. The net effect of reduced or absent diaphragmatic and intercostal muscle function is a partial or complete loss of ventilatory capacity, and a mode of ventilation referred to as *paradoxical abdominal breathing* may be observed.

The chest wall is normally expanded during inspiration, but the opposite is noted in the presence of reduced or absent diaphragmatic and intercostal muscle function. Thoracic and abdominal muscle function is more or less lost if the SCI is located at the level of C5 and above; ventilation is then nearly completely dependent on diaphragm function. Minimal movement of the chest wall and passive inspiratory/expiratory movements of the flaccid abdominal wall characterize diaphragmatic breathing.

It is thus of greatest importance to establish adequate oxygenation in order to counteract the consequences of secondary pathophysiological events. Some authors have proposed prophylactic intubation and assisted ventilation for patients with high cervical lesions. This measure is motivated by the need to avoid respiratory fatigue and insufficiency in patients showing diminished breathing capacity. Clinical symptoms such as agitation, disorientation, anxiety, and decreased breathing capacity (verified by arterial blood gases) determine the need for

TABLE 7.1 Conditions and measures related to respiratory insufficiency.

Conditions	Measures
Respiratory insufficiency due to paralysis of the diaphragm and respiratory accessory muscles	Support ventilation (either by utilizing the bag/valve mask or intubation, alternatively tracheostomy with assisted ventilation)
Impaired cough function and accumulation of mucus, with signs of anxiety, disorientation, and agitation indicate respiratory insufficiency	As above and "assisted cough" using manual compression of the chest and careful suction of secretions. Ventilator assisted ventilation, careful suction of secretions and repeated manual compressions of the chest.
Inadequate ventilation as reflected in arterial blood gases	Aim at correction to PO_2 >12 kPa and PCO_2 4,5–5,5 kPa

intubation and assisted ventilation. Orotracheal intubation is, if intubation indeed is required, most frequently preferred over nasotracheal intubation.

Insertion of the tube is performed in the same manner as at the scene of the accident (see Chapter 6), with the anterior part of the rigid cervical collar opened and a second individual stabilizing the neck during the maneuver. (The similar two-person procedure is used when a gastric tube is inserted to prevent aspiration pneumonia.)

Arterial blood gases are measured frequently to guarantee the patient optimal ventilation. Oxygenation is adequate if the PO_2 is 100 mm Hg (12 kPa) or higher and the PCO_2 is less than 45 mm Hg or between 4.5 and 5.5 kPa. Intubation is usually required if the PO_2 is less than 70 mm Hg (~ 9 kPa) measured on room air, or if the PCO_2 rises above 45 mm Hg (~6 kPa).

Cardiovascular Considerations

Spinal cord blood flow is affected by injuries to and bleeding in other organ systems (Tables 6.1 and 7.2) in addition to the alterations seen in the injured spinal cord area itself. The initial mechanical impact, as well as subsequent vasospasm, causes local changes in spinal cord blood flow. Both these mechanisms are partly responsible for the loss of spinal cord blood flow autoregulation (see Chapter 4). The influence of the sympathetic nervous systems is lost if SCI occurs above the level of T6. The loss of sympathetic outflow results

TABLE 7.2 Systemic and local (spinal cord) causes of reduced spinal cord blood flow.

Systemic Level	Spinal Cord Level
Injuries and bleeding in other organ systems	Loss of microcirculation (e.g., due to vasospasm)
Neurogenic shock: Hypotension and bradycardia Reduced total heart volume Hypothermia	Loss of microvascular autoregulation

in an unopposed parasympathetic influence, and neurogenic shock develops as a consequence of this "autosympathectomy." This condition is characterized by dysrhythmias, bradycardia, insufficient central blood return, and reduced perfusion pressure due to a decrease in mean arterial pressure (systemic hypotension). The resistance of the peripheral vessels is reduced as a result of the vasodilatation, and blood accumulates in peripheral vessels of the extremities. The loss of autoregulation and the systemic hypotension thus results in reduced spinal cord blood flow. This decrease in blood flow constitutes the prerequisite for subsequent spinal cord ischemia and the ultimate destruction of nervous tissue.

The hypotension (systolic blood pressure <70 mm Hg) seen after SCI could, as previously mentioned, be part of the symptoms related to neurogenic shock. However, it may also appear as a consequence of hypovolemic shock caused by abdominal, chest, and/or fracture bleeding. Other forms of shock, such as cardiogenic shock due to myocardial infarction and septic shock as a consequence of bacteriemia, are also seen on rare occasions.

The treatment of neurogenic and hypovolemic shock differs. Incorrect treatment of neurogenic shock using the principles applicable to hypovolemic shock results in an accumulation of fluid in the spinal cord and edema, followed by an accelerating development of secondary pathophysiological events. The presence of certain symptoms may help differentiate these two conditions (Table 6.6).

Hypotension in patients with an isolated injury to the spinal cord is thus not due to hypovolemia but rather due to a redistribution of blood from the central to the peripheral system (neurogenic shock). It has been shown that a systolic blood pressure below approximately 90 mm Hg increases morbidity and mortality following SCI. The blood pressure must therefore be maintained aggressively to assure adequate blood flow to the spinal cord during the first hours to days following injury (Table 7.3). A central venous catheter (CVC) for registration of the central venous pressure and vascular access, and a Foley catheter (FC) for urine drainage are inserted initially. Urine output is a valuable parameter to separate hypovolemic shock from the neurogenic shock.

TABLE 7.3 Cardiovascular management.

Insert CVC and Foley catheter. Place the patient in Trendelenburg position.

Try to verify the correct shock diagnosis by excluding or confirming hypovolemia as the cause of hypotension.

Try to optimize the spinal cord blood flow in order to counteract the loss of autoregulation.

Optimal spinal cord blood flow is reached by maintaining a sufficient systolic blood pressure (at least 90 mm Hg, but preferably 110 mm Hg).

Treat the SCI patient with crystalloids initially until hypovolemic shock has been excluded. Neurogenic shock is treated according to similar principles as for traumatic brain injury. Add colloid solution and vasopressors to achieve a maximal systolic blood pressure.

The patient should be placed in the Trendelenburg position, regardless of the type of shock, in order to increase the reflow of the peripherally distributed blood and improve the circulation. The Trendelenburg position is especially effective if the patient suffers from neurogenic shock.

The standard treatment for shock is to deliver crystalloid (isotonic) solutions, such as Ringer's lactate, although some controversy exists regarding the choice of fluid replacement. The presence of neurogenic shock should be suspected as soon as all relevant investigations have been performed and injuries to other organ systems have been excluded, and especially if fluid replacement with crystalloid solutions is ineffective in restoring systemic blood pressure. It is of utmost importance to identify neurogenic shock as soon as possible, since the continued administration of crystalloid solutions to these patients will result in an accumulation of fluid in the extracellular space. A risk of a rapid, over-compensating fluid delivery exists since, as a rule, crystalloid solutions are administered in a volume approximately four times exceeding a suspected blood loss. This fluid overload may lead to spinal cord as well as pulmonary edema.

Thus, the principles of fluid replacement in SCI follow those for brain injury as soon as neurogenic shock has been diagnosed. The total fluid volume delivery must be maintained at a maximum of 2.5 L during the first 24-hour period. Colloid solutions, such as albumin, dextran, or starch- and gelatin-based preparations, are administrated as needed. These solutions contain larger molecules compared to isotonic solutions. These larger molecules remain within the blood vessels and help to draw back extravasated fluid, thus resulting in improved cardiovascular function and spinal cord blood flow.

Bradycardia triggered by neurogenic shock is initially treated with atropine, whereas hypotension associated with this condition is usually treated with vasopressors, such as dopamine, and if needed, dobutamine.

Neurological Examination

A detailed neurological examination is vital following initial resuscitation. The neurological evaluation should be performed repeatedly throughout the early posttraumatic phase, in order to detect alterations in neurological status.

The American Spinal Injury Association (ASIA) standards of neurological and functional classification of SCI are considered the most accepted guidelines for assessment of neurological function (a detailed description is presented in Chapter 8). Examination according to ASIA standards makes it possible to determine the neurological level of injury, characterize remaining neurological function below the level of injury, and evaluate for the completeness of the lesion (including the various neuroanatomical syndromes of incomplete injury). The possibility of detecting changes in neurological function is considered especially important. The examination is easy to repeat, and enables a reliable prognosis in the early stage following injury. The ASIA uniform standards also facilitate communication between all units treating the SCI patient. The standards are also of substantial value in the field of future research.

The neurological evaluation is hampered by factors such as concurrent brain injury or altered degree of consciousness due to drugs or excessive intake of alcohol. In addition, the prognostic possibility for regaining function may be hidden by the presence of spinal shock. Peripheral nerve injuries or damage to the brachial plexus, as well as immobilized extremities due to fractures, may further complicate the interpretation of the neurological examination. Nonetheless, the value of performing a careful neurological examination of sensory and motor function, especially at sacral levels, cannot be overemphasized. It is not unusual to detect spared sacral function among signs of an otherwise complete injury. This finding may result in an altered treatment strategy, since the lesion is, in such cases, regarded as incomplete and the prognosis is considered better than that for complete lesions.

Radiological Evaluation

Once the initial goal of optimal respiratory and cardiovascular management is achieved, radiological investigations may be directed toward areas of interest, guided by the findings of the clinical neurological evaluation. In the acute stage, however, most imaging studies will encompass the entire spinal column.

The purpose of the neurological examination is to not only localize the level of lesion, but most importantly to detect signs of deterioration or improvement in function. In the face of multiple vertebral injuries, the neurological examination serves to determine the level of the SCI. New developments in the field of radiology have improved the ability to visualize posttraumatic changes to both the spinal column and the spinal cord, and optimal treatment depends strongly on a precise radiographic assessment of the injured area. The available techniques are plain radiographs, computed tomography (CT), and magnetic resonance imaging (MRI). The indications, advantages, and disadvantages using these methods are presented in Chapter 8. The three techniques are exemplified in Figure 7.1A–C, illustrating a fracture through the base of the

dens, a so-called type 2 odontoid fracture. The three figures illustrate a similar injury as visualized by plain radiographs, CT including reconstruction images, and MRI. The MRI demonstrates spinal cord edema as a sign of a severe injury to the spinal cord.

Pharmacological Treatment

The use of drugs in the treatment of the spinal cord lesion is a relatively recent phenomenon. As we learn more about the mechanisms of secondary injury in SCI, pharmacotherapy continues to be refined to the acute stage following injury. These so-called neuroprotective pharmacological treatments aim to reduce or reverse the actions of secondary pathophysiological events (see the section "Biochemical Changes," in Chapter 4 and see Chapter 9 for more details of the pharmacological treatment of SCI).

Surgical Decision Making

The final cornerstone in the management of the SCI patient is surgical decision-making. The choice between surgical intervention or conservative (nonsurgical) treatment in the management of fractures and/or ligamentous injuries must be evaluated carefully, and a detailed review of possible treatment approaches for the cervical, thoracic, and lumbar spine is presented in Chapters 10 through 15. Here, we describe treatment options assuming a hypothetical SCI with a simultaneous fracture and/or ligamentous injury.

In deciding on a treatment plan, it is important to distinguish between injuries that result only in fractures and/or ligamentous damage and those that also primarily involve the spinal cord. The indications for surgery, depending on the severity of the injury, may be either orthopedic, neurosurgical, or both.

Orthopedic treatment of the skeletal and/or ligamentous injury is focused on reposition and stabilization of the injured segment. Neurosurgical interventions are undertaken to reduce compression of the spinal cord caused by fracture fragments, blood, disk material, and/or ligamentous tissue.

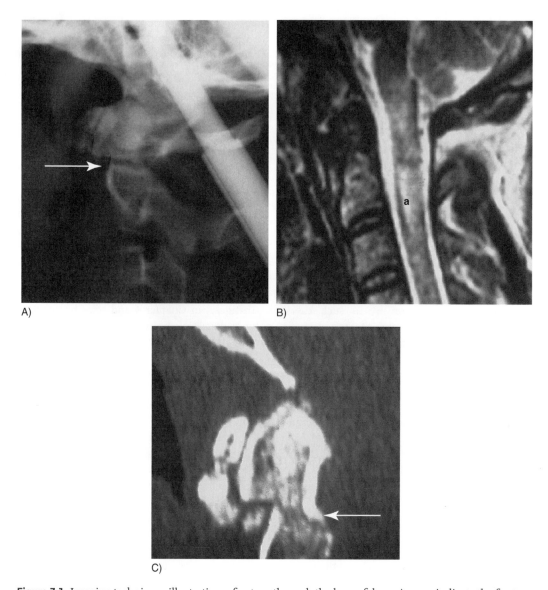

A)

B)

C)

Figure 7.1 Imaging techniques illustrating a fracture through the base of dens. Arrows indicate the fracture line. A: Plain radiographs B: Magnetic resonance imaging (MRI); *a*, spinal cord edema C: Computed tomography (CT) scan.

General Considerations: Conservative Versus Surgical Treatment

Impairment of neurological function usually indicates the presence of a concomittant severe injury to the spinal column and/or ligaments. Such lesions are typically regarded as mechanically unstable if they occur simultaneously with a spinal cord lesion. Exceptions, such as in many

instances of the central cord syndrome, occur among elderly patients with spinal stenosis and a mild hyperextension trauma. Ligamentous injuries in the upper part of the cervical spine without a concomitant fracture, on the other hand, may occur in tandem with a lesion to the spinal cord, thus indicating instability in the affected spinal column segment(s). As has been discussed extensively elsewhere in this book, controversy exists as to whether injuries to the spinal column and ligamentous structures should be treated surgically or conservatively.

Conservative treatment of SCI, still commonly used in for example in Great Britain, is based on Sir Ludwig Guttmann's principles of postural reduction. According to these principles, patients are treated with bed rest, with or without traction, until pain is relieved. This is followed by the use of various cervical collars for 6–12 weeks. Surgical treatment may be considered in later stages, if a remaining spinal deformity proves to be unstable and/or a progressive neurological deterioration is detected. The conservative treatment of injuries to the upper cervical spine includes an external orthosis such as the Halo-vest (see Chapter 15). The Halo approach is currently used in the treatment of over 60% of cervical spine injuries. As long as the fracture is kept in acceptable alignment, this treatment is preferable if no concurrent SCI is present. However, the Halo treatment may, according to some authors, delay rehabilitation among patients with an injury to the spinal cord. Among patients without a simultaneous injury to the spinal cord, orthoses are also used in 75% of thoracolumbar injuries.

Controversies persist regarding the benefits of surgical decompression of the spinal cord and restoration of spinal column alignment following trauma, as well as regarding the timing of surgery. Animal experimental studies show that continuing compression from bone, blood, or intervertebral disk material increases the severity of neurological deterioration, and this increase is time-dependent. It has also been shown that early removal of the foreign material results in less ultimate neurological deficits. Similar circumstances should logically apply to humans, but no scientific data exists proving that early decompression and stabilization is preferable to nonsurgical treatment in humans. On the other hand, neither has it strictly been scientifically proven that conservative treatment is more efficacious. Given the nature of the disorder, such studies are difficult to undertake. Current trends in the treatment of SCI patients, however, tend to involve an increase in surgical interventions and less interest in conservative approaches.

Guidelines for Surgical Intervention

Certain trends regarding surgical decision-making can be discerned in the literature despite considerable disagreement. The indications for surgical treatment are presented in Table 7.4, although the choice of treatment for any particular patient is heavily influenced by a variety of circumstances. Because, by strict scientific criteria, neither surgical nor nonsurgical treatment has been shown to be preferable regarding neurological restoration following SCI, the authors present, in Table 7.5 their interpretation of the recommendations found in the literature. Surgical intervention is indicated if the patient exhibits an ongoing neurological deterioration in combination with radiologically verified compression of the spinal cord. Early surgical decompression of the spinal cord is most often recommended if the patient suffers from an incomplete lesion and the radiological examination reveals a concomitant compression of the spinal cord caused by bony fragments, blood, and/or disk material. Consensus is lacking regarding surgical intervention in patients with complete lesions showing radiologically verified compression of the spinal cord.

There are additional relative indications for surgical intervention. Patients with fractures and/or ligamentous injuries at the cervical level, in combination with a SCI and a concurrent compression of the cervical roots, could serve as an example of such an indication. In such cases, the primary goal of the surgical intervention is not to restore spinal cord function per se, but rather to save nerve root function. An improved nerve root

---

TABLE 7.4 Goals of surgical treatment in SCI patients.

Restore spinal column alignment and stability
Facilitate early mobilization
Reduce pain from spinal column lesions
Minimize hospital length of stay
Prevent secondary complications (e.g. pain, deformity, and neurological deterioration)

TABLE 7.5 Guidelines for surgical and conservative (non-surgical) treatment of SCI patients.

	Surgical Treatment	Conservative Treatment
Neurological deterioration	Yes	No
Neurological improvement	No	Yes
Neurological level of lesion	Caudal	Cranial
Radiological evaluation	Instability	No instability
Spinal cord compression evident on CT/MRI	Yes	No
Spinal cord changes on MRI	Contusion	Edema
Age	Younger	Older
Attitudes of the surgeon I	Believer in the relevance of secondary injury mechanisms	Non-believer in the relevance of secondary injury mechanisms
Attitudes of the surgeon II	Judges the risk for surgical complications as acceptable	Judges the risk for surgical complications as unacceptably

function in even one single segment may result in a clinically important improvement in neurological function among tetraplegic patients. Surgery is unnecessary in the incompletely injured patient, provided he shows signs of neurological improvement in the initial stage after injury. Surgical intervention may be considered in such a patient, however, if expected neurological improvement fails to evolve and the present degree of impairment is unacceptable. An elderly patient with degenerative changes in the spinal column suffering from a central cord syndrome could serve as an example in which delayed surgical intervention (within days) may be indicated. This group of patients is quite often also suffering from severe neuropathic pain in the upper extremities. Early decompression has empirically been shown to significantly reduce the degree of pain.

Spinal stabilization is advocated if the plain radiograph reveals fractures involving both the anterior and posterior columns (see Chapter 10). MRI changes (e.g., spinal cord contusion and compression) indicate a need for surgical intervention, whereas conservative treatment is preferable if the MRI shows only spinal cord edema without accompanying signs of mechanical compression of the spinal cord (Fig. 7.2).

In the final analysis, the attitude of the consulting surgeon is important: A more

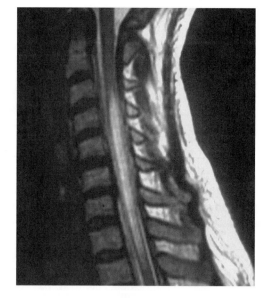

Figure 7.2 Spinal cord edema without signs of spinal cord compression.

active approach towards surgical intervention is expected if the surgeon believes in the theory of secondary injury in SCI and also considers the surgical risk for neurological and other complications (Table 7.6) as acceptable. Excellent information regarding complications may be found in data from NASCIS II and from a

TABLE 7.6 Possible surgical complications
of the anterior approach at the
cervical level.

Neurological deterioration
Vascular injuries (e.g., to the vertebral artery)
N. recurrens damage with vocal cord paresis
Esophageal perforation
Tracheal perforation
Horner syndrome
Pneumothorax
Infection

manuscript presented by Wilberger and coworkers
(see "Suggested Reading"). These two studies
present complications related to nonsurgical
(NASCIS II), early (<24 hours), and late (>24
hours) surgical intervention. The incidence of
complications such as pneumonia, pulmonary
embolism, deep venous thrombosis (DVT), and
pressure ulcers was reduced up to 50% in the
group treated with early surgical intervention as
compared to the other two treatment groups.
Neurological deterioration related to surgical intervention was reported to occur in 0% and 2.5% in
the early and late surgical groups, respectively. The
risks of complications related to surgical treatment
are reduced, according to current opinion, if
surgery is performed as early as possible.
However, surgical intervention to the spine
should take secondary priority if injuries to other
vital organ systems require immediate surgical
attention.

In summary, no conclusive scientific documentation exists regarding the beneficial effect
of surgery on neurological recovery after decompression of the spinal cord, restoration of the
spinal alignment, and stabilization of the injured
segment in the early stage following injury.
Wilberger and coworkers presented trends
toward improved results following early intervention, but these findings cannot be considered
conclusive. As all studies advocating either surgical or nonsurgical treatments are retrospective,
the issue of surgical treatment will not be settled
until prospective studies of high scientific quality
are performed. However, the results from
animal experimental studies strongly support
early surgical intervention.

ADDITIONAL INTENSIVE CARE MEASURES

Deep Venous Thrombosis

Vasodilatation and accumulation of blood
peripherally increase the risk of DVT, especially in the lower extremities. Up to 80% or
more of patients with complete lesions have
been reported to develop DVT, whereas the
Model SCI System presented an overall incidence of 13.6% among inpatients during the
acute stage following SCI. The incidence of
DVT is highest 7–10 days post injury. The
prevention of DVT comprises elastic stockings
and/or pneumatic devices that pump blood
from the periphery to the central system.
Anticoagulant prophylaxis, typically with low-
molecular-weight heparin (LMWH), is frequently used. Passive movements and early
mobilization are other important preventative
options. Intravenous infusions in paretic or
paralyzed extremities should be avoided. A
central venous catheter, for delivery use, is
preferred in tetraplegic patients during the
intensive care period. It is usually difficult
to confirm the presence of DVT by bedside
examination. The three classic signs of
DVT—a tense/swollen calf, a positive
Homan sign, and an increase in calf temperature—are sometimes difficult to detect in the
SCI patient. Invasive venograms or ultrasound are thus performed to confirm the
diagnosis. Conventional anticoagulation treatment is recommended, either with intravenous heparin or subcutaneous LMWH once
the diagnosis is confirmed.

Pulmonary Embolism

Vigilance must be high for symptoms associated with pulmonary embolism (PE). Classic
hallmarks such as chest pain, dyspnea, and
tachycardia may be absent due to changes in
the autonomic outflow. Pain perception may be
reduced as a result of disturbances in the transmission of sensory impulses, and pneumonia
and intubation may mask PE. CT of the chest
reveals the diagnosis. The treatment is identical to that of DVT, although this condition
is regarded as more severe.

Gastrointestinal and Nutritional Measures

Acute disturbance of autonomic control of intestinal function, in combination with the hormonal response to stress and the possible presence of abdominal trauma, result in digestive dysfunction and a reduced uptake of nutrients. Acute, paralytic ileus and gastroparesis results in an accumulation of large volumes of intestinal fluid.

This accumulation of fluid contributes to hypovolemia and electrolyte disturbances, and reflux of gastric content may lead to aspiration pneumonia. It is therefore of great importance to relieve the stomach of excess fluid, especially if the patient exhibits paralytic ileus, using naso/orogastric tubes. Many authorities also advocate continuous drainage of the stomach in order to counteract reflux and pneumonia. The symptoms of paralytic ileus usually resolve within 2–3 weeks.

Stress- and steroid-mediated gastric ulcers occur frequently in the acute stage. Symptoms such as hematemesis, referred pain to the shoulder region, tachycardia, and diffuse abdominal discomfort may indicate the presence of gastric ulcers. These symptoms are sometimes masked among SCI patients, and one must be vigilant for the presence of gastric ulcers. Monitoring the acid level of gastric contents is used in some institutions, and prophylactic therapy, usually antacids or H_2-blockers, is given. Treatment of verified gastric ulcers follows current routines.

Total parenteral nutrition (TPN) and/or enteral nutrition should be initiated as soon as possible following injury. TPN, preferably through a central venous catheter, should replace the peripheral administration of fluids as soon as possible, with the administration of TPN usually starting within 24–48 hours following injury. Enteral nutrition is initiated as soon as bowel sounds are audible and the patient starts to pass gas. Pancreatitis is often associated with paralytic ileus, probably caused by an unbalanced parasympathetic stimulation resulting in spasm of the sphincter of Oddi and an increase in amylase production. Among patients suffering from pancreatitis, TPN is continued until amylase values are normalized. Evacuation of the bowels should be performed on a regular basis since constipation will delay post injury return of bowel peristalsis.

Bladder Care

The nerve supply of the bladder is blocked during the period of spinal shock, and the bladder is thus unable to empty by reflex. An urethral catheter must be inserted within the first 2–3 hours after injury. Bladder distension must be avoided due to the risk of autonomic dysreflexia. Permanent bladder dysfunction (e.g., detrusor damage and reflux) may occur if the bladder remains distended. The indwelling catheter is replaced by intermittent catheterization as soon as the patient's general condition is stabilized. Intermittent catheterization will reduce the rate of bacteriuria, which is important since urinary tract infection is probably the most frequent complication of the post acute period.

Pressure Ulcer Prevention

Skin care is an early priority and should start immediately following injury. The patient must be turned every 2 hours during the acute stage. Areas of bony prominence vulnerable to pressure ulcers, such as the sacral and trochanter regions, must be particularly protected from unnecessary pressure. Mattresses containing air, water, or foam should be used to minimize pressure to sensitive areas.

Contracture Prevention

A contracture denotes a shortening of a muscle, tendon, or ligament. The prevention of wrist contractures is especially important following injury. Patients should be offered range-of-motion exercise programs and orthotic devices.

ACKNOWLEDGMENTS

The authors would like to express their gratitude to our colleague Staffan Pålsson, Department of Anesthesiology, Norrtälje Hospital, Sweden, and ATLS nurse Ragnhild Klum, Department of Anesthesiology, Akademiska Sjukhuset, Uppsala, Sweden, for valuable contributions in the creation of this chapter.

Suggested Reading

Al Eissa S, Reed JG, Kortbeek JB, Salo PT. Airway compromise secondary to upper cervical spine injury. *J Trauma* 2009;67(4):692–696.

Apuzzo MJL, ed. Management of acute spinal cord injuries in an intensive care unit or other monitored setting. *Neurosurgery* 2002;50(3 Suppl):S51–S57.

Apuzzo MJL, ed. Radiographic assessment of the cervical spine in symptomatic patients. *Neurosurgery* 2002;50 (3 Suppl):S36–S43.

Apuzzo MJL, ed. Blood pressure management after acute spinal cord injury. *Neurosurgery* 2002;50(3 Suppl):S58–S62.

Apuzzo MJL, ed. Pharmacological therapy after acute cervical spinal cord injury. *Neurosurgery* 2002;50(3 Suppl): S63–S72.

Apuzzo MJL, ed. Deep vein thrombosis and thromboembolism in patients with cervical spinal cord injuries. *Neurosurgery* 2002;50(3 Suppl):S73–S80.

Apuzzo MJL, ed. Nutritional support after spinal cord injury. *Neurosurgery*. 2002;50(3 Suppl):S81–84.

Barboi C, Peruzzi WT. Acute medical management of spinal cord injury. In: Lin VW, ed., *Spinal Cord Medicine Demos Medical Publishing*. New York, USA: Principles and Practice, 2003:113–123.

Bellomo R. Fluid resuscitation: colloids vs. crystalloids. *Blood Purif* 2002;20(3):239–242. Review.

Berlly M, Shem K. Respiratory management during the first five days after spinal cord injury. *J Spinal Cord Med* 2007;30(4):309–318. Review.

Bracken MB, Shepard MJ, Collins WF, et al. A randomized, controlled trial of methylprednisolone or naloxone in the treatment of acute spinal-cord injury. Results of the Second National Acute Spinal Cord Injury Study. *N Engl J Med* 1990;322(20):1405–1411.

Casha S, Christie S. A systematic review of intensive cardiopulmonary management after spinal cord injury. *J Neurotrauma* 2009;December 23 (Epub ahead of print).

Chen D, Apple DF Jr., Hudson LM, Bode R. Medical complications during acute rehabilitation following spinal cord injury—current experience of the Model Systems. *Arch Phys Med Rehabil* 1999;80(11):1397–1401.

Chen L, Yang H, Yang T, et al. Effectiveness of surgical treatment for traumatic central cord syndrome. *J Neurosurg Spine* 2009;10(1):3–8.

Delmarter RB, Coyle J. Acute management of spinal cord injury. *J Am Acad Orthop Surg* 1999;7(3):166–175.

Fehlings MG, Sekhon LH, Tator C. The role and timing of decompression in acute spinal cord injury: what do we know? What should we do? *Spine* 2001;26(24 Suppl): S101–10. Review.

Furlan JC, Fehlings MG. Cardiovascular complications after acute spinal cord injury: pathophysiology, diagnosis, and management. *Neurosurg Focus* 2008;25(5): E13.

Guest JD, Sonntag VKH. Patient selection and timing of surgical intervention. In: Tator CH, Benzel CH, eds.,

Contemporary Management of Spinal Cord Injury: From Impact to Rehabilitation. Park Ridge IL: American Association of Neurological Surgeons, 2000:109–122.

Holtz A. Early management after acute traumatic spinal cord injury. *Ups J Med Sci* 1995;100(2):93–123. Review.

Krassioukov A, Warburton DE, Teasell R, Eng JJ. A systematic review of the management of autonomic dysreflexia after spinal cord injury. *Arch Pys Med Rehabil* 2009;90(4):682–695.

Krassioukov A, Eng JJ, Warburton DE, Teasell R. A systematic review of the management of orthostatic hypotension after spinal cord injury. *Arch Pys Med Rehabil* 2009;90(5):876–885.

La Rosa G, Conti A, Cardali S, et al. Does early decompression improve neurological outcome of spinal cord injured patients? Appraisal of the literature using a meta-analytical approach. *Spinal Cord* 2004;42 (9):503–512. Review.

McBride DQ, Rodts GE. Intensive care of patients with spinal trauma. *Neurosurg Clin N Am* 1994;5(4):755–766. Review.

McKinley WO, Gittler MS, Kirshblum SC, et al. Spinal cord injury medicine. 2. Medical complications after spinal cord injury: Identification and management. *Arch Phys Med Rehabil* 2002;83(3 Suppl 1):S58–64, S90–98. Review.

Miyanji F, Furlan JC, Aarabi B, et al. Acute cervical traumatic spinal cord injury: MR imaging findings correlated with neurologic outcome—prospective study with 100 consecutive patients. *Radiology* 2007;243(3): 820–7. Epub 2007 April 12.

Muzevich KM, Voils SA. Role of vasopressor administration in patients with acute neurologic injury. *Neurocrit Care* 2009;11(1):112–119. Epub 2009 April 22. Review.

Ploumis A, Ponnappan RK, Maltenfort MG, et al. Thromboprophylaxis in patients with acute spinal injuries: an evidence-based analysis. *J Bone Joint Surg Am* 2009;91(11):2568–2576. Review.

Raslan AM, Fields JD, Bhardwaj A. Prophylaxis for venous thrombo-embolism in neurocritical care: a critical appraisal. *Neurocrit Care* 2009;December 22.

Rowan CJ, Gillanders LK, Paice RL, Judson JA. Is early enteral feeding safe in patients who have suffered spinal cord injury? *Injury* 2004;35(3):238–242. Review.

Sassoon CSH. Respiratory dysfunction in spinal cord disorders. Rosa boken p:155–167.

Schinkel C, Anastasiadis AP. The timing of spinal stabilization in polytrauma and in patients with spinal cord injury. *Curr Opin Crit Care* 2008;14(6):685–689.

Tator CH, Rowed DW, Schwartz ML, et al. Management of acute spinal cord injuries. *Can J Surg* 1984;27 (3):289–293.

Tator CH, Fehlings MG, Thorpe K, Taylor W. Current use and timing of spinal surgery for management of acute spinal surgery for management of acute spinal cord injury in North America: results of a retrospective multicenter study. *J Neurosurg Spine* 1999;91 (1):12–18.

Teasell RW, Arnold JM, Krassioukov A, Delaney GA. Cardiovascular consequences of loss of supraspinal control of the sympathetic nervous system after spinal cord injury. *Arch Phys Med Rehabil* 2000;81(4):506–516. Review.

Urdaneta F, Layon AJ. Respiratory complications in patients with traumatic cervical spine injuries: case report and review of the literature. *J Clin Anesth* 2003;15(5):398–405.

Vale FL, Burns J, Jackson AB, Hadley MN. Combined medical and surgical treatment after acute spinal cord injury: results of a prospective pilot study to assess the merits of aggressive medical resuscitation and blood pressure management. *J Neurosurg* 1997;87 (2):239–246.

Wilberger JE. Diagnosis and management of spinal cord trauma. *J Neurotrauma* 1991;(8) Suppl 1:S21–28.

Winslow C, Rozovsky J. Effect of spinal cord injury on the respiratory system. *Am J Phys Med Rehabil* 2003;82 (10):803–814. Review.

8 Diagnostic Methods

CLINICAL ASSESSMENT AND CLASSIFICATION ACCORDING TO ASIA

The *International Standards for Neurological and Functional Classification of SCI*, developed by the American Spinal Injury Association (ASIA) (Fig. 8.1), are often used for clinical neurological classification of focal spinal cord lesions, especially traumatic myelopathies. They provide a standardized quantitative description of the neurological level of injury and sensorimotor function above and below this level. However, an examination conducted according to ASIA only furnishes part of the clinically relevant information and therefore is not intended to replace a complete neurological exam. Moreover, assessment conducted according to ASIA is not designed to address diffuse, multifocal, and/or pathway-specific lesions. Conventional neurological examination is preferable in such cases. This chapter presents an overview of the ASIA classification system. For further details please refer to the specific manuals available.

Assessment

Sensory Function

Sensory examination comprises testing of what are known as *key points* in each of the 28 dermatomes on both the left and right sides of the body (Fig. 8.2). The key points correspond with a defined area of skin in each dermatome where overlapping innervation to adjacent dermatomes is at a minimum, thereby making these areas most suitable for testing the function of each specific dermatome. The dermatomes extend from level C2 to S5, where S4 and S5 are considered as one dermatome. Each key point, including the anal/perianal region, is tested for light touch (with a cotton tip applicator or similar object) and pain (using a pin or similar object). Sensory function is graded as follows: normal = 2; impaired/distorted = 1; absent = 0; not testable = NT. The latter may be due to amputation or a cast covering the area. In most cases, testing of sensory function is not too difficult. However, some pitfalls may be mentioned:

- During pain testing with a pin, should the patient perceive touch *without* any pain component, the pain sensation should be graded as absent within the relevant dermatome.
- Should a painful stimulus be perceived as *stronger* when testing a specific dermatome compared with testing a dermatome with normal sensation (such as on the face or other location well above the level of injury), sensitivity to pain should be graded as impaired/distorted within the relevant dermatome.
- If during sensory testing of a dermatome the patient should perceive stimulation with *both* light touch and pin-prick as painful, thus lacking the ability to differentiate a blunt from a sharp stimulus, sensation to pain should be graded as distorted or absent in the relevant dermatome.
- Should the patient experience *any* sensory perception, regardless of type, in response to light touch and pin-prick in the anal region, the injury should be classified as incomplete; otherwise as complete.
- *The definition of complete versus incomplete injury is based solely on the presence or absence of sensory function (and/or motor function = voluntary sphincter contraction) in the anal region, regardless of the presence or absence otherwise of*

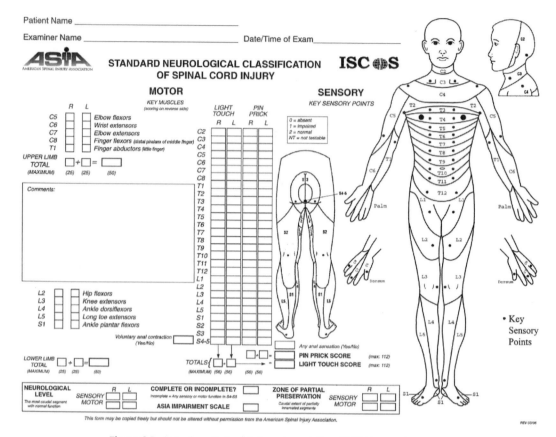

Figure 8.1 American Spinal Injury Association (ASIA) questionnaire.

sensorimotor residual function below the level of injury.

- The T3 dermatome is the most difficult one to assess, because of the considerable individual variation in how far down along the anterior chest wall the adjoining C4 dermatome extends. For this reason, sensory function in the T3 dermatome should be graded as absent if sensation within the T1 and T2 dermatomes is absent, even when sensation appears to be present within the T3 dermatome, only to become absent once again in the T4 dermatome.

The summation of points for pain and light touch, respectively, is given for the left and right sides of the body (maximum of 56 for each side) in addition to a total sum (maximum of 112 for each modality).

Motor Function

Motor function testing according to ASIA encompasses 10 myotomes, specifically C5–T1 and L2–S1, corresponding to the five *key muscles* each in the left and right arms and left and right legs (Fig. 8.2).

Voluntary muscle function is graded for each muscle as follows:

0 = Total paralysis
1 = Palpable or visible muscle contraction
2 = Active movement through full range of motion with gravity eliminated (i.e., when the extremity or its extremity segment is relieved of weight)
3 = Active movement through full range of motion against gravity
4 = Active movement through full range of motion against moderate resistance

5 = Active movement through full range of motion against full (normal) resistance

5* = The patient succeeds in overcoming sufficient resistance to movement for muscle strength to be considered normal, assuming that simultaneous mobility-inhibiting factors could be eliminated (e.g., pain inhibition)

NT = Not testable; the muscle cannot be assessed due to amputation, casting, ankylosis or simultaneous plexus injury, or peripheral nerve damage

- The most difficult key muscle to assess in the upper extremities is the triceps (Fig. 8.3). When testing this muscle, it is essential to maintain a horizontal forearm position across the chest (with patient lying supine). Patients with weak or absent triceps function often unintentionally "cheat" by externally rotating the shoulder in order to passively extend the elbow.
- When testing the deep finger flexors, the wrist and proximal phalanges must be stabilized in order to isolate the muscle. Finger flexion may otherwise result passively from a

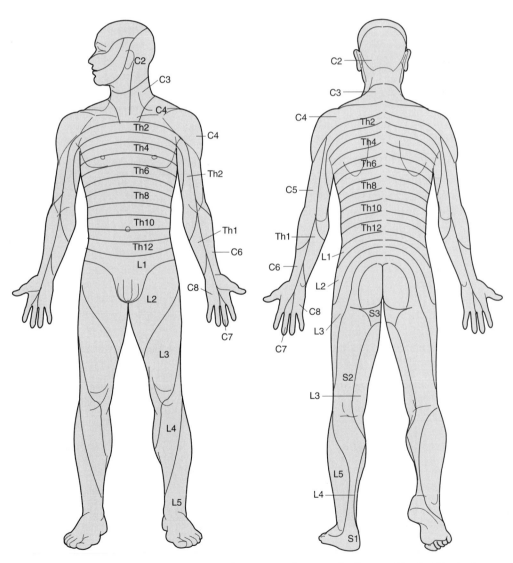

Figure 8.2 Segmental skin innervation (dermatome chart) on the front and back of the body.

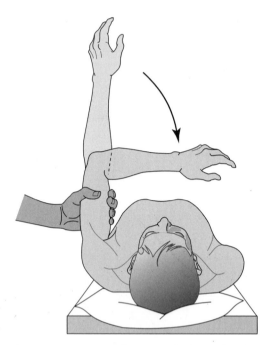

Figure 8.3 Testing of triceps function for the purpose of isolating muscle activity during elbow extension.

tenodesis effect; in other words, by passive tension on the flexor tendon with wrist extension.
• Special care must also be given to examining the finger abductors. Among patients who have the ability to actively extend their fingers, such extension may lead to a degree of simultaneous finger abduction. The fingers should therefore be placed in extended position and the abductors should be both observed and palpated while testing the abductor digiti minimi muscle (Fig. 8.4).
• Additional interference during motor function testing may be caused by movements elicited by reflex contractions and/or muscle spasms; that is, involuntary movements. When a spastic, involuntary muscle contraction is superimposed on a voluntary contraction, it may be difficult or impossible to assess the degree to which the strength of contraction may be attributed to voluntary or reflex motor function.

These are just a few of many examples of practical problems that may decrease validity and reliability when testing according to ASIA.

The sum of motor function points is given for the left and right side (maximum of 50, respectively) and as a total (maximum of 100).

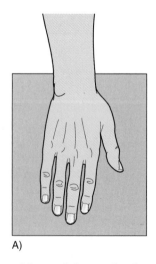

A)

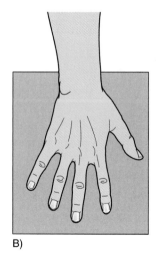

B)

Figure 8.4 Testing of finger abductors for the purpose of isolating muscle activity while spreading the fingers.

Classification

Classification according to ASIA is based on four components:

- Neurologic level of lesion
- Complete or incomplete lesion
- ASIA Impairment Scale Grade
- Zone of partial preservation (ZPP) for complete lesions

Neurological Level of Lesion

The following three concepts are used to determine neurological level of lesion:

- *Neurological level of lesion*: The most caudal spinal cord segment with normal sensory *and* motor function
- *Sensory level*: The most caudal spinal cord segment with normal *sensory* function (light touch *and* pain)
- *Motor level*: The most caudal spinal cord segment with normal *motor* function.

When determining the neurological level of lesion, "normal" motor function is operationally defined as including, in addition to grade 5, also grade 3 or 4 motor function in the myotome, but only on condition that the key muscles at the level *immediately* above are graded as normal; in other words, as grade 5. Note that neurological level of lesion must be differentiated from *skeletal* level of lesion. The skeletal level of lesion refers to the location of the injury on the *spinal column*, whereas the neurological level of lesion refers to the location on the *spinal cord*. In the cervical spine, these levels correspond fairly well, but the more caudal the injury, the greater the discrepancy. As mentioned earlier, this is related to the fact that the spinal cord ends at the level of the L1 vertebra in adults and is thus significantly shorter than the spinal column (see Chapter 3).

Complete or Incomplete Lesion

The criteria for *complete* and *incomplete lesion* are based, as described earlier, on the presence or absence of what is known as *sacral sparing*—preserved sensory and/or voluntary motor function within the sacral segments. A lesion is defined as being complete if neither motor nor sensory residual function is present in the lowest sacral segments. Conversely, a lesion is incomplete if motor and/or sensory residual function is present in the lowest sacral segments.

ASIA Impairment Scale Grade

The ASIA Impairment Scale (AIS) is a modification of the previously used Frankel Scale. In AIS, infralesional function is graded on a 5-point scale from A to E:

- *Grade A*: A complete lesion according to the above definition
- *Grade B*: An incomplete lesion, in which sensory but not motor function is preserved below the neurological level
- *Grade C*: An incomplete lesion, in which motor function is preserved below the neurological level of lesion and more than half of the key muscles below the neurological level have a muscle grade of less than 3
- *Grade D*: An incomplete lesion, in which motor function is preserved below the neurological level and at least half of key muscles below the neurological level have a muscle grade of 3 or better
- *Grade E*: "Normal" function, in the sense that voluntary motor and sensory function are normal throughout the body. However, note that a patient with this grade could very well have significant residual symptoms such as neuropathic pain, spasticity, incontinence, and/or erectile dysfunction.

Zone of Partial Preservation

Note that classification according to grades B, C, or D in all cases presume the presence of motor and/or sensory residual function in segments S4–S5. Otherwise the lesion is classified as complete (ASIA Grade A), and the residual motor and/or sensory function below the level of lesion is instead described as a *zone of partial preservation* (ZPP). The ZPP thus denotes the spinal cord segment(s) below the neurological level of lesion where sensory and/or motor resi-dual function is present *in a patient with a complete lesion, by definition.*

RADIOLOGIC WORKUP FOR SPINAL COLUMN TRAUMA

The purpose of the neurological examination is to record the current neurological status and any deterioration or improvement over time, as well as to locate the level of lesion so that radiologic workup can be aimed at the suspected level of lesion. As diagnostic imaging is undergoing rapid development, of all chapters in this book, the description of radiologic workup is likely to become outdated first.

To ensure that the patient with a SCI receives optimal treatment, we depend on an accurate radiologic diagnosis of the injured area. A large number of techniques are available, and in this chapter we discuss the most common diagnostic imaging methods currently available: conventional x-ray, computed tomography (CT), and magnetic resonance imaging (MRI), where the latter does not involve ionizing radiation. See Figure 7.1, which compares the use of these three techniques.

Following trauma, many conceivable scenarios can arise that may influence the choice of diagnostic procedure. Spinal column trauma must be considered in relation to other injuries, which may mean that the radiologic workup varies, even if spinal status is similar from patient to patient.

For example, in acute minimal cervical spine trauma with no medical history of head injury, where the patient is alert and neurologically intact, and suspicion of fracture is low, a conventional cervical spine x-ray is recommended as an initial screening method.

However, in a patient who by history has suffered a concussion and has neck pain, the recommendation is to analyze possible injury to the cervical spine with a CT, on condition that a CT scanner with spiral technology is available. In patients with concussion, a CT of both the head and cervical spine is preferable to a plain x-ray of the cervical spine and CT of the head. The advantage of this strategy is faster patient management, since unnecessary transfers and movements are avoided in a patient with a potentially unstable neck injury. The CT examination also provides superior imaging, compared with conventional x-ray. The disadvantage is a larger radiation dose, but this is justifiable on condition that the indication for the radiographic examination is correct. In patients exposed to high-energy trauma with or without head injury or suspicion of an injury to some other vital part of the body, such as the thorax or abdomen, a cervical spine examination is included in the trauma CT protocol used routinely for this patient group. The trauma CT examination includes the head, cervical spine, thorax, and abdomen, as well as the thoracic and lumbar spine down to and including the symphysis (i.e., the pelvis is included in the examination). Consequently, no conventional x-ray of the thoracic and lumbar spine is necessary in trauma patients.

Conventional X-ray

The conventional radiographic examination includes four projections, starting with a lateral view of the cervical spine (Fig. 8.5). The principle governing assessment of this examination is that all seven cervical vertebrae must be visualized, along with the upper portion of the T1 vertebral body. If the transition between the C7 and T1 vertebral bodies cannot be adequately visualized, a so-called *swimmer's view* is obtained, which entails lifting one arm up over the head (on the same side as the x-ray cassette) while pulling the opposite arm down and simultaneously gently rotating the shoulders to eliminate them from the field of view. This method significantly improves visualization of the relevant level.

When reviewing the lateral cervical spine, four lordotic lines are of importance (Fig. 8.6). The anterior vertebral body line, which corresponds to the anterior longitudinal ligament, follows the anterior margin of the vertebral bodies in a relatively soft, flowing line. In addition, there are two similar lines behind the vertebral bodies, of which the anterior line corresponds to the posterior longitudinal ligament and simultaneously to the anterior wall of the spinal canal, while the other corresponds to the

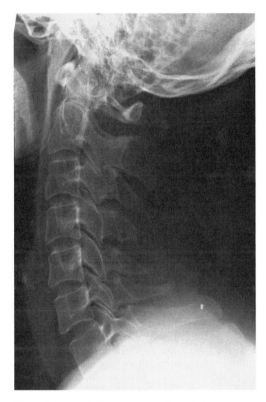

Figure 8.5 Cervical spine x-ray, lateral view.

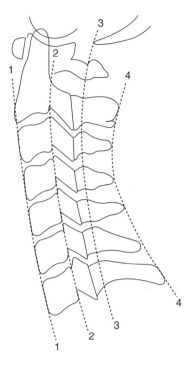

Figure 8.6 Drawing based on cervical spine x-ray, lateral view, in which the four lines of reference are marked.

posterior wall of the spinal canal. Finally, a fourth line can be drawn along the posterior tips of the spinous processes. When evaluating the lateral cervical spine, the prevertebral soft tissues are also important, since vertebral fractures may cause soft-tissue swelling anterior to the vertebral bodies. Prevertebral soft-tissue swelling is difficult to assess in intubated patients and in children.

After assessment of the lateral cervical spine, the examination continues with an *open mouth view* (Fig. 8.7). This projection is used to assess levels C1 and C2. The conventional frontal image (Fig. 8.8) provides some information about the position of the spinous processes and possible rotational malpositioning of joints, whereas an oblique lateral view (Fig. 8.9) is used to assess the pedicles, foramina, and facet joints.

Examination of the thoracic and lumbar spine only includes lateral projections and anteroposterior images (frontal views).

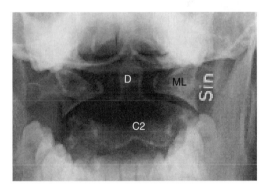

Figure 8.7 Open mouth view. The top of the dens (*D*), the C2 vertebral body (*C2*), and the C1 lateral mass of atlas (*ML*) are labeled.

The possibility of encountering multiple fractures increases greatly once one fracture is found, and the general rule of thumb is therefore to carry out CT imaging of the entire spinal column in cases of high-energy trauma.

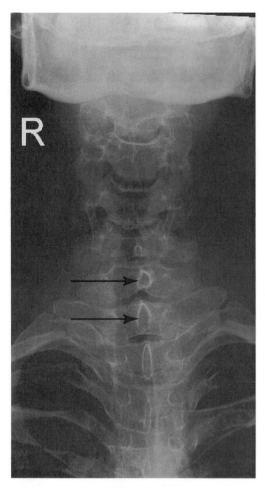

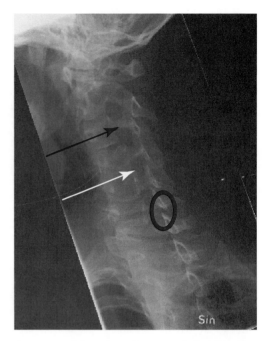

Figure 8.9 Oblique lateral view. Pedicle (*red arrow*), intervertebral foramen (*white arrow*) and facet joint (*red ring*).

Figure 8.8 Frontal image. The spinous processes (*arrows*) are visualized.

Indications for flexion/extension radiography are controversial. In this procedure, lateral images are taken of the cervical spine in flexion and extension, and the patient is first asked to flex the cervical spine and then to hyperextend it as much as possible. This examination is never to be recommended in emergency situations. The usefulness of the examination is limited by decreased mobility caused by pain-triggered muscle spasms; in addition, flexion and extension entail a risk of provoking a medullary lesion in case of spinal instability. However, flexion/extension x-rays may be done 10–14 days after the trauma, when the patient is pain-free or the pain is well-controlled. It is essential for the patient to make a thorough attempt at achieving full range of movement in the cervical spine at the time of the examination.

Computed Tomography Scan

CT is a radiographic examination that involves the use of an x-ray camera that rotates around the patient. The machine can be thought of as a large clothes dryer into which the patient is slowly introduced while lying on the examination table. The x-ray–emitting tube is mounted on a rotating wheel and a detector is mounted on the opposite side of the wheel. Since one image is generated for each 10 degrees of rotation, 36 slices of the spinal column can be examined during one complete 360-degree rotation. X-ray absorption varies among different tissues. Bone and blood have high absorption or attenuation and are seen as white structures, whereas spinal fluid and air, which have the lowest absorption, are seen as dark or black structures, respectively. CT technology is developing rapidly; currently, the fastest machines take 32-image slices in less than 1 second. Thus, the head, cervical spine, thorax, and abdomen can be examined in less than 1 minute. The new spiral CT scanners take continuous images and allow for considerably improved reconstruction in two and three planes.

The image slice thickness can be reduced to 1 mm, which allows reconstructions to be made in all planes with a resolution equal to that of the image slices. The radiation dose associated with a CT of the cervical spine is about 10 times greater than in a conventional cervical spine x-ray, assuming that the latter can be done without the need to retake any pictures. The new CT machines will be able to cut the radiation dose in half. CT examinations are particularly useful when assessing skeletal structures (Figs. 8.10–8.13), but CT technology is unable to depict soft tissues as good as MRI. Fractures and facet joint abnormalities are rarely missed. CT may have an even greater advantage in assessing the transition between C7 and T1, for which conventional x-rays may be inadequate. It is important to note that CT should *not* be used as a screening test to substitute for clinical assessment. Finally, it should be observed that CT is not suitable for imaging intraspinal soft-tissue changes.

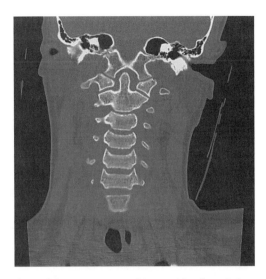

Figure 8.11 Reconstructed image. The frontal plane from a spiral computed tomography (CT) scan.

Magnetic Resonance Imaging

MRI is not actually a radiographic technique, since the technology is based on a strong magnetic field and radio waves. Until MRI technology was introduced, no radiologic examination could detect small lesions in spinal cord tissue.

MRI provides outstanding morphological information. Herniated disks, hemorrhages, and bone fragments that may impinge on the spinal cord can be visualized using this

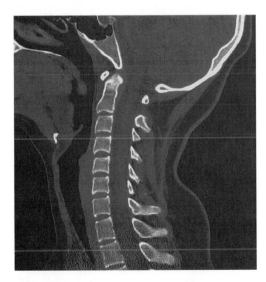

Figure 8.10 Computed tomography (CT) spiral scan in the form of a reconstructed midline image. The four lordotic lines can be superimposed, just as in conventional x-ray (compare to Fig. 8.5).

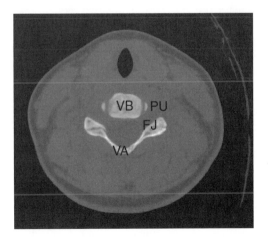

Figure 8.12 Computed tomography (CT) slice. Vertebral body (*VB*), processus uncinatus (*PU*), facet joint (*FJ*), and vertebral arch (*VA*).

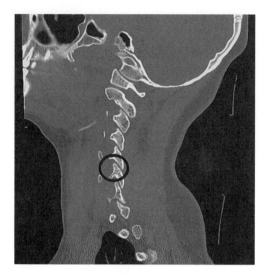

Figure 8.13 Sagittal reconstruction image in which the facet joints are clearly visible.

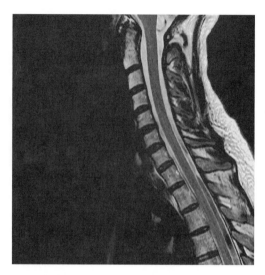

Figure 8.14 Sagittal magnetic resonance image (MRI). Image clearly shows the contents of the spinal canal. In this T2-weighted sequence, the spinal cord is depicted as gray and the spinal fluid as white.

technique. However, the main advantage of MRI is the ability to visualize hemorrhages and edema, as well as other changes within spinal cord tissue. Even excellent visualization of the skeleton is now possible, and luxations of the facet joints can be demonstrated using this technique.

MRI is usually carried out with sagittal and axial projections (Figs. 8.14 and 8.15). T2-weighted and proton density–weighted images are best suited to demonstrate soft-tissue injuries in and around the spinal cord. In T2-weighted studies, the most commonly used sequence, the spinal fluid is depicted as white, as is acute spinal cord edema (see Fig. 7.2). The appearance of hemorrhages is time-dependent following trauma, since different hemoglobin metabolites show different attenuation.

The extent of bleeding and edema also provides some indication of the severity of injury and therefore also about prognosis. Schaefer and coworkers presented a classification system to elucidate the appearance of T2-weighted images in SCI and how they relate to prognosis (Table 8.1).

In summary, MRI examination is now the best option for answering most questions about spinal column and spinal cord anatomy and pathophysiology. The need for CT to

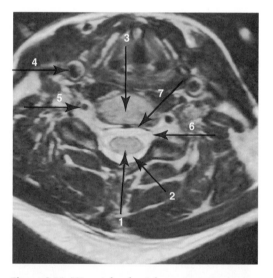

Figure 8.15 T2-weighted axial magnetic resonance image (MRI). Image showing multiple structures apart from the spinal cord (*1*), cerebrospinal fluid (*2*), and vertebral body (*3*). The carotid (*4*) and vertebral (*5*) arteries, as well as the nerve root (*6*) are clearly visualized. The posterior longitudinal ligament (*7*), resembling the wings of a bird, is attached at the midline.

TABLE 8.1 Relationship between MRI appearance (T2-weighted) and prognosis according to Schaefer.

	Appearance	Prognosis
Type 1	Hypointense (dark) changes in the spinal cord corresponding to intramedullary hematoma.	Associated with severe neurological deficits and poor prognosis
Type 2	Hyperintense (light) changes within the spinal cord corresponding to edema without focal hemorrhage. The edema extends beyond the height of one vertebral body from the level of injury.	Motor recovery possible
Type 3	Same as type 2, but the edema extends less than the height of one vertebral body from the level of injury.	This patient group has the least neurologic deficit and the best prognosis.

image details within the actual area of injury continues to decrease as the quality of MRI imaging improves, as is illustrated by this MRI sequence of the facet joints (Fig. 8.16).

MRI cannot be carried out on patients who have magnetically active implants, such as pacemakers and older osteosynthesis materials. Otherwise, the only disadvantages of MRI are the lack of round-the-clock availability in some facilities, time requirements, and practical problems associated with monitoring respiratory and cardiovascular function while the examination is being conducted.

ACKNOWLEDGMENTS

The authors wish to extend their thanks to Dr. Mårten Annertz, Neuroradiology section, University Hospital in Lund, for his invaluable help in providing and describing the radiographic material presented in this chapter.

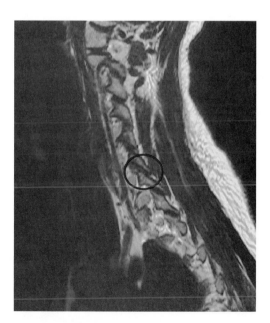

Figure 8.16 Sagittal magnetic resonance image (MRI). Image illustrating the normal position of the facet joints (*red ring*).

Suggested Reading

Anderson K, Aito S, Atkins M, et al. Functional recovery outcome measures work group. Functional recovery measures for spinal cord injury: an evidence-based review for clinical practice and research. *J Spinal Cord Med* 2008;31(2):133–144.

Bono CM, Vaccaro AR, Fehlings M, et al. Measurement techniques for lower cervical spine injuries: consensus statement of the Spine Trauma Study Group. *Spine (Phila Pa 1976)* 2006;1;31(5):603–609.

Bono CM, Vaccaro AR, Fehlings M, et al. Measurement techniques for upper cervical spine injuries: consensus statement of the Spine Trauma Study Group. *Spine (Phila Pa 1976)* 2007;1;32(5):593–600.

Flander AE, Croul SE. Spinal trauma. In: Atlas SW, ed., *Magnetic Resonance Imaging of the Brain and Spine* Philadelphia: Lippincott, Williams and Wilkins, 2002:1769–1825.

Furlan JC, Noonan V, Singh A, Fehlings M. Assessment of impairment in patients with acute traumatic spinal cord injury: a systematic review of the literature. *J Neurotrauma* 2009;December 23.

Grauer JN, Vaccaro AR, Lee JY, et al. The timing and influence of MRI on the management of patients with cervical facet dislocations remains highly variable: a survey of members of the Spine Trauma Study Group. *J Spinal Disord Tech* 2009;22(2):96–99. Comment in: *Surg Neurol* 2009 July;72(1):4–5.

Harris JH, Mirvis SE. The Radiology of Acute Cervical Spine Trauma, 3rd ed. Baltimore: Williams & Willkins, 1996.

Lammertse D, Dungan D, Dreisbach J, et al. Neuroimaging in traumatic spinal cord injury: an evidence-based review for clinical practice and research. *J Spinal Cord Med* 2007;30(3):205–214. Review.

Levi R. The Stockholm spinal cord injury study: medical, economical and psycho-social outcomes in a prevalence population (doctoral dissertation). Stockholm: Karolinska Institutet, 1996.

McGraw JK. *Interventional Radiology of the Spine.* New York: Humana Press, 2004.

Miyanji F, Furlan JC, Aarabi B, et al. Acute cervical traumatic spinal cord injury: MR imaging findings correlated with neurologic outcome—prospective study with 100 consecutive patients. *Radiology* 2007;243(3): 820–827. Epub 2007 April 12.

Parizel PM, van der Zijden T, Gaudino S, et al. Trauma of the spine and spinal cord: imaging strategies. *Eur Spine J* 2009;2. Epub ahead of print.

Ross JS, M Brant-Zawadzki, Chen MZ, Moore KR. *Diagnostic Imaging: Spine.* New York: Elsevier, 2004.

Swischuk LE. *Imaging of the Cervical Spine in Children.* New York: Springer-Verlag, 2002.

Tator C. Epidemiology and general characteristics of the spinal cord-injured patient. In: Tator CH, Benzel CH, eds., *Contemporary Management of Spinal Cord Injury: From Impact to Rehabilitation.* Park Ridge, IL: American Association of Neurological Surgeons, 2000:15–19.

Internet

www.internetmedicin.se Search by specialty at the upper left. Click on "Neurokirurgi" [Neurosurgery] and then "Halsryggsskador (med eller utan ryggmärgsskador)" [Cervical spine injuries (with or without spinal cord injuries)].

Model SCI Care Systems report statistics from 15% of the spinal cord injury population. Via search engine: National Spinal Cord Injury Statistical Center. The first hit describes UAB's National Spinal Cord Injury Statistical Center. Go to the Model Spinal Cord Injury Care Systems site for a wealth of interesting statistics.

Other

National Spinal Cord Injury Database. The best reference is the November 1999 issue of *Archives of Physical Medicine and Rehabilitation.* See *Archives of Physical Medicine and Rehabilitation* November 1999;80(11): 1363.

9 Pharmacological Treatment

The importance of secondary pathophysiologic injury mechanisms related to trauma have led to a search for *neuroprotection*—ways to protect spinal cord tissue from the ramifications of these mechanisms. Table 34.1 reviews the different drugs that have been tested and that have positively influenced such secondary processes.

Four substances in particular have been promising during laboratory testing and in clinical trials. These include two types of corticosteroids (methylprednisolone and tirilazad mesylate), naloxone and GM-1-ganglioside. Methylprednisolone and GM-1-ganglioside have undergone the most thorough clinical testing. The other two substances have been assessed in clinical studies, in which they were compared with methylprednisolone without demonstrating any beneficial effect.

This chapter mainly focuses on drugs with the potential to improve neurological outcome after SCI. Clinical drug treatment of patients with SCI, by contrast, focuses on symptomatic relief, prophylaxis, and treatment of SCI-related complications. These treatments are described in their respective sections. Additionally, an overview of the pharmacological spectrum in acute and post-acute SCI care is illustrated by a table at the end of this chapter.

METHYLPREDNISOLONE

The synthetic glucocorticosteroid methylprednisolone sodium succinate (MPSS) has been thoroughly studied in both animal experiments and clinical trials. In animal trials, MPSS (see Table 34.2) stabilized membrane structures following trauma, decreased inflammatory response, prevented lipid peroxidation, counteracted a reduction of blood flow to the spinal cord and thereby reduced subsequent ischemia, prevented intracellular uptake of calcium, positively influenced energy metabolism, and finally, improved neurological function in experimental animals.

Following these favorable results in the laboratory, clinical trials of MPSS were initiated. The pharmacological properties of methylprednisolone require that both a bolus dose and an infusion be given as combination therapy in order to achieve the best results from the medication, and it is essential that treatment be initiated as soon as possible after trauma. The efficacy of MPSS was tested in three clinical trials, the National Acute SCI Studies (NASCIS) 1, 2, and 3. In NASCIS 1 a 1,000 mg bolus was administered, followed with 1,000 mg/day for 10 days in one patient group, while a second group was given a 100 mg bolus and an equally large daily dose for an additional 10 days. This study, presented in 1984, showed no difference in neurological recovery between the two groups, but no control group was included. Additional animal studies then showed that the dose of methylprednisolone given in this study was too low. The subsequent multicenter NASCIS 2 study administered significantly higher doses of methylprednisolone by initiating treatment with a bolus dose of 30 mg/kg, followed by an infusion of 5.4 mg/kg/hour for 23 hours. This study also included two other patient groups who received naloxone and placebo. In all, 487 patients were studied. According to the authors, the 1-year follow-up, which was presented in 1992, showed statistically significant improvement in motor score by American Spinal Injury Association (ASIA) criteria. In this study, all patients who demonstrated motor improvement were given MPSS within 8 hours following injury. Strong criticism, both methodological and statistical in nature, was aimed at the NASCIS 2 study. The major criticism was that NASCIS 2 only assessed gains in motor score according to ASIA, but not in abilities according to, e.g., Functional Independent Measure (FIM).

Patients who sustained bullet wounds and were treated with intravenous steroids demonstrated no neurological improvement compared with the placebo group.

In the third NASCIS study, which was published in 1997, FIM was added. In NASCIS 3, patients in all three groups were administered the same bolus dose of methylprednisolone as in NASCIS 2. The patients were then divided into three groups. One group received the same dose of MPSS infusion as in NASCIS 2 for 23 hours, another group for 48 hours, and the third group received the lazaroid tirilazad for 48 hours (2.5 mg/kg bolus every 6 hours).

Lazaroids are synthetic nonglucocorticoid steroids. Experimentally, they have been found to be more potent than methylprednisolone in counter-acting iron-dependent lipid peroxidation. Animal experiments have also shown that the lazaroid tirilazad has an effect on neurological recovery, and the hypothesis is that tirilazad not only counteracts lipid peroxidation on the microvascular level, but also decreases post-traumatic ischemia. Nor does Tirilazad have the negative effects of methylprednisolone, such as immunosuppression and hyperglycemia.

The 1-year follow-up of NASCIS 3 was published in 1998, and the authors concluded that if treatment began within 3 hours of injury, a similar motor improvement was obtained 1 year after the trauma, regardless of whether the patient was treated for 24 or 48 hours. If treatment began within 3–8 hours of the trauma, outcome was better when treatment continued for 48 hours. If treatment was initiated more than 8 hours after the injury, improvement in motor function was less than that seen in the placebo group in the NASCIS 2 study. The group of patients who received tirilazad for 48 hours demonstrated the same pattern of improvement as those patients who received MPSS infusion for 24 hours, but

with fewer side effects. Since these patients received a bolus of MPSS, the effect of tirilazad as such was difficult to assess and therefore no definite conclusion about the effect of this drug could be drawn.

In summary, the NASCIS study authors recommend continuing treatment for 24 hours if treatment is initiated within 3 hours of the injury and continuing treatment for 48 hours if treatment is initiated within 3–8 hours of the injury. The recommendation of the authors to use methylprednisolone for 48 hours is based solely on the motor score according to ASIA, since no significant improvement in FIM could be demonstrated. NASCIS 3 was also the target of much criticism (from Hugenholtz and colleagues [2002], among others). Reviewers expressed a number of critical viewpoints on how the study was conducted and interpreted, and their criticism was directed at the same principles as in NASCIS 2. Despite the NASCIS studies, there is still no consensus on whether methylprednisolone has a significant benefit on neurological recovery. Also of relevance to this discussion is the fact that administration of cortisone for 48 hours is associated with a higher risk of side effects such as pneumonia, sepsis, and respiratory complications than is treatment for 24 hours, even though the difference in the complication rate did not reach statistical significance. Other side effects associated with administration of methylprednisolone include aggravation of diabetes, immunosuppression, increased risk of infections, impaired wound healing, and increased risk of bleeding ulcers.

According to Hugenholtz, the use of steroids in SCI can be summarized by stating that high-dose infusion with methylprednisolone that begins within 8 hours of injury is *not* to be considered as "standard therapy" or as a "treatment guideline," but rather as a "possible optional treatment." This reflects the general opinion about steroid therapy, which is also in line with the scientific review published in the journal *Neurosurgery* in 2002. Table 9.1 shows the treatment protocol at one Swedish center using Solu-Medrol[R] in the acute phase.

TABLE 9.1 Flow chart for treatment with Solu-Medrol®.

Solu-Medrol® (methylprednisolone) Infusion

Indications:
Acute spinal cord trauma.

Properties:
Animal experiments studies have shown that the substance counteracted several of the secondary mechanisms of injury that arise after trauma. According to the National Acute SCI clinical studies 2 and 3 (NASCIS 2 and NASCIS 3), the drug has a beneficial effect on motor recovery after SCI.

Duration of treatment
If the treatment/bolus dose is initiated within 3 hours post injury, then treatment should continue for 24 hours.
If the treatment/bolus dose is initiated within 3–8 hours post injury the treating physician will decide whether an additional 24 hours of treatment (total of 48 hours) is indicated.

Contraindications:
Cauda equina syndrome, penetrating injuries, presence of serious life-threatening disease, pregnancy, drug abuse, and ongoing steroid therapy.
Patients younger than 13 years should not be treated with Solu-Medrol®.

Preparation and treatment using bolus dose:
Bolus dose:
Administer as soon as possible, though no later than 8 hours after the injury, 2g Solu-Medrol® bolus dose, regardless of patient weight.
Dissolve Solu-Medrol® 2 g in the benzyl alcohol that comes with it (about 30 mL).
Add the premixed 30 mL Solu-Medrol® solution to 20 mL of normal saline (9 mg/mL) which will then correspond to 50 mL premixed Solu-Medrol ® infusion solution.
Administer the entire 50 mL volume as an infusion over 15 minutes.

Infusion rate: 3 mL/minute or 180 mL/hour.

Turn off the infusion for 45 minutes:
Maintain venous access for 45 minutes prior to initiating continuous infusion.

Preparation and treatment using continuous infusion:
45 minutes after finishing bolus dose, begin continuous infusion of Solu-Medrol® at a rate of 5.4 mg/kg body weight/hour.
The table below indicates the recommended maintenance dose of Solu-Medrol in mg in relation to patient weight, to be administered per twelve hours. The table specifies this treatment duration since the shelf-life of this preparation is only 12 hours.
Solu-Medrol® is available in 125 mg, 500 mg, 1000 mg, and 2000 mg packaging.
Infusion rate: 3 mL/minute or 180 mL/hour

Table for 12 hours of treatment (expressed in mg) with Solu-Medrol R

Patient weight	50 kg	60 kg	70 kg	80 kg	90 kg	100 kg
Maintenance dose Solu-Medrol® in mg/12 hours	3250	3750	4500	5000	5750	6500
Aspirate this volume from 100 mL normal saline 9 mg/mL	25	35	45	55	65	75
Add this volume Solu-Medrol® solution	50	60	70	80	90	100

Dissolve the required amount of Solu-Medrol® for 12 hours in the benzyl alcohol that comes with it. Use a 100 mL infusion solution of normal saline (9 mg/mL) (contents in soft plastic bag).
  Then aspirate the corresponding volume of normal saline (9 mg/mL) infusion solution given by the table above.
  Next add the volume of Solu-Medrol® solution given in the table above to the remaining normal saline solution.
  The total volume of the infusion, regardless of weight, will be 125 mL (appropriate volume even for overweight patients)
Infusion rate: 11 mL per hour

From Bracken MB:, Shepard MJ, Collins WF and coworkers: A randomized controlled trial of methylprednisolone or naloxone in the treatment of acute SCI. New England Journal of Medicine 1990;322:1405–1411.Bracken MB, Shepard MJ, Holford TR, Leo-Summers L, Aldrich E, Fazl M, et al. Administration of methyl prednisolone for 24 or 48 hours or tirilazad mesylate for 48 hours in the treatment of acute SCI. Results of the Third National Acute SCI Randomized Controlled Trial. National Acute SCI Study. JAMA 1997;277(20):1597–604, with permission.

GM-1-GANGLIOSIDE

Gangliosides are complex glycolipids that are primarily found in the phospholipid-containing outer layer of the cell membrane. In animal experiments, the substance has been shown to stimulate the growth of neurons in injured tissue and to increase the quantity of surviving axons (i.e., those axons that pass through the injured area intact), which facilitates recovery of motor function distal to the injury. Gangliosides also appear to inhibit cell destruction by counteracting the neurotoxic effect of excitatory amino acids, but do not limit the physiological effects of excitatory amino acids on calcium channels. Thus, gangliosides comprise a main component of the cell's external double lipid layer, and exogenous gangliosides are believed to attach to this lipid membrane and cause effects similar to those produced by endogenous substances.

After Geisler and coworkers presented a small clinical study involving 34 patients in 1991, the same research group initiated a multicenter study of gangliosides the following year. After administering the specified steroid therapy according to the NASCIS 2 protocol, the patients in this study were then given various doses of GM-1 gangliosides for 56 days. The patients received standard medical treatment. The study was able to show a trend toward neurological improvement, but this did not reach statistical significance. The improvement noted was in muscles that were initially totally paralyzed but which regained useful motor function, rather than in an increase of strength in paretic muscles. Improvement in the lower extremities was greater than in the upper extremities, which is consistent with the fact that the white substance passing through the lesion area contains those structures in which GM-1 exerts its greatest effect.

According to general recommendations, GM-1 gangliosides remain a "treatment option," even though clinical efficacy has not been demonstrated.

OTHER PHARMACOLOGICAL TREATMENT

Clinical pharmacotherapy in SCI primarily targets symptomatic relief, prophylaxis for various complicating disorders, and/or treatment of manifest SCI-related complications. To illustrate the fact that pharmacological treatment for traumatic SCI is not merely a question of whether or not to use cortisone, please refer to a sampling of common medications given to one patient treated at the intensive care unit during the first months following SCI (Table 9.2).

TABLE 9.2 Pharmacological treatment given to a patient during the three first months after a SCI.

Intensive Care Period

Actrapid
Albumin
Alvedon (Tylenol)
Artonil (Zantac)
Tylenol with codeine
Diprivan
Dormicum
Ephedrine
Packed RBCs
Esmeron (Zemuron)
Fentanyl
Glucose
Clexane
Lactulose
Morphine
Meronem
Movicol
Norepinephrine
Octostim
Sodium Pentothal
Rehydrex
Ringer's acetate
Rifadin
Robinul
Solu-Medrol
Tracrium
Trandate
Zantac

Rehabilitation Period (in addition to above)

Duroferon
Forlax
Omeprazole
Propavan (Largon)
Zopiclone

Suggested Reading

Apuzzo MJL, ed. Pharmacological therapy after acute cervical spinal cord injury. *Neurosurgery* 2002;50 (3 Suppl):S63–S72. [This manuscript contains an extensive and still relevant bibliography of 51 articles that essentially cover all research and development within the field of pharmacotherapy.]

Baptiste DC, Fehlings MG. Pharmacological approaches to repair the injured spinal cord. *J Neurotrauma* 2006;23(3–4):318–334.

Baptiste DC, Fehlings MG. Emerging drugs for spinal cord injury. *Expert Opin Emerg Drugs* 2008;13(1): 63–80. Review.

Bracken MB, Shepard MJ, Holford TR, et al. Administration of methylprednisolone for 24 or 48 hours or tirilazad mesylate for 48 hours in the treatment of acute spinal cord injury. Results of the Third National Acute Spinal Cord Injury Randomized Controlled Trial. National Acute Spinal Cord Injury Study. *JAMA* 1997;277(20): 1597–1604.

Bracken MB, Holford TR. Neurological and functional status 1 year after acute spinal cord injury: estimates of functional recovery in National Acute Spinal Cord Injury Study II from results modeled in National Acute Spinal Cord Injury Study III. *J Neurosurg Spine* 2002;96(3):259–266.

Geisler FH, Coleman WP, Grieco G, Poonian D; Sygen Study Group. The Sygen multicenter acute spinal cord injury study. *Spine* 2001;26(24 Suppl):S87–98.

Hawryluk GW, Rowland J, Kwon BK, Fehlings MG. Protection and repair of the injured spinal cord: a review of completed, ongoing, and planned clinical trials for acute spinal cord injury. *Neurosurg Focus* 2008;25(5):E14. Review.

Tsutsumi S, Ueta T, Shiba K, et al. Effects of the second national acute spinal cord injury study of high-dose methylprednisolone therapy on acute cervical spinal cord injury-results in spinal injuries center. *Spine* (*Phila Pa 1976*) 2006;15;31(26):2992–2996. Discussion 2997.

Internet

www.aans.org Search on the word "neuroprotection" to access Tator CH, Fehlings MG. Review of clinical trials of neuroprotection in acute spinal cord injury. *Neurosurg Focus* 1999;6(1):Article 8.

Other

The following two references present conflicting views of methylprednisolone, the most controversial SCI treatment, the first in favor of and the second against the use of this steroid in acute SCI.

Bracken MB, Aldrich EF, Men DM, et al. Clinical measurement, statistical analysis, and risk-benefit: controversies From trials of spinal injury. *J Trauma* 2000;48(3):558–561.

Hugenholtz H, Cass DE, Dvorak MF, et al. High-dose methylprednisolone for acute closed spinal cord injury: only a treatment option. *Can J Neuron Sci* 2002;29(3):227–235. Review.

Overview of Specific Injuries to the Spinal Column and Ligaments

The incidence of spinal column fractures and/or ligamentous injuries is estimated at 2–5 per 1,000 individuals. The number of individuals treated for a spinal column injury is thus at least 100 times higher than the number of individuals afflicted by traumatic SCI.

Chapters 10–15 present detailed surveys of injuries to the spinal column and ligaments. Fractures and ligamentous injuries of the upper and lower cervical spinal column are described in Chapters 11 and 12, respectively. These chapters also contain an overview of the treatment options in injuries to the cervical spine. The surgical techniques used to treat these injuries are described in Chapter 13.

Classification and treatment of thoracolumbar fractures is presented in Chapter 14. Nonsurgical treatment is presented in Chapter 15. We have chosen to present the use of orthoses in one chapter since the principles of such treatment are, in many respects, similar for the entire spinal column.

Our review of surgical and nonsurgical treatments is based on the literature and discussions with colleagues within this field. We are well aware of differing treatment principles among various countries and trauma centers. The text thus should be viewed as merely presenting options rather than definitive guidelines.

Initially, we wish to introduce the terms *motion segment* and *anatomic plane*, and also briefly review some biomechanical aspects of

the spinal column. (All references relating to Chapters 10–15 are shown at the end of this chapter.)

MOTION SEGMENT

A motion segment contains two adjacent vertebral bodies including their facet joints, ligamentous structures, and the interposed intervertebral disk (Fig. 10.1).

ANATOMICAL PLANE

Anatomical or reference planes are used to illustrate the extent of an injury. Three anatomical planes are illustrated in Figure 10.2. The *frontal* or *coronal plane* divides the body into an anterior and posterior part. The *sagittal plane* splits the body vertically into a left and a right side; consequently, sagittal images contain sequences viewed from the side. The *transversal plane* divides the body into an upper (rostral) and a lower (caudal) part. Transverse images are also called *axial images*. The anatomical planes cross each other at 90-degree angles and can thus be used as a coordinate system to describe the direction of movements in spinal cord trauma.

BIOMECHANICS

The nomenclature presented here is often used when injuries to the spinal column and ligaments are described. The right-handed

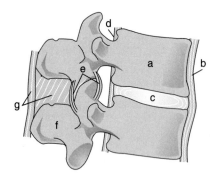

Figure 10.1 Illustration of a motion segment. *a*, vertebral body; *b*, anterior longitudinal ligament; *c*, intervertebral disk; *d*, posterior longitudinal ligament; *e*, facet joint; *f*, spinous process; *g*, posterior ligament structures.

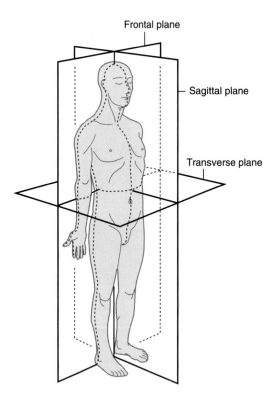

Figure 10.2 The anatomical planes.

Cartesian system is most frequently used when three-dimensional biomechanical aspects of spine must be explained (Fig. 10.3A,B). Briefly,

the Cartesian system contains three axes: x, y, and z.

Figure 10.4A,B illustrates the motion directions in the coordinate system with the x-axis running from dorsal to ventral (anteroposterior), the y-axis from left to right (mediolateral), and the z-axis from rostral to caudal.

The load on the spinal column in connection with trauma is made up of external forces (F) and moments (M) (Table 10.1). The forces in this three-dimensional coordinate axis system are translational or linear (i.e., along axes), while the moments are rotational (i.e., around axes) (Fig. 10.3A,B).

Three types of loads are seen in the sagittal plane. The shear force (FX) runs in an anteroposterior direction and causes a translational movement. Forces in the axial direction (FZ) may either result in a compression or distraction force, whereas a bending moment results in a flexion or extension movement (MY).

The loads occurring outside the sagittal plane are the translational forces in the mediolateral or opposite direction (FY), the left to right or reverse lateral bending moment (MX), and the right or left axial rotation moment (MZ).

The impact of a trauma may result in displacement of the spinal column. The displacement is initially seen as a translation of the vertebral bodies in an anteroposterior and/or lateral direction or as a change in the height of the vertebral bodies. Rotational displacement results in changed angles to the injured vertebral body, such as hyperflexion/hyperextension and axial rotation.

Figure 10.5A,B shows the effects of a flexion-extension trauma that illustrates the descriptions of the various loads just described. Compression of the anterior and distraction of the posterior structures are seen when the spinal column sustains an isolated flexion-bending movement. The cranially located vertebral body is displaced anteriorly and, consequently, a translation movement takes place. The opposite (Fig. 10.5B) is seen following an isolated extension-bending movement.

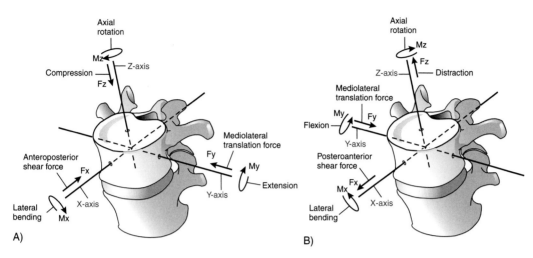

Figure 10.3 A,B: Schematic overview of the three-dimensional axes/coordinates and the different loads that may occur in a trauma to the spinal column.

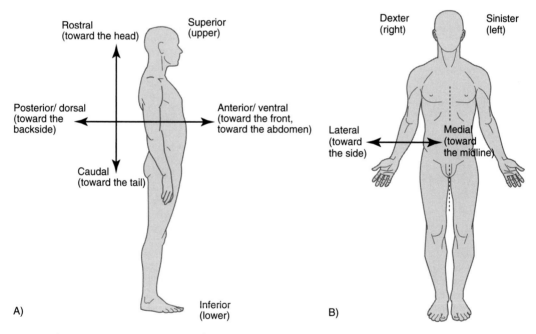

Figure 10.4 A,B: Description of moments located inside and outside of the sagittal plane.

TABLE 10.1 Forces and moments involved in trauma to the spinal column.

Forces	Moments
Translation force along the x-axis (anteriorly or posteriorly)	Lateral bending moment around the x-axis
Compression–distraction force along the z-axis (axial)	Rotation moment around z-axis
Translation force along the y-axis (medially or laterally)	Flexion–extension bending moment around the y-axis

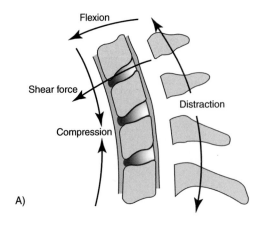

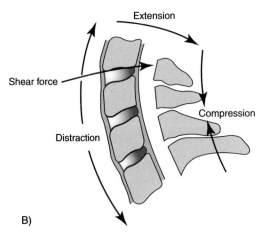

Figure 10.5 Course of events following (A) flexion and (B) extension bending moment, respectively.

Suggested Reading

Aebi M, Thalgott JS, Webb JK. *AO ASIF Principles in Spine Surgery.* New York: Springer Verlag, 1998.

Allen BL, Ferguson RL, Lehmann TR, O'Brian RP. A mechanistic classification of closed indirect fractures and dislocations of the lower cervical spine. *Spine* 1982;(1):1–27.

Anderson LD, D'Alonzo RT. Fractures of the odontoid process of the axis. *J Bone Joint Surg* 1974;56:1663–1674.

Anderson PA, Montesano PX. Morphology and treatment of occipital condyle fractures. *Spine* 1988;13:731–736.

Baldwin NG, Van Buskirk CS. Surgical techniques: Lumbosacral and sacropelvic fixation. In: Tator CH, Benzel CH, eds., *Contemporary Management of Spinal Cord Injury: From Impact to Rehabilitation.* Park Ridge, IL: American Association of Neurological Surgeons, 2000:189–198.

Benzel EC. Spinal orthotics. In: Menezes AH, Sonntag VKH, eds., *Principles of Spinal Surgery.* New York: McGraw-Hill, 1996:181–190.

Benzel EC. *Spine Surgery: Techniques, Complication Avoidance, and Management.* New York: Elsevier Churchill Livingstone, 2005.

Bridwell KH, Anderson PA, Boden SD, et al. What's new in spine surgery. *J Bone Joint Surg Am* 2009;91(7):1822–1834.

Brooks AL, Jenkins EB. Atlanto-axial arthrodesis by the wedge compression method. *J Bone Joint Surg* 1978;60A:279–284.

Cooper PR. Stabilization of fractures and dislocations of the lower cervical spine. In: Cooper PR, ed., *Management of Post-traumatic Spinal Instability.* Park Ridge, IL: American Association of Neurological Surgeons, 1990:111–133.

Crockard AH, Peterson D. Surgical techniques: Craniocervical junction. In: Tator CH, Benzel CH, eds., *Contemporary Management of Spinal Cord Injury: From Impact to Rehabilitation.* Park Ridge, IL: American Association of Neurological Surgeons, 2000:123–132.

Denis F. The three column spine and its significance in the classification of acute thoracolumbar spinal injuries. *Spine* 1983:8:817–831.

Dvorak MF, Fisher CG, Fehlings MG, et al. The surgical approach to subaxial cervical spine injuries: an evidence-based algorithm based on the SLIC classification system. *Spine (Phila Pa 1976)* 2007;1;32(23):2620–2629.

Elgafy H, Bellabarba C. Three-column ligamentous extension injury of the thoracic spine: a case report and review of the literature. *Spine (Phila Pa 1976)* 2007;1;32(25):E785–E788. Review.

Eichler ME, Stillerman CB, Roy RS. Surgical techniques: Cervical spine stabilization. In: Tator CH, Benzel CH, eds., *Contemporary Management of Spinal Cord Injury: From Impact to Rehabilitation.* Park Ridge, IL: American Association of Neurological Surgeons, 2000:133–172.

Fielding JW, Hawkins RJ. Atlanto-axial rotatory fixation. (Fixed rotatory subluxation of the atlantoaxial joint). *J Bone Surg* 1977;59:37–44.

Frymoyer JW, Wiesel SW. *The Adult & Pediatric Spine,* 3rd ed. Philadelphia: Lippincott Williams & Wilkins, 2004.

Fujimura Y, Nishi Y, Kobayashi K. Classification and treatment of axis body fractures. *J Orthop Trauma* 1996;10:536–540.

Gokaslan ZL, McCormick P. Surgical techniques: Thoracic and lumbar. In: Tator CH, Benzel CH, eds., *Contemporary Management of Spinal Cord Injury: From Impact to Rehabilitation.* Park Ridge, IL: American Association of Neurological Surgeons, 2000:173–187.

Henriques T. *Biomechanical and Clinical Aspect on Fixation Techniques in the Cervical Spine.* Uppsala: Uppsala University, 2003.

Holdsworth FW. Fractures and dislocations of the spine. *J Bone Joint Surg* 1963;45-B:6–20.

Hostler D, Colburn D, Seitz SR. A comparison of three cervical immobilization devices. *Prehosp Emerg Care* 2009;13(2):256–260.

Levine AM, Edwards CC. The management of traumatic spondylolisthesis of the axis. *J Bone Joint Surg Am* 1985;67:217–226.

Lind B, Sihlbom H, Nordwall A. Forces and motions across the neck in patients treated with halo-vest. *Spine* 1988;13:162–167.

Magerl F, Aebi M, Gertzbein SD, Harms J, Nazarian S. A comprehensive classification of thoracic and lumbar injuries. *Eur Spine J* 1994;3:184–201.

Magerl F, Seemn P-S. Stable posterior fusion of the atlas and axis by transarticular screw fixation. In: Kehr P, Werdner PA, eds., *Cervical Spine I*. New York: Springer-Verlag, 1987:322–327.

Menezes AH, Sonntag VKH. *Principles of Spinal Surgery*. New York: McGraw-Hill, 1996.

Nassr A, Lee JY, Dvorak MF, et al. Variations in surgical treatment of cervical facet dislocations. *Spine* 2008; 33(7):E188–E193, *Eur Spine J* 2009;September 2 (Epub ahead of print).

Nicoll EA. Fractures of the dorso-lumbar spine. *J Bone Joint Surg* 1949;31-B:376–394.

Omeis I, Duggal N, Rubano J, et al. Surgical treatment of C2 fractures in the elderly: a multicenter retrospective analysis. *J Spinal Disord Tech* 2009;22(2): 91–95.

Panjabi MM, White III AA. Basic biomechanics of the spine. *Neurosurg* 1980;7(1):76–93.

Patel AA, Dailey A, Brodke DS, et al. Spine trauma study group. Subaxial cervical spine trauma classification: the subaxial injury classification system and case examples. *Neurosurg Focus* 2008; 25(5):E8.

Patel AA, Dailey A, Brodke DS, et al. Spine Trauma Study Group. Thoracolumbar spine trauma classification: the thoracolumbar injury classification and severity score system and case examples. *J Neurosurg Spine* 2009;10(3):201–206.

Smith HE, Vaccaro AR, Maltenfort M, et al. Trends in surgical management for type II odontoid fracture: 20 years of experience at a regional spinal cord injury center. *Orthopedics* 2008;31(7):650.

Traynelis VC, Marano GD, Dunker RO, et al. Traumatic atlantooccipital dislocation. Case report. *J Neurosurg* 1986;65:863–870.

White AA, Panjabi MM. *Clinical Biomechanics of the Spine*, 2nd ed. Philadelphia: JB Lippincott, 1990.

11 Upper Cervical Spine Fractures and Ligament Injuries (C0–C2)

Injuries to the upper cervical spine (or the occipitoatlantoaxial [C0–C2] joints) occur following trauma to the head and neck region. A broad variety of neurological complications are seen as a result of fractures and ligamentous injuries in this area. Death may occur due to respiratory insufficiency in cases with concomitant injury to the cervical spinal cord. However, most injuries in the upper cervical spine do not result in any neurological deficits because of the relatively large diameter of the spinal canal and also because most of the fractures in this region expand rather than narrow the spinal canal.

C0–C2 fractures represent about 10–15% of all cervical spine fractures. An isolated axis fracture is the most common type of injury of the upper cervical spine. In one large epidemiological study, isolated axis fractures constituted 71% (294 patients) of 414 patients presenting with fractures to this region. Seventeen percent (70 patients) in the same study were fractures of the atlas and the remaining 12% (50 patients) involved both C1 and C2 vertebrae. It should be observed that 50% of atlas fractures are associated with a fracture of the axis. Fractures of the atlas represent only 1–3% of all fractures of the spinal column, but they are responsible for 20% of all fatal injuries. These deaths usually occur at the scene of the accident, before any prehospital care is available.

ANATOMICAL OVERVIEW

The occiput, atlas, and axis form a biomechanical unit in which the atlas serves as a sort of "washer" to buffer the forces between the stiff occipital condyles (i.e., the skull base) and the mobile axis vertebra (i.e., the cervical spine).

Several ligaments and other structures maintain stability of the upper cervical spine

(Figs. 11.1–11.4). The principal stabilizing structures in the craniovertebral junction are the facet joint capsules of C0–C1, the anterior and posterior atlantooccipital membranes, and the two lateral atlantooccipital membranes (not illustrated). The transverse ligament is the strongest stabilizing ligament of C1 and holds C1 to the skull base through the ascending part of the cruciform ligament. The skull base is stabilized to C2 mainly by the tectorial membrane (occipitoaxial ligament) and the paired alar ligaments. The tectorial membrane prevents hyperextension in the upper cervical region, and the paired alar ligaments prevent excessive rotation and lateral bending between C0 and C1.

The atlas is a unique vertebra in that it has neither a vertebral body nor intervertebral disks in contact with the adjacent occiput and axis (Fig. 11.4). The muscles are attached at the tubercles located in the middle of the cylindrically shaped arches. The ovally shaped lateral masses, viewed from above, articulate with the occipital condyles in a "ball-and-socket" configuration (Figs. 11.1, 11.4). The tops of the lateral masses are concave, and fit well with the oval occipital condyles. The ball-and-socket configuration results in virtually no axial rotation in the C0–C1 joints, and in a limited degree of flexion, extension, and lateral bending. The articulating surfaces between atlas and axis are biconvex, resulting in the opposite pattern of movement when compared to the C0–C1 joints. The axial rotatory capacity is extensive whereas flexion, extension, and lateral bending movements are very limited.

Two principal stabilizing ligaments lay between C1 and C2. The strongest stabilizer, the transverse ligament, runs between the medially located tubercles of the lateral masses. This ligament acts as a "seat belt" by attaching the dens to the posterior

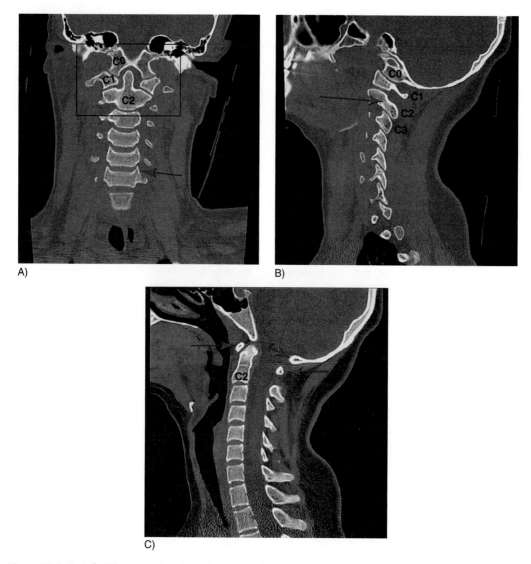

Figure 11.1 Spiral CT scans showing the cervical spine. A: Coronal reconstruction illustrating the occipito-atlantal-axial unit. The relationships between C0–C1, C1–C2, and most importantly, C2–C3 are shown in this image. The *red arrow* indicates the uncinate process (processus uncinatus). B: Sagittal view through the articulating joints a few centimeters from the midline (paramedian view) demonstrating the "ball-and-socket" configuration between the C0 and C1 joint and the biconvex C1–C2 joint. Observe the C2–C3 joint that is considered a "normal" joint in the cervical column. The structure between the C1–C2 and C2–C3 joints (*arrow*) is the pars interarticularis. C: Midline sagittal section illustrating the relationship between the top of dens (C2), foramen magnum (*double arrow*), and the anterior and posterior arches of C1 (single arrows).

surface of the anterior arch of the atlas. The alar ligaments extend between occiput and the tip of the dens and surround C1 between the occiput and C2 (Figs. 11.1–11.3). The ligament prevents wide rotation and lateral bending of CI.

No universally accepted classification of fractures and ligamentous injuries exists in this region. Classifications similar to those of the thoracic and lumbar spine are not applicable because of the very specific anatomical

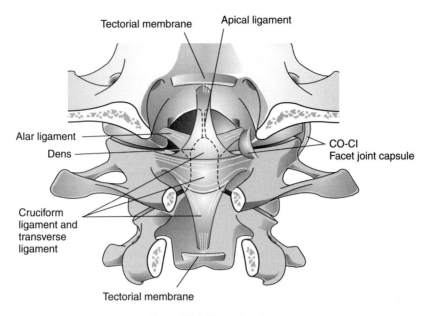

Tectorial membrane

Apical ligament

Alar ligament

Dens

CO-Cl
Facet joint capsule

Cruciform ligament and transverse ligament

Tectorial membrane

Figure 11.2 Posterior view.

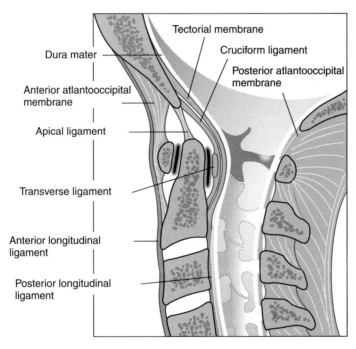

Dura mater

Anterior atlantooccipital membrane

Apical ligament

Transverse ligament

Anterior longitudinal ligament

Posterior longitudinal ligament

Tectorial membrane

Cruciform ligament

Posterior atlantooccipital membrane

Figure 11.3 Lateral view.

and biomechanical conditions and the great variety of injuries. The loading mechanisms behind many of the fractures and ligament injuries in this region are complex and difficult to reconstruct. Here we present a broad overview of injuries in this region and their standards of treatment (Table 11.1). Specific surgical and nonsurgical treatments for these injuries are presented in Chapters 13 and 15, respectively.

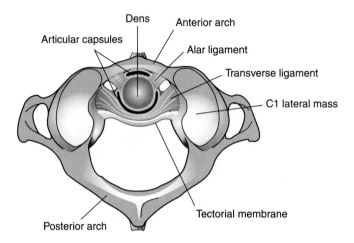

Figure 11.4 Shows transverse section through atlas.

TABLE 11.1 Injuries to the upper cervical spine: classification and treatment options.

	Reducing the malalignement	Non-surgical treatment	Surgical treatment
Occipital condyle fractures			
Type I and II		Soft or hard cervical collars	
Type III		Hard cervical collar or Halo vest	Occipito-cervical fusion if instability is present
Atlanto-occipital dislocation	Avoid traction but try to reponate the dislocation	Halo vest	Occipito-cervical fusion if significant malalignment
Atlas fractures			
Isolated ring fractures		Soft or hard cervical collar for 6–8 weeks	
Jefferson fracture			
Minor dislocation <7 mm		Cervical collar, cervico-thoracic orthosis or Halo-vest	Fusion C0–CII if ongoing dislocation despite non-surgical treatment
Major dislocation >7 mm		Halo-vest	Fusion C0–CII if ongoing dislocation despite non-surgical treatment
Lateral mass fracture			
Non-dislocated		Cervical collar 6–8 weeks	
Comminute		Halo-vest	
Transverse ligament rupture			Fusion CI–CII
Axis fractures			
Odontoid fractures			
Type I		Hard cervical collar if atlanto-axial instability has been excluded	

Table 11.1 (continued)

	Reducing the malalignment	Non-surgical treatment	Surgical treatment
Type II		Hard cervical collar	Anterior internal fixation (screw technique)
		Halo-vest for 10–12 weeks	Fusion CI–CII
Type III		Halo-vest in most cases	Fusion CI–CII
Traumatic spondylolisthesis			
Type I		Hard cervical collar	
Type II	Yes	Halo-vest – if successful reduction of malalignment	Posterior fusion if unacceptable malalignment or increased malalignment during Halo-vest treatment
Type II a	Yes	See type II	See type II
Type III	Yes	Halo-vest following wire techniques	Fusion using plate or wire techniques
Nonodontoid-nonhangman's fractures			According to the principles of atlanto-axial instability
"Tear drop" fracture	Yes		Posterior fusion
Atlanto-axial instability			
Anterior instability			
with fracture			According the principles of each fracture
without fracture			
		Hard cervical collar – if the transverse ligament is intact	
			Fusion CI–CII if the transverse ligament is ruptured
Rotational instability			
Type I		Hard cervical collar for 4–6 weeks	Fusion CI–CII if re-dislocation occur
Type II–III			Fusion CI–CII

OCCIPITAL CONDYLE FRACTURES

Occipital condyle fractures are rare. They usually occur as isolated fractures following compression force, axial rotation, and lateral bending moment. Occipital condyle fractures are associated with blunt head injuries as a result of the axial force running from the crown to the mandible. The risk of sustaining a fracture of the skull base including the occipital condyles increases, thus, when the cervical column is pressed toward the stiff and fixed cranium.

Diagnosis and Classification

Plain radiographs rarely capture these fractures. Computed tomography (CT) imaging is required, and the visualization of the fractures is enhanced by two- and three-dimensional reconstruction. The radiological investigation

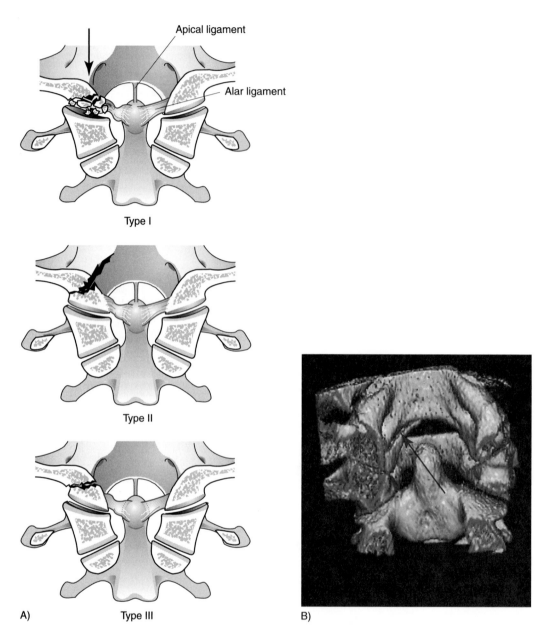

Figure 11.5 Occipital condyle fractures. A: Occipital condyle fractures type I–III. B: Computed tomography (CT) reconstruction of a right-sided type II fracture (*arrow* describes the fracture line).

regarding instability is focused on the alar ligament and the tectorial membrane (Fig. 11.5). Anderson and Montesano have classified occipital condyle fractures into three types. Type I refers to a comminute fracture (i.e., containing several fragments) with neither significant displacement of bone into the foramen magnum nor signs of avulsion of the alar ligament. The type II fracture is an extension of a linear skull-base fracture; and type III is an avulsion fracture of the occipital condyle as a result of the tension force of the alar ligament.

Treatment

The choice of treatment depends on circumstances, such as the presence of a uni- or bilateral occipital condyle fracture, other fractures/

ligamentous injuries in the upper cervical spine, and/or the presence of neurological impairment. Typically, there is no need for surgical treatment of occipital condyle fractures, since they usually heal without complications. Types I and II are considered stable and are treated with external immobilization (e.g., 8–12 weeks in a cervical soft or hard collar). Halo-vest treatment may be an alternative in the type III injuries, because of an increased risk of instability. Unstable type III fractures may be part of an occipitocervical instability and are then treated by occipital–cervical fusion.

ATLANTOOCCIPITAL DISLOCATION

Atlantooccipital dislocation constitutes approximately 1% of all injuries to the upper cervical spine. They are typically fatal and are most common among children. The injury mechanism involves multiple components such as hyperextension and hyperflexion bending moments. The pattern of deceleration–acceleration as a cause of this type of injury resembles the injury mechanism associated with whiplash injuries. Most of the supportive structures stabilizing the craniocervical junction are damaged, particularly the alar ligaments and tectorial membrane, resulting in forward dislocation of the occipital condyles in relation to the lateral masses of atlas (Fig. 11.6).

Diagnosis and Classification

Atlantooccipital dislocations may not be visualized on plain radiographs. Indirect signs, such as retropharyngeal hematoma and emphysema located anterior to the spinal column, indicate concomitant damage to the posterior pharyngeal wall. Magnetic resonance imaging (MRI) reveals clival hematoma and changed signals in, for instance, the alar ligament (Fig. 11.7). The distance and degree of displacement between the foramen magnum and atlas can be assessed by two- and three-dimensional CT reconstructions (Fig. 11.8). The relationship between the cranium and upper cervical spine can be assessed using the Powers index. The Powers index is the ratio between the length of two lines. One line measures the distance between the basion and the posterior arch of the atlas (BC); the second line describes the distance between the opisthion and the anterior arch of the atlas (OC). The mean ratio (BC/OC) in normal individuals is 0.77. Values of 1.0 or greater suggest an atlantooccipital dislocation.

According to Traynelis and coworkers, atlantooccipital dislocations are divided into type I (anterior dislocation), type II (vertical dislocation), and type III (posterior dislocation; Fig. 11.9). Atlantooccipital dislocations are, as previously mentioned, associated with injuries to the cranium and face. Concomitant damage to the brainstem may explain the relatively high mortality associated with this type of injury. Atlantooccipital dislocations are most frequently seen in child pedestrians who have been struck by cars. The horizontal placement of the articulating joints between C0 and C1 in children facilitates the gliding of these joints.

Treatment

The choice of treatment of atlantooccipital dislocations depends on the severity of the ligamentous injuries. Traction is generally contraindicated. The spinal cord may be stretched during this procedure, resulting in further risk of cord injury. A hard cervical collar should be used until final treatment is decided. Minor dislocations, also among children, are treated with a halo-vest orthosis. Gross misalignments and injuries that are considered ligamentous are usually managed with an occipital–cervical fusion.

ATLAS FRACTURES

Atlas fractures occur following axial force or vertical compression acting on the vertex of the skull. The force is transmitted caudally, and the occipital condyles become pressed against the lateral masses of atlas. The most famous type of atlas fractures is the *Jefferson fracture*, after the researcher who classified these fractures based on their appearance and the degree of involvement of the alar and transverse ligaments.

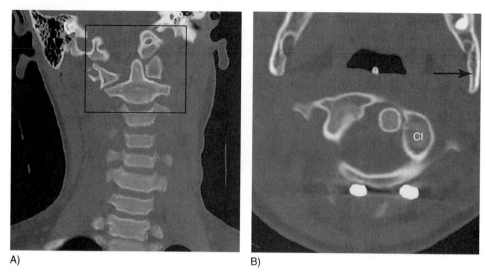

A)   B)

Figure 11.6 Spiral computed tomography (CT) scan. Frontal reconstruction illustrating a displacement at the level of C0 and C1 (particularly on the right side). The reconstruction is performed exactly in a straight position in relation to C2. A: A bilateral displacement of the joints is seen at the level of C1 and CII. The appearance of the right and left lateral masses differs and these findings show that C1 is rotated in relation to C1 (compare to Figure 11.4). B: The axial view also shows that C1 is rotated in relation to ramus mandibulae (*arrow*). The vertebral body of C2 is uninjured (compare to Figure 11.1A).

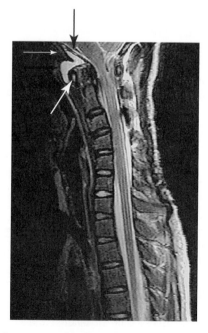

Figure 11.7 T2-weighted magnetic resonance image (MRI). Image illustrates a hematoma with high-density signals in the C0–C1 region. The *thin white arrow* indicates clivus, the *thin red horizontal arrow* points to the hematoma, and the *thick vertical red arrow* shows the tectorial membrane. The membrane is disconnected from the caudal part of the clivus by the hematoma. The hematoma reaches to the front of atlas (the *thick white arrow* points out the arch of atlas).

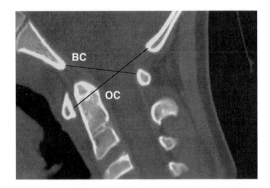

Figure 11.8 Computed tomography (CT) reconstruction used to calculate the Powers index.

Atlas fractures may be classified as follows:

> Isolated ring fractures (arch fractures)
> Jefferson fracture:
>
> > With minor dislocation
> > With severe dislocation (Spence distance
> > >7 mm indicate ligament injuries)
>
> Lateral mass fracture without dislocation
> Comminute lateral mass fractures
> Transverse ligament rupture

Isolated arch fractures actually consist of two fracture lines, either two anterior, two posterior, or one fracture on both the anterior and posterior arches (Fig. 11.11). The *Jefferson fracture* is composed of two fractures on each of the two arches (Fig. 11.12A,B). The transverse ligament is considered to be injured if the lateral masses are separated by 7 mm or more (i.e., the Spence distance is ≥7 mm) (Fig. 11.13).

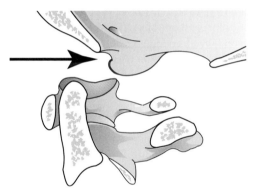

Figure 11.9 Atlanto-occipital posterior dislocation (seen from the side) of the occipital condyles (*black arrow*) in relation to C1.

Diagnosis and Classification

Plain radiographs obtained in sagittal and open-mouth projections (Fig. 11.10) may reveal an atlas fracture. It is possible to identify fractures of the posterior arch, prevertebral swelling, and an increase in diastasis (>3 mm) between the dens and atlas using plain radiographs obtained with sagittal views. Open-mouth projections are useful to detect fractures and dislocations of the lateral masses. CT delineates the morphology of the fractures and MRI reveals injuries to the ligaments.

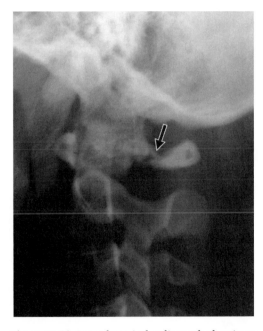

Figure 11.10 Lateral cervical radiograph showing a nondislocated fracture through the posterior arch of atlas (*arrow*).

Treatment

Isolated arch fractures are treated by external stabilization, as with hard cervical collars. Jefferson fractures with a Spence distance of less than 7 mm may be treated with either hard cervical collars, a Halo-vest, or a cervicothoracic orthosis for 6–12 weeks. A rigid external fixation, such as a Halo-vest, should always be used if the Spence distance is equal to or exceeds 7 mm. A Halo-vest is then applied for 10–12 weeks, after which time flexion-extension radiography is performed. Surgery should be considered if a dislocation of 3.5 mm or more remains between C1 and C2 following the conservative treatment period. Nondisplaced fractures of the lateral masses are treated with a hard cervical collar for 6–8 weeks.

Comminuted lateral mass fractures (Fig. 11.14) involving the tubercle (i.e., the attachment of the transverse ligament) require, as a minimum, treatment with a Halo-vest. Surgery is indicated if the transverse ligament is ruptured.

Isolated fractures of the lateral mass and isolated ruptures of the transverse ligament are extremely rare.

AXIS FRACTURES

Fractures of the axis have a very dramatic background, mainly because of their association with

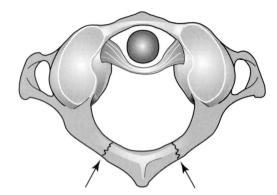

Figure 11.11 Double fracture of the posterior arch of C1.

hanging. "Hangman's fracture" was previously identified with all fractures of the axis but, according to current classifications, this fracture only represent one of several fracture types of the second vertebra (Fig. 11.15).

The "drop" method of hanging was probably introduced to Britain in the 5th century by German invaders. The original penalty "hanged by the neck until dead" usually entailed strangulation, but in the mid 1800s the method of hanging changed and the ensuing punishment was better described as "death by SCI." Fredric Wood-Jones, director of London School of Medicine for Women investigated victims hanged with the knot placed subaurally and submentally, respectively. The subaurally

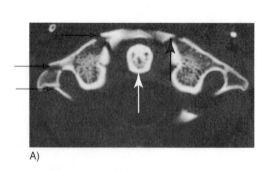

A)

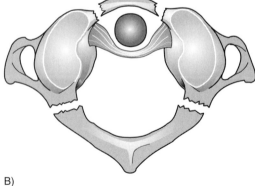

B)

Figure 11.12 A: Axial computed tomography (CT) of C1 illustrating a Jefferson fracture. Multiple fractures of the atlas ring are seen but only a minor dislocation occurs. The *white arrow* in the middle points at the dens axis. The posterior arch of atlas is not included in this view. B: A classical Jefferson fracture with altogether four fracture lines.

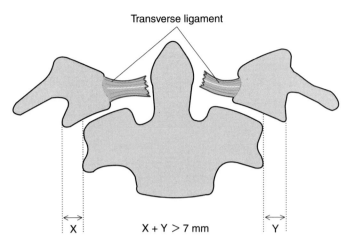

Figure 11.13 The distances x and y shows a dislocation between the inferior articular surface of C1 and the superior articular surface of C2. The vertebral body of C1 is increased in width, and the transverse ligament is considered ruptured if the Spence distance (the sum of x and y) is equal to or exceeds 7 mm.

located knot, placed below the angle of the jaw and mastoid process, resulted in a force through the skull base as the victim was dropped. This mode of knot placement had been used since the Roman era and resulted in disruptions of the cranial base but no fractures of the cervical spine. The submentally placed knot, however, resulted in instant death, as demonstrated by Captain C. F. Fraser, superintendent at the Rangoon Central Jail. He donated five skeletons to Wood-Jones, and the

examination of the skulls revealed no disruptions of the skull base but fractures of the cervical spine. The submental knot position was used from then on, because it produced a quick and thus "humane" death. Biomechanically, the use of the submental knot resulted in a distraction force and hyperextension, leading morphologically to a separation of the arch of axis from the vertebral body (i.e., a traumatic spondylolisthesis). The hangman's fracture, according to current

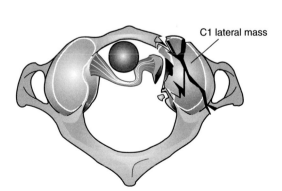

Figure 11.14 A lateral mass fracture without dislocation. The attachment of the transverse ligament is affected by the fracture.

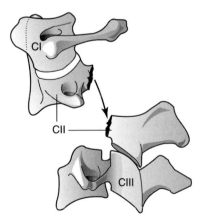

Figure 11.15 Hangman's fracture. The fracture extends through the pars interarticularis of C2, and the vertebral body of C2 is separated from the vertebral arch and posterior structures of axis.

classifications, denotes a traumatic spondylolisthesis of the axis as a result of an axial force in combination with a hyperextension movement. Thus the term remains in current classifications although this fracture type does not resemble the morphology seen after hangings.

Fractures of the axis are, typically, associated with older individuals. These fractures are often caused by low-energy trauma, as osteoporosis frequently occurs among the elderly. Approximately 50% of cervical fractures in patients 65 years and older are C2 fractures. Special attention must therefore be given to such fractures among this group of patients.

Fractures of axis represent approximately 20% of cervical column fractures. They are classified as odontoid (50%), hangman's (25%), and vertebral (i.e., neither odontoid nor hangman; 25%) fractures.

Odontoid Fractures

Odontoid fractures are caused by a combination of axial compression and horizontal shear forces. Blunt trauma toward the cranium and fall accidents are common causes among the elderly and younger population, respectively.

Diagnosis and Classification

Odontoid fractures may be overlooked easily, especially if nondislocated, and where plain radiographs are used in the acute setting. CT, using thin slices and reconstruction images, better demonstrates these fractures, which are subdivided according to Anderson and d'Alonzo into three types (Fig. 11.16).

Type I fractures are uncommon. They are usually oblique and located at the tip of the dens. They are considered avulsion injuries located at the attachment of the alar ligament to the odontoid process. This type of fracture may be associated with craniocervical instability because of the damage to the alar ligament. Type II fractures are the most common. They are located at the junction of the odontoid process and the vertebra of C2 (Figs. 11.17 and 11.18). This fracture has a high incidence of nonunion (65% if dislocation is >6 mm) probably caused by stoppage of the blood supply. The cross-sectional area of cancellous

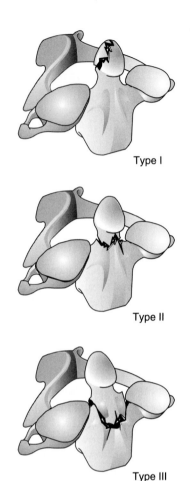

Figure 11.16 Odontoid fractures types I, II, and III.

bone is very limited at the fracture site and the presence of soft-tissue material may, by becoming interposed at the fracture surfaces, also contribute to nonunion. Type III fractures engage the vertebral body itself. The fracture area is large, and this fracture type usually heals without problems (Fig. 11.19).

Treatment

Almost all type I odontoid fractures heal without problems. However, one must consider the possibility of a coexisting atlantooccipital dislocation before choosing treatment for this stable type of fracture. The standard treatment is, after injuries to the alar ligament have been excluded, a hard cervical collar for 6 weeks. Surgical fusion of

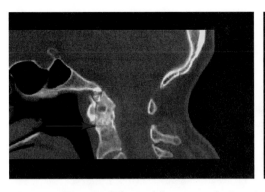
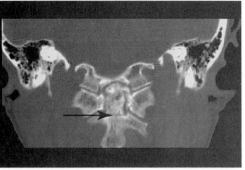

Figure 11.17 A nondislocated fracture at the junction of the vertebral body and the odontoid process.

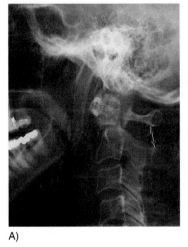
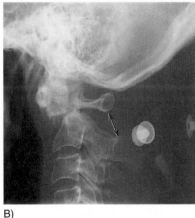

A)   B)

Figure 11.18 A: A type II fracture with approximately 5 mm anterior dislocation of the odontoid process/ atlas complex in relation to the vertebral body of C2. Observe the anterior dislocation of the posterior arch of CI in relation to the vertebral body of CII. B: The same type of fracture. The dislocation here, however, is considerably more substantial. The posterior arch of C1 is also displaced anteriorly, resulting in a further narrowing of the spinal canal (the *double arrow* shows the distance between the posterior arch of C1 and the posterior superior edge of C2).

C1–C2 may be performed if a ligamentous injury is detected.

Treatment of type II fractures is based on the patient's age, the appearance of the fracture, and the presence of concurrent injuries. There is an increased risk of nonunion (pseudarthrosis) if the dislocation between the odontoid process and the vertebral body of C2 is equal to or exceeds 6 mm.

Stabilizing treatment for type II fractures is considered necessary. The stabilizing measures are either nonoperative using a hard cervical collar (in dislocations of <6 mm) or a Halo-vest, whereas surgical treatment is required in some cases. Some studies indicate a high frequency of nonunion among patients treated with Halo-vest. Two possibilities of surgical treatment for this fracture type are available if the fractures do not heal, anterior or posterior internal fixation. The disadvantage of posterior internal fixation is the abolishment of all movement between C1 and C2. This results in a rotational reduction of about 50% in the cervical

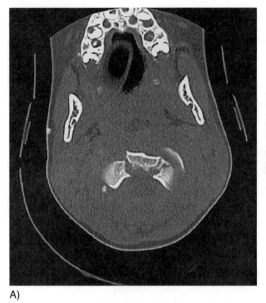
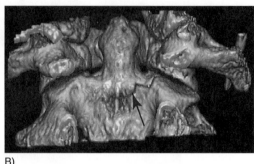

A)   B)

Figure 11.19 Odontoid fracture type III. Computed tomography (CT) axial (A) and frontal (B) reconstruction images are obtained through the vertebral body of C2 (the *arrow* in B shows the fracture line).

spine. The advantage of the anterior internal fixation is the preservation of the full ability to rotate.

Noncomminuted type II fractures dislocated less than 5 mm and located perpendicular to the odontoid process are usually treated with a Halo-vest for 10–12 weeks. Plain radiographs or CT scans are regularly performed during this period. Anterior fixation, using odontoid screws, is a common alternative. The screws offer instant rigid fixation, allow healing, and preserve rotation between atlas and axis. A hard cervical collar offers an additional treatment possibility among very old osteoporotic patients.

Patients exhibiting fractures with a high risk for nonunion may be considered candidates for surgical intervention. Fractures dislocated 6 mm or more with an oblique fracture line in the anteroposterior view or with a comminute appearance are usually treated by internal fixation. Patients showing signs of SCI and/or chest injury are also usually candidates for surgical intervention.

Type III fractures almost always heal if treated with a Halo-vest. A hard cervical collar

is a treatment option in rare cases. Surgical management with internal fixation may be used if the Halo-vest treatment fails. These rare cases are treated with a posterior fusion between C1 and C2.

Traumatic Spondylolisthesis (Hangman's Fracture)

This type of fracture usually results from an axial force and hyperextension bending moment. The pars interarticularis of C2, also known as the pedicle or isthmus, is one of the weakest structures of the cervical spine (Fig. 11.1B). A bilateral fracture through the pars interarticularis constitutes the prerequisite for Hangman's fractures.

Diagnosis and Classification

Sagittal plain radiographs may capture a hangman's fracture, although CT gives a more exact depiction of the fracture morphology. Traumatic spondylolisthesis is classified, according to Levine and Rhyne, into four subgroups. This classification is based on the morphology of the fracture, as well as on the angulation and

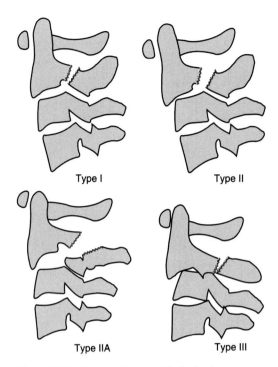

Type I   Type II

Type IIA   Type III

Figure 11.20 Traumatic spondylolisthesis.

dislocation of C2 in relation to C3. Type I engages the pars interarticularis at the junction between the pedicle and the arch of C2 (Fig. 11.20). An anterior translation of less than 3 mm without any concurrent angulation is typical in this type of fracture, and no surrounding structures are usually involved.

A type II fracture is caused by a flexion bending moment in addition to an initial axial force and a hyperextension bending moment. This results in damage to the intervertebral disk and ligamentous structures. A dislocation of 4 mm or more of C2 in relation to C3 is seen, but no signs of abnormal angulation are present (Fig. 11.20).

An oblique fracture line characterizes type IIA fractures. A dislocation is present as is the case in type II fractures. The obliquity of the fracture line increases the risk of forward angulation of the vertebral body and dens in relation to the vertebral arch.

Three variations of type III fractures have been described. The characteristic feature is the combination of fractures through the facet joints of C2 and C3 and a simultaneous fracture of the arch. The facet joint injuries are probably caused

by a flexion bending moment and a distraction force, in addition to the initial loading. This fracture is characterized by a significant dislocation and forward angulation, as well as by an increased distance from the posterior part of the disk and facet joint dislocations.

Treatment

Type I fractures (Fig. 11.21) are considered stable and are thus treated with a hard cervical collar for 6–8 weeks (Table 11.1). Type II fractures are regarded as unstable. The Halo-vest normally offers adequate immobilization and restored alignment. Type II fractures usually heal without problems. The treatment of the type IIA fractures is more controversial. The management is the same as that of type II, provided an adequate reduction of the dislocation is achieved. However, internal fixation is used if the initial misalignment is unacceptable and if the dislocation and/or the forward angulation increases during nonsurgical treatment. An anterior or posterior fusion of C2 and C3 is then needed.

The unusual type III fracture is typically treated by open reduction since closed reduction usually fails to restore alignment. A posterior approach combined with an open reduction of the misalignment and a subsequent internal fixation is the most frequent treatment. The facet joint dislocation is reduced manually. The internal fixation is performed using various screw techniques in combination with plates or rods. The screws used to fix the plate or rods also keep the fracture through the pars interarticularis in place, which is a great advantage. However, damage to the vertebral arteries is a risk when using the screw technique. Halo-vest external fixation is recommended as an additional treatment if the less-rigid wiring technique is used for fixation.

Nonodontoid/Nonhangman's Fractures

Nonodontoid/nonhangman's fractures of the C2 body are classified according to Fujimura (1966) into four subtypes. All fractures in this group are localized in the C2 body beneath the odontoid process. Type I represents the so-called "tear-drop fracture" caused by severe hyperextension-bending moment that results

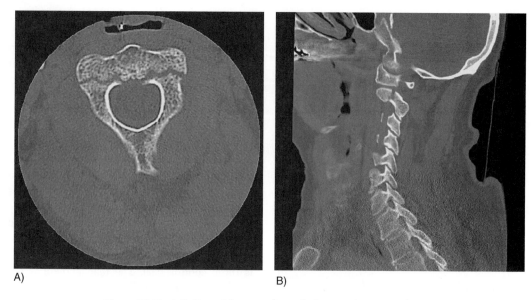

A)   B)

Figure 11.21 A,B: Type I fracture through the pars interarticularis.

in avulsion of the anterior inferior corner of the C2 vertebral body. Type II resembles the type III odontoid fracture (Fig. 11.16) but is localized further back on the C2 body. Type III is a burst fracture of the C2 body, and type IV is a sagittally oriented vertical split fracture through the body of C2. This fracture is considered unstable.

Treatment

Treatment of this fracture group is based on the degree of dislocation between the atlas and axis. Fractures considered stable are treated with a hard cervical collar, whereas unstable fractures are initially managed with a Halo-vest. The fracture area of spongy bone is large, which results in a high percentage of healing. Surgical treatment is required in the management of the type I fracture and also if alignment is impossible to obtain in the other types of fractures treated nonsurgically. A posterior fusion is then usually performed between C2 and C3.

Atlantoaxial Instability

Atlantoaxial instability (AAI) is characterized by an excessive (i.e., nonphysiological) movement at the junction between atlas and axis as a result of

bony or ligamentous damage. AAI is defined as an atlantodens interval (ADI; i.e., the distance between the odontoid process and the posterior border of the anterior arch of the atlas) of more than 3 mm in adults and of more than 5 mm in children, as measured by plain radiographs. Instability may result in displacement in all directions. Translation of the vertebral arch of the atlas in relation to the dens (anteroposterior translation) and rotation of the atlas relative to the axis (rotatory displacement) are the most common types of atlantoaxial instability. The strong transverse ligament and the facet capsules normally maintain the integrity of the atlantoaxial articulation. A rupture of the transverse ligament results in the most common types of AAI mentioned. The most severe types of instability, such as a vertical displacement, also require disruption of the alar ligament and tectorial membrane, resulting in a widening of the C1–C2 facet joints.

Diagnosis and Treatment

AAI is typically seen on plain lateral flexion-extension radiographs, although the interpretation of atlantoaxial rotatory displacement is more difficult using this technique. An atlantoaxial distance of greater than 4–5 mm, as demonstrated by lateral radiographs, is indicative of anteroposterior instability. Two- and three-dimensional CT reconstructions, however, detect avulsion fractures engaging the transverse ligament. An increased distance between the lateral mass and the dens of more than 2 mm indicates instability. MRI may reveal hematoma and ligamentous damage.

The most common causes of AAI are:

Anteroposterior instability:
- Rupture of the transverse ligament
- Odontoid fractures
- Unstable Jefferson fractures
- Associated occipitocervical instability (rupture of the alar ligament)

Rotatory displacement:
- Facet subluxation (type I)
- Rupture of the transverse ligament (displacement of 3–5 mm; type II)
- Rupture of the transverse and alar ligaments (displacement of >5 mm; type III)

Treatment

AAI is by definition an unstable situation, which in most cases requires immediate treatment. A hard cervical collar is used if there are no signs of fracture of C1 or C2 and if the transverse ligament is intact. Lateral flexion-extension radiographs are performed at the end of the treatment period. Internal fixation must be considered if signs of instability remain. Patients with ruptures of the transverse ligament require surgical treatment.

Rotatory displacements are extremely rare. The type I rotatory displacement only requires a hard cervical collar if the displacement is corrected and remains in alignment during a treatment period of 4–6 weeks. Surgical treatment is indicated if a redislocation occurs during the period of conservative treatment. Rotatory displacement of type II and III generally requires surgical treatment (i.e., fusion of C1 and C2).

ACKNOWLEDGMENTS

The authors would like to express their gratitude to Associate Professor Leif Anderberg, Department of Neurosurgery, University Hospital, Lund for excellent advice in the creation of Chapters 10–13.

12 Lower Cervical Spine Fractures and Ligament Injuries (C3–C7)

The so-called lower or subaxial injuries of the cervical spine involve the levels between C3 and C7. These injuries are quite common; about 75% of all injuries to the cervical spine are located subaxially. Advanced imaging using computed tomography (CT) and magnetic resonance imaging (MRI) has improved the possibility of early diagnosis. In 1982, Allen and Fergusson presented a classification of subaxial injuries based on mechanism of injury. Six subgroups are distinguished:

- Compression-flexion
- Vertical compression
- Distraction-flexion
- Compression-extension
- Distraction-extension
- Lateral flexion

Because this "multi-subgroup" classification was developed before CT and MRI were available, it presents many difficulties when applied to daily clinical practice. Therefore, we have chosen to follow a simplified classification, developed by Cooper and coworkers, that includes only five subgroups. Cooper's classification contains only one group with an extension injury mechanism, and the lateral-flexion group of the Allen and Fergusson classification has been excluded. Penetrating injuries, a separate group according to Cooper's classification, will be discussed in Chapter 18. An anatomical overview, as well as the concept of "instability," will be presented prior to the discussion of individual fracture types grouped according to Cooper's classification scheme.

ANATOMICAL OVERVIEW

The vertebral bodies of the lower cervical spine are ovally shaped and sloped in a forward and downward direction (Fig. 11.1C). They are all similar in shape but increase in size caudally. The spinous processes are directed back and downward. The spinous process of C7 (the vertebra prominens) is the largest of all spinous processes. Unlike all other bifid spinous processes, the spinous process of C7 has only one part at the apex. The upper surfaces of the vertebral bodies are concave due to the presence of bony ridges, the *uncinate processes* (Fig. 11.1A). The lower articular facet joint surfaces of the upper vertebral body cover the upper articular surfaces of the lower vertebral bodies (Fig. 12.1). The intervertebral disk, located between two adjacent vertebral bodies, absorbs force during vertical compression. Aging results in reduced disk water content and secondarily to reduced disk height. The facet joints must then carry an increased load, which leads to accelerated cervical spine degeneration. The process of aging results in a narrowing of the spinal canal as a consequence of the expansion of disk material and ligament structures, and bone spurs (osteophytes) at the margin of the vertebral bodies. Spinal stenosis (i.e., narrowing of the spinal canal) may contribute to neurological symptoms following trauma to the cervical spine. This is most frequently observed following extension bending loads among elderly patients.

The anterior longitudinal ligament is firmly attached to the vertebral bodies at the level of the

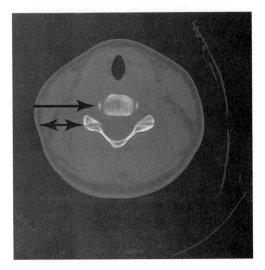

Figure 12.1 Axial computed tomography (CT). A vertebral body at the level of the lower cartilaginous endplate. The uncinate processes belonging to the vertebra located below is seen lateral to the vertebral body (*arrow*). An uninjured intervertebral joint (facet joint) is indicated with the *double arrow*.

disks and cartilaginous end plates and not to the vertebral bodies itself (Fig. 12.2). The anterior longitudinal ligament prevents hyperextension of the cervical spine following extension loads; that is, it maintains stability during extension bending moments. The posterior longitudinal ligament is located on the posterior surfaces of vertebral bodies. It is attached to the vertebral

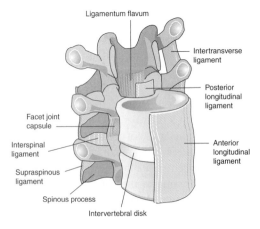

Figure 12.2 Major support structures of the spinal column.

bodies in a similar mode as the anterior longitudinal ligament. The posterior ligament likewise prevents hyperextension. The ligamentum flavum constitutes the third major ligament of the cervical spine. It covers the posterior wall of the spinal canal and ties the vertebral arches together. The facet joint capsules, the intra- and supraspinous ligaments, and the nuchal ligament are structures also contributing to stability in the motion segments. These structures predominantly prevent hyperflexion bending moments and translation in the anteroposterior direction.

The vertebral arteries pass through the vertebral foramina in the lower cervical spine. Nerve roots pass just behind the vessels. An increased risk of damage to the arteries exists when the vertebral foramina are narrowed by bony spurs, as is the case among elderly people with spondyloarthrosis (Fig. 12.3).

THE CONCEPT OF INSTABILITY

Stability is here defined as the ability of the supporting elements of the spinal column to tolerate normal loads without leading to major deformity, neurological dysfunction, and/or incapacitating pain. Instability may occur acutely, as when the vertebral column is unable to offer protection to the spinal cord at the moment of injury. Instability may also come about subacutely, resulting in increased neurological deterioration and/or pain in the post-acute period. Finally, instability may develop many years after the initial trauma and result in symptoms similar to those experienced in the post-acute period. Various attempts have been made to operationalize instability. Two different subdivisions are used in clinical practice: the two- and three-column spine concepts by White and Panjabi and by Denis, respectively.

The Two-column Spine Concept

This concept is based on the following principles (Fig. 12.4):

- The *anterior column* consists of the posterior longitudinal ligament and all structures located anterior to this ligament,

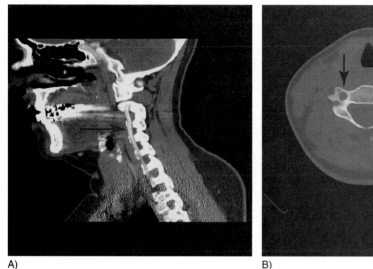
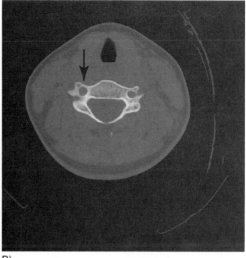

A) B)

Figure 12.3 Imaging of (A) the vertebral artery and (B) the vertebral foramina.

including the vertebral body. The soft-tissue components (the so-called anterior ligament complex) comprise the anterior longitudinal ligament, the intervertebral disk, and the posterior longitudinal ligament in each motion segment of two adjacent vertebrae.

• The *posterior column* consists of all structures behind the posterior longitudinal ligament, including the vertebral arches, facet joints, and posterior ligamentous complex.

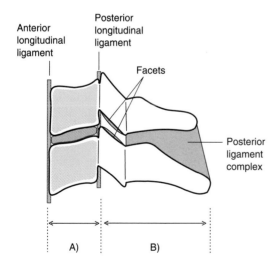

Figure 12.4 The two-column spine concept. A: anterior column; B: posterior column.

Instability is operationalized according to the White and Panjabis checklist (Table 12.1). A fracture is considered unstable if the totla score >5.

TABLE 12.1 Diagnostic checklist of clinical instability in the middle and lower cervical spine (scoring points within parenthesis).

Anterior elements damaged or unable to function (2)
Posterior elements damaged or unable to function (2)
Sagittal plane translation (flexion/ extension x-rays) >3.5 mm (4)
Relative sagittal plane angulation (resting x-rays) >11 degrees (2)
Abnormal disk narrowing (1)
Developmentally narrow spinal canal (1)
Spinal cord damage (2)
Nerve root damage (1)
Dangerous loading anticipated (1)

The Three-column Spine Concept

The three-column spine concept offers an alternative classification. This concept was initially designed by Denis to classify fractures in the thoracic and lumbar spine. It is, however, also quite frequently used when instability in the lower cervical spine is discussed (Fig. 12.5). According to this concept, the *anterior column* contains the anterior longitudinal ligament, the anterior part of the

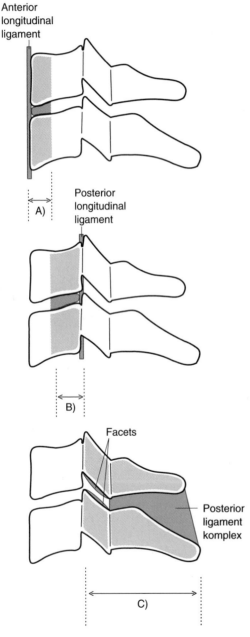

Anterior longitudinal ligament

Posterior longitudinal ligament

A)

B)

Facets

Posterior ligament komplex

C)

Figure 12.5 The three-column-spine concept. A: anterior column; B: middle column; C: posterior column.

intervertebral disk, and the vertebral body. The *middle column* is formed by the posterior part of the intervertebral disk, the vertebral body, and the posterior longitudinal ligament. Thus, the anterior and middle column in Denis' classification corresponds to the anterior column in the concept of White and Panjabi. The *posterior column* is identical in both of these concepts.

Instability is, according to the three-column spine concept, operationalized as a failure of two or three of the three columns.

A fracture is always instable if the middle column is damaged, since damage to this column always involves additional failure, either of the anterior or posterior column or both. Neither classification has been evaluated scientifically, so should therefore only be considered as heuristic means to facilitate the choice of treatment.

FRACTURE CLASSIFICATION

Closed fractures in the lower cervical spine may, as previously mentioned, be divided into four subgroups: flexion-dislocation injuries, flexion-compression injuries, compression-burst injuries, and extension injuries.

Flexion-Dislocation Injuries (Facet Joint Dislocations of Varying Severity)

Flexion-dislocation injuries comprise about 40% of the injuries of the lower cervical spine and 10% of all injuries to the spinal column. This type of injuries occurs following a variety of forces and moments, such as rotation, flexion, and tension. The main load is directed through the occiput, usually with the cervical spine in a flexed position. As a result of the load, the head continues to move forward and upward by its own weight. The posterior elements are elongated and the anterior elements are compressed as a consequence of these movements.

Damage to the posterior structures is always seen in this type of injury but, typically, no significant damage occurs in the vertebral body itself. Flexion-dislocation injuries are divided into four degrees of severity: facet subluxation,

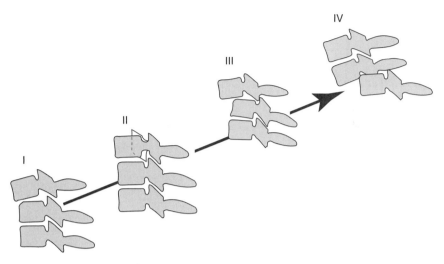

Figure 12.6 Flexion-dislocation injuries. The empty square behind the facet joint in type II illustrates a unilateral facet dislocation.

unilateral facet dislocation, bilateral facet dislocation, and floating vertebrae (Fig. 12.6).

Facet subluxation

In simple facet subluxation, an increase in the distance occurs between adjacent spinous processes (Figs. 12.6; I, 12.7). An injury to the posterior ligament complex results in a facet subluxation if the neck bends forward. The increase in distance between the two adjacent spinous processes is denoted as a *flexion sprain*. This type of injury may be difficult to visualize in the acute stage of injury. The flexion/extension radiography is hampered by impaired motion due to presence of pain and reflexogenic cervical muscle spasm, but are of greatest value usually 10–14 days after trauma, when pain has decreased and the range of movement is acceptable. MRI will, in most cases, confirm the presence of injuries to the posterior ligaments and should be used if the result is inconclusive using plain lateral flexion-extension radiographs.

Treatment. This less-complicated type of flexion-dislocation injury is either treated with hard cervical collar, Halo-vest, or internal fixation (Table 12.2). Lateral flexion-extension radiographs must be performed routinely 6–8 weeks after injury if nonsurgical treatment is chosen. The treatment of choice is usually,

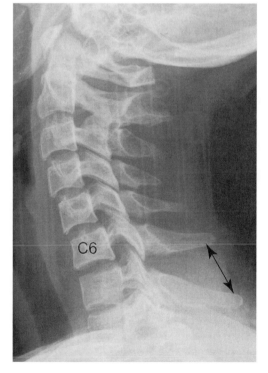

Figure 12.7 Flexion sprain injury. The distance between the spinous processes of C6 and C7 is increased (*double arrow*). A minor translation is also seen in the C6–C7 facet joint.

TABLE 12.2 Treatment guidelines following injuries to the lower cervical spine.

	Narrowing of the Spinal Cord	Posterior Ligament Injuries	Treatment
Flexion-dislocation injuries			
"Flexion-sprain injury"	No	Yes	Hard cervical collar; Halo-vest treatment; surgery
Unilateral facet dislocation	Yes	Yes	Halo-vest treatment; surgery
Bilateral facet dislocation	Yes	Yes	Surgery
Floating vertebra	Yes	Yes	Surgery
Flexion-compression injuries			
Reduction of vertebral			
body height			
<30%	No	No	Hard cervical collar
>30%	No	No	Hard cervical collar; Halo-vest; surgery
>30%	Yes	Yes	Anterior + (if necessary) posterior internal fixation
>30%	No	Yes	Anterior or posterior internal fixation
Compression-burst fractures			
Type I	No		Hard cervical collar
Type II	No		Hard cervical collar
Type III	Yes		Surgery
	No		Halo-vest treatment
Extension injuries			
Distraction-extension			
Type I			Hard cervical collar/surgery
Type II			Surgery
Compression-extension			
Type I			Hard cervical collar
Type II			Hard cervical collar/surgery
Type V			Surgery
Mb Bechterew	Yes	Yes	a) Anterior internal fixation and fusion followed by
			b) optional treatment with posterior internal fixation and fusion or Halo-vest

however, internal fixation performed to prevent uni- or bilateral facet dislocations, as well as to prevent development of chronic pain and neurological sequelae.

Unilateral Facet Dislocation

Damage to the posterior ligamentous structures following trauma ranges from partial to complete (Figs. 12.6; II, 12.8 and 12.9). The articulating surfaces are exposed completely if a unilateral facet dislocation occurs. This is known as the *nude facet* or *inverted hamburger sign*.

Treatment. Two out of three patients with unilateral facet dislocation show signs of incomplete SCI or root symptoms. A unilateral facet dislocation should, as a rule, be reduced in order

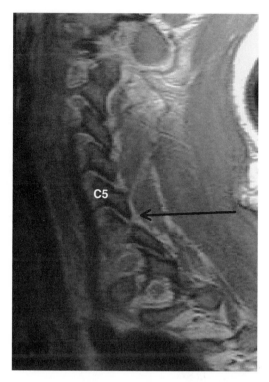

Figure 12.8 Unilateral facet dislocation. Sagittal MRI illustrating locked facets between C5 and C6 (see *arrow*). The articulating surfaces of the facet joint have thus entirely slid apart.

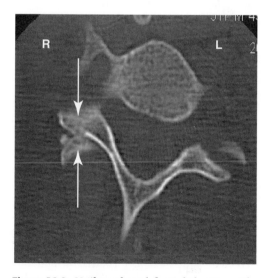

Figure 12.9 Unilateral total facet dislocation. The two articulating surfaces (indicated by two *arrows*) of the right-sided facet joint have totally slid apart. The congruity of the left facet joint is altered but no dislocation is seen.

to avoid subsequent pain. Halo-vest treatment for 3 months is used, if reduction is achieved by closed reduction. This is standard treatment in the absence of neurological symptoms in some centers. The Halo-vest treatment may also be used if closed reduction fails. An unsuccessful reduction may be acceptable despite a higher risk of developing pain.

Open reduction and internal fixation is, however, typically the preferred choice. The presence of extruded disk material and/or hematoma compressing the spinal cord determines whether an anterior or posterior approach is preferable. A reduction of the dislocation in the presence of compressing disk material may increase the risk of neurological sequelae. Thus, an anterior approach is used in the presence of compromising disk material, and removal of the extruded disk material is the first step in the surgical procedure. This is followed by a reduction of the dislocation, and the procedure ends with an anterior internal fixation and fusion. A posterior approach may serve as an alternative if no signs of disk extrusion are seen on the MRI. The posterior approach may include either an open reduction of the facet dislocation or, as an alternative, a removal of the dislocated facet to relieve the pressure on the spinal cord and/or nerve root. Either procedure should be followed by posterior fusion and internal fixation.

Bilateral Facet Dislocation

In bilateral facet dislocation injury, lateral radiographs will reveal a displacement of the vertebral body corresponding to 50% or more of the sagittal diameter (Figs. 12.6; III, 12.10), and a facet dislocation will be seen bilaterally (Fig. 12.11). Damage to the posterior ligamentous complex and bony fractures of the lamina and facet joints are frequently visualized. The upper anterior corner of the lower vertebra may be rounded off, indicating failure of the anterior column. The typical levels where bilateral facet dislocations occur are C5–C6 and C6–C7. Two out of three such patients prove to have a complete SCI, with morphological signs of damage to both the anterior and posterior column, thus fulfilling criteria of spinal instability. Bilateral facet dislocation represents a type of injury most often associated with extruded or

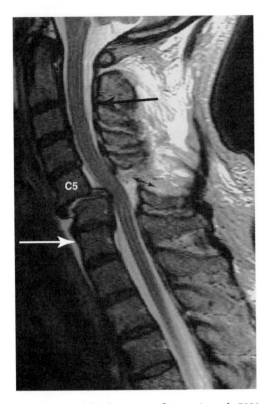

Figure 12.10 A displacement of approximately 50% of the sagittal diameter of the vertebral body is visualized on this T2-weighted midline image. The intervertebral disk below the body of C5 is ruptured (causing a high signal), but no traumatic extrusion of the intervertebral disk is seen. The distance between the spinous processes of C5 and C6 is substantially increased and the *double arrow* indicates the location of a rupture of the posterior ligamentous structures. The ligaments are black on the T2-weighted images (as indicated by a *single red arrow*) reaching from the foramen magnum to the level of dislocation. The black structure returns at the lower level of C6 and continues caudally. Please also observe the small prevertebral bleed (high signal in front of vertebrae C6 and C7, *white arrow*).

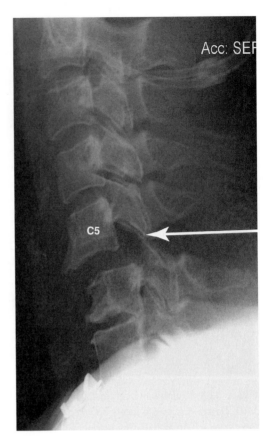

Figure 12.11 Lateral radiographs illustrating a locked facet (*white arrow*) on the same patient.

herniated disks. The presence of intervertebral disk material that compromises the spinal cord, as seen on MRI, influences the choice of subsequent treatment.

Treatment. Closed manual reduction followed by Halo-vest treatment was historically used in such cases. However, this method has largely been abandoned due to the risk of increased neurological deterioration and even death during the maneuver as a result of additional compression of the spinal cord caused by the extruded disk material. Traction treatment is also still used in some cases. Such treatment should be initiated (if used) as soon as possible. Typically, 5 kg is applied to start. A .5 kg of weight is added for each level below C2. Thus, 7 kg is used as an initial traction weight following a dislocation at the C6 and C7 level. About 20 kg is usually considered the maximum weight, but higher loads have been reported in the literature. The risk of nonunion of the fusion and redislocation is reported as relatively high if the Halo-vest is used in isolation. Patients should be offered surgical treatment in cases of redislocation during Halo-vest treatment or in cases of nonunion.

Compression of the spinal cord caused by disk material may increase, as previously mentioned, during the reduction procedures and cause severe damage to the spinal cord and further neurological deterioration. Due to this risk, reduction methods during the initial stage of management have given way to surgery as the treatment of choice in nearly all cases of bilateral facet dislocations. Most centers advocate both anterior and posterior internal fixation and fusion since there is typically evidence of damage to all columns. An anterior removal of the intervertebral disk material to minimize the risk of further neurological deterioration precedes the open reduction and the subsequent anterior and posterior internal fixation and fusion; for details see Chapter 13.

Floating Vertebra

Dislocations corresponding to the length of an entire vertebral body or a motion segment showing extreme mobility are denoted *floating vertebrae* (see Fig. 12.6; IV). The treatment is identical to that used in bilateral facet dislocation.

Flexion-Compression Injuries

The load resulting in a flexion-compression injury is directed downward and forward, thus, an oblique, axially directed load is required to produce this type of injury. Flexion-compression injuries represent 20% of injuries to the lower cervical spine. A compression of the anterior portion of the vertebral body is seen on lateral radiographs, while the height of the posterior portion of the vertebral body remains intact. The distance between the spinous processes is increased following a severe compression of the vertebral body, as a sign of damage to the posterior ligament structures (Fig. 12.12). The simplest type of flexion-compression injury shows a minor compression at the upper anterior corner of the vertebral body (grade I). The next degree of severity involves a more obliquely shaped anterior edge, with a more pronounced compression of the vertebral body resulting in a beak-like shape (grade II). A fracture of the beak is seen in grade III (teardrop appearance). Grade IV has the fractured beak of grade III, but a dislocation of the posterior wall of the vertebral body of less than 3 mm into the spinal canal is also noticed (Fig. 12.13). The posterior part of the

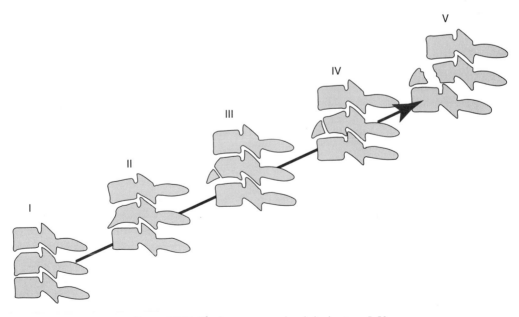

Figure 12.12 Flexion-compression injuries type I–V.

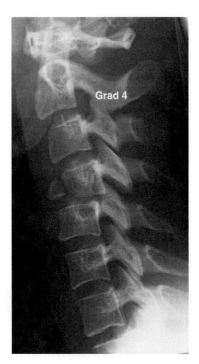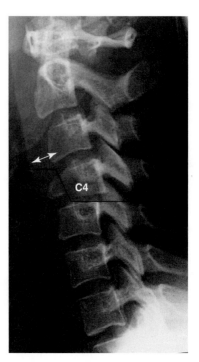

Figure 12.13 Flexion-compression injury grade IV without and with arrow and fracture line. The double-arrow shows the prevertebral soft-tissue shadow. The *red line* indicates the course of a flexion teardrop fracture involving C3 and C4. The teardrop fragment is attached to the C5 vertebral body via the anterior longitudinal ligament. An additional ligamentous injury must be present at the level of C3 and C4. The fracture traverses the posterior two-thirds of the intervertebral disk, through the posterior part of the spinal canal and finally between the spinous processes of C4 and C5. The vertebral body of C4 is dislocated a few millimeters in relation to CV.

vertebral body is dislocated into the spinal canal in the most severe type of injury, grade V, and the distance between the articulating facet joint surfaces is increased. Locked facets, a characteristic sign of flexion-dislocation injuries, are not observed in flexion-compression injuries.

Treatment

The fracture is considered stable if the compression of the vertebral body is less than one-third and no signs of spinal canal narrowing are seen. Conservative treatment for 8–12 weeks is recommended. The indication for surgery gets stronger in proportion to the severity of the flexion-compression injuries. The degree of spinal canal narrowing (due to bony material in the spinal canal) and compression of the spinal cord, the

presence of ligamentous injuries, and the severity of the neurological deterioration is of importance in fracture management if the vertebral body height is reduced by more than one-third.

Surgical treatment is the method of choice in the presence of posterior ligament injuries and/or significant bony compression of the spinal cord.

Compression-Burst Injuries

The compression-burst fractures take the place of vertical compression fractures in the classification of Allen and Ferguson (Figs. 12.14 and 12.15). This type of injury is caused by axial compression, with the load affecting the center of the vertebral body while the spinal column is in a neutral position. The posterior part of the

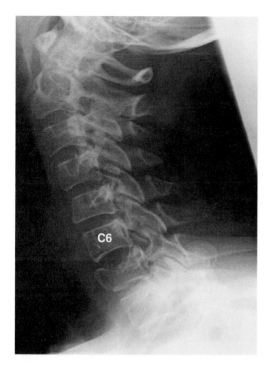

Figure 12.14 Grade II compression-burst fracture (C7 vertebral body).

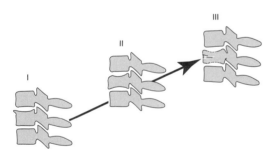

Figure 12.15 Compression-burst fractures.

vertebral body is also involved in the compression-burst fracture, and the vertebral body is split into several fragments (comminuted) resulting in compression of the spinal cord in the most severe cases.

The least severe type of compression-burst fractures involves one of the two cartilaginous end plates, and the fracture is visualized through that end plate (grade I). Fractures are seen in both end plates in grade II. The most severe degree of compression-burst fractures, grade

III, are additionally characterized by fragmentation of the central part of the vertebral body (Fig. 12.16). The fragmentation may result in a subsequent dislocation of bony components into the spinal canal and clinical signs of spinal cord compression.

Treatment

Burst fractures involve the posterior part of the vertebral body, in addition to the damage seen in the anterior part. The ligamentous structures are intact and the vertebral column is stable in the least severe forms of burst fractures. Conservative treatment using a hard cervical collar is recommended in those cases. Grade III compression

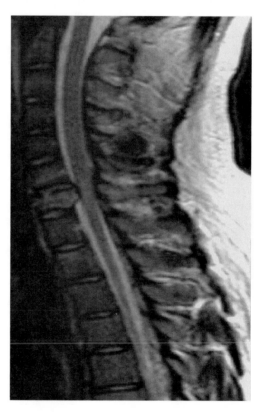

Figure 12.16 T2-weighted magnetic resonance image (MRI). Image shows a significant compression of the C7 vertebral body (grade III). Observe the curved shape of the extrusion of the vertebral body into the spinal canal. The anterior cerebrospinal fluid space is obliterated and a discrete edema of the spinal cord can also be observed at the level of injury.

burst fracture is considered unstable and surgical treatment is usually required. An anterior decompression followed by fusion and internal fixation is recommended if a significant compression of the spinal cord is present. Halo-vest treatment is optional if the spinal cord is unaffected by the vertebral body. Some authors recommend an anterior as well as posterior fusion if all three columns are damaged.

Extension Injuries

Extension injuries are seen following distraction (Fig. 12.17) or compression (Figs. 12.19 and 12.20). Elderly people with spondylosis are particularly vulnerable to this type of injury, and a high incidence of spinal cord involvement is observed in this group (Fig. 12.18). Avulsion of an anteriorly located fragment is seen in younger individuals, in addition to damage to either the anterior or posterior structures.

Distraction-Extension

Two types of injury are seen if a distraction force is added to the initial extension bending moment (Fig. 12.17). The least complicated type of injury (grade I) involves damage to the anterior longitudinal ligament and a widening of the anterior intervertebral disk space is seen. Complicated injuries (grade II) also include damage to the posterior ligament complex, resulting in a posterior dislocation of the upper vertebral body into the spinal canal.

Treatment. Grade I distraction-extension injuries are usually seen among elderly people with

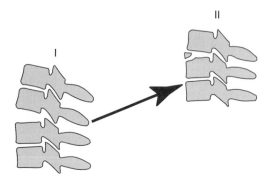

Figure 12.17 Distraction extension injuries.

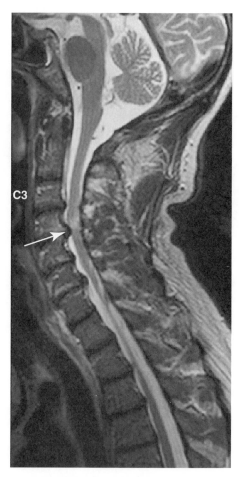

Figure 12.18 T2-weighted midline magnetic resonance image (MRI). Image shows severe spondylosis including encroaching degenerative changes between C3 and C4. The cerebrospinal fluid (CSF) space is completely obliterated at the level of C4 and C5, and an area of high signal, compatible with a spinal cord contusion is seen within the spinal cord (*arrow*). The already narrowed spinal canal (spinal stenosis) has probably been further encroached during the moment of injury.

degenerative spondylosis. Choice of treatment is controversial and depends on the severity of neurological deterioration. Conservative treatment is typically recommended in the acute stage, but surgical intervention should be performed if the patient shows increased neurological deterioration. Anterior decompression followed by fusion and fixation is required in

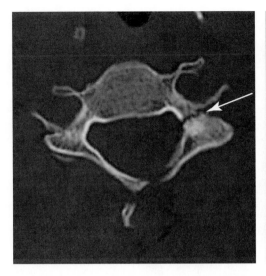
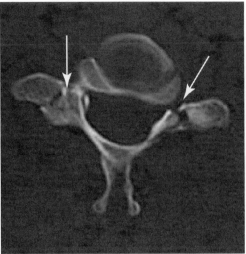

Figure 12.19 Left axial CT scan. Image illustrates a unilateral fracture and the right image a bilateral vertebral arch fracture, most obvious seen on the left side.

those cases. Surgical treatment is usually indicated for severe grade II injuries.

Compression-Extension

The two least complicated levels in a five-level scale of compression-extension injuries include fractures at one (unilateral; grade I) or two (bilateral; grade II) locations on the vertebral arch, as illustrated by the axial CT images in Figure 12.19. The most severe type of injury (grade V) includes fractures at two locations on the vertebral arch and an anterior dislocation of the vertebral body. Ligamentous injuries occur posteriorly between the injured vertebra and the vertebra located above and anteriorly between the injured vertebra and the vertebra located below (arrows in Fig. 12.20).

Treatment. Unilateral compression-extension injury (grade I) is treated conservatively using a hard cervical collar. A bilateral fracture of the vertebral arch (grade II) is usually treated in the same fashion. However, it is highly recommended that an additional CT scan be performed after 8 weeks, at the end of the conservative treatment period. Surgical treatment is required if the CT reveals a dislocation of the vertebral body, and should be considered initially in those cases in which the fracture lines extend through the facet joints on both sides. The most severe compression-extension fractures are managed surgically.

Bechterew Disease

Bechterew disease (ankylosing spondylitis) is a chronic inflammatory disorder affecting predominantly the sacroiliac joints and the spinal column. Onset typically occurs between ages 16 and 35, and affects predominantly males. Bechterew disease shares many characteristics with other autoimmune spondyloarthropathies. Ankylosing spondylitis is associated with arthritis in

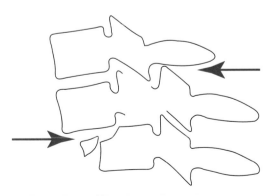

Figure 12.20 Compression extension injury grade V.

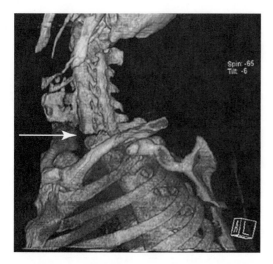

Figure 12.21 Bechterew disease. Computed tomography (CT) reconstruction images showing a horizontal fracture in the lower part of the cervical spine. The *arrow* points out the fracture line.

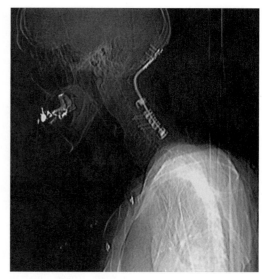

Figure 12.22 Lateral radiograph. Image illustrates a posterior fusion, ranging from occiput to the upper part of the thoracic spine.

multiple joints; inflammatory bowel disease, such as Crohn disease and ulcerative colitis; psoriasis; and Reiter disease. Genetic factors are considered to be partly responsible, and most patients carry the HLA-B27 gene. Radiological examination of the spine and sacroiliac joints reveals characteristic signs also in early stages of the disease. The inflammatory process affects the spinal column and anterior longitudinal ligament, causing chronic pain, stiffness, and gradual ossification of these structures. As this ossification creates bridges between adjacent vertebral bodies, pain eventually ceases when bony fusions are fully established between vertebral bodies. This ossification (fusion) is denoted *ankylosis*. Movement between vertebral bodies also ceases as fusion is established and thus pain disappears. The ankylosis affects the entire cervical column, resulting in complete rigidity and a "bamboo spine" appearance on radiological examinations. The biomechanical properties of the spine will become altered, and the head is now attached to a uniform, stiff lever. The ankylotic area is particularly vulnerable to trauma, and the cervical column may quite easily be fractured (Fig. 12.21).

Treatment

Treatment of cervical spine fractures both in the absence and presence of SCI in patients with Bechterew disease, requires specific considerations for surgical management. Because the "bamboo" configuration of the cervical column creates larger forces than normal on every motion segment, standard treatment with anterior fusion and internal fixation will not be sufficient to withstand these forces. The method of choice is usually to continue the anterior internal fixation and fusion with a posterior internal fixation ranging from occiput to T1 or T2 (Fig. 12.22). The patient is free to mobilize, and a hard cervical collar is also used during the first postoperative period. Halo-vest treatment for 3 months is an alternative to posterior surgical intervention. Halo-vest treatment is used if the patient's general condition does not admit two surgical interventions, if spinal deformity prevents the patient from being placed in a prone position, and/or finally, if a correction of the deformity during the posterior approach increases the risk of SCI.

Surgical Management of Injuries to the Cervical Spine

FUSION AND INTERNAL FIXATION TECHNIQUES

The goals of surgical management following traumatic injuries to the cervical spine are to decompress the spinal cord, restore cervical column deformities, and achieve acute and long-term stability of the motion segment. The use of instrumentation offers immediate stability to the injured spine, and is further maintained until bony fusion is established or the healing process of the ligamentous structures is completed. The vertebral bodies of the cervical spine resembles ring-shaped objects that must be reattached to form an aligned column again following damage. Spinal fixation devices may be placed at one, two, or three locations on each vertebra in the damaged motion segment (i.e., one-, two-, or three point fixation; Fig. 13.1).

The anterior and posterior approaches to explore the cervical spine will also be illustrated in connection with presentation of the spinal stabilization techniques.

UPPER CERVICAL SPINE

Posterior Approach to the Cervical Spine

The posteriorly located craniocervical junction and cervical spine is reached with the patient placed in a prone position, with the head fixed to a Mayfield head rest (Fig. 13.2). The vertebral bodies are identified using the C-arch process. The procedure starts with a midline skin incision from the protuberantia occipitalis externa to the spinous process of C7. The fascia, nuchal ligament, and posterior neck muscles are separated in the midline with electrocautery, after which the spinous processes are palpable (Fig. 13.3).

The paraspinal muscle groups are then loosened from the vertebral arches and retracted as laterally as possible without involving or damaging the vertebral arteries (see Chapter 12; Fig. 12.3). The paraspinal muscles are held laterally using self-retaining retractors and an adequate exposure of the vertebral arches is achieved. Removal of the vertebral arch (laminectomy) is the first step of the decompression and/or instrumentation procedure. Presence of vertebral arch fractures and suspected damage to the dura motivates this procedure (Fig. 13.4; also see same figure in Color Plate section). The dura is visualized after removal of the vertebral arches, and this step precedes fusion and instrumentation. Bone chips are usually harvested from the posterior iliac crest but the bone collected from the laminectomy may, in some cases, yield sufficient bone material to perform the fusion. Tricortical bone (three of four sides of the transplant consist of cortical bone; Fig. 13.5A) is most frequently collected from the posterior iliac crest. The transplant is usually 3–4 cm in length. Before starting the internal instrumentation procedure, this transplant is shaped to fit the space between the vertebral arches of the injured motion segment, usually C1 and C2.

Internal Instrumentation Techniques

In 1939, Gallie introduced a posterior technique using wire and bone harvested from the posterior iliac crest (Fig. 13.5B). However, a high incidence of nonfusion was reported using this technique. Several other one-point fixations have therefore been developed in order to improve the fusion rate. These techniques include the use of double wires and pieces of bone (Brooks-Jenkins) and sublaminar hook fixation

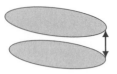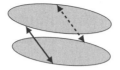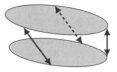

Figure 13.1 One-, two-, and three-point fixation. (Courtesy of T. Henriques, M.D.)

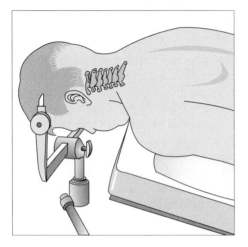

Figure 13.2 Prone position during the posterior approach.

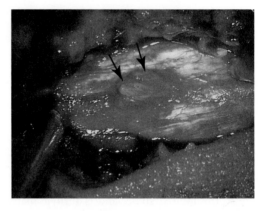

Figure 13.4 Dural tear in the lumbar region showing extradurally located nerve roots (*black arrows*). See also Color Plate Fig. 13.4.

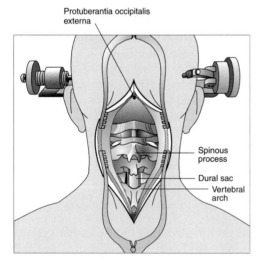

Protuberantia occipitalis externa

Spinous process

Dural sac

Vertebral arch

Figure 13.3 Exposure of the spinous processes, vertebral arch, and dura.

(Hallifax). In 1979, Magerl introduced the transarticular screw fixation technique. This procedure, in combination with the posterior wire technique between the levels of C1 and C2,

fulfilled the three-point fixation criteria. The combination of transarticular screw fixation and wire techniques is probably the most frequently used posterior internal fixation technique.

Screw fixation of the processus odontoideum is the only anterior internal fixation technique. All other internal fixation techniques are performed following a posterior approach. We have chosen to present various techniques but not correlate them to injury types, since treatment is not uniform among different trauma centers.

Posterior Stabilization

Wire Techniques

In 1939, Gallie introduced a new wiring and bony grafting procedure using one sublaminar wire and bone from the iliac crest for dorsal atlantoaxial fusion. However, this technique offered practically no rotational stability (Fig. 13.5B) and was later modified by Brooks and Jenkins. They used two sublaminar wires applied on each side of C1 and C2, underneath

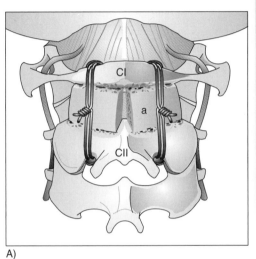

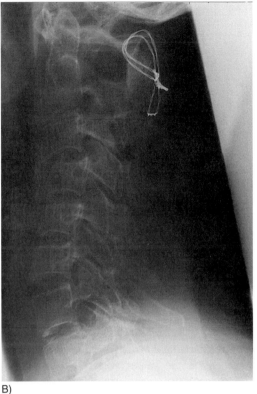

Figure 13.5 A: Wire technique according to Brooks and Jenkins. Tricortical bone is used as fusion material. B: Plain radiograph obtained sagittally showing the location of the wire following fixation according to Gallie.

the lamina, and two unicortical grafts from the iliac crest as fusion material. This technique provides solid rotational, flexional, and extensional stability (Fig. 13.5A).

Facet Screw Fixation

Transarticular screw fixation stabilizes the motion segment between C1 and C2. The screws are applied following a special drilling technique through C2 that results in a compression of the articular surfaces of the two vertebras and a relatively stable fixation (Fig. 13.6).

Combination Techniques

Some centers use a combination of C1–C2 facet screw fixation and interspinous wiring techniques together with bone grafts to provide later fusion (Fig. 13.7).

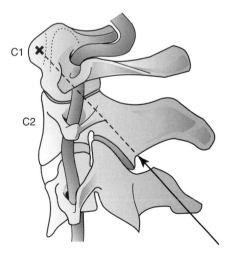

Figure 13.6 Transarticular screw placement.

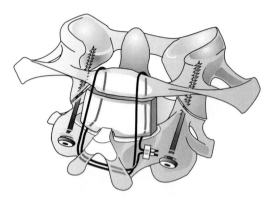

Figure 13.7 Combination of C1 and C2 wire and transarticular screw fixation techniques.

Intralaminar Clamps (Hooks)

The intralaminar clamp technique for fixation of the atlantoaxial motion segment is rarely used (Fig. 13.8). A graft is initially placed between the lamina to prevent extension and to offer rotational stability. Hooks are then fastened on the upper surface of atlas and the undersurface of the axis, posteriorly to the graft.

Occipitocervical Fixation

A variety of metal implants for occipitocervical fixation are available (Fig. 13.9). Devices such as plates and rods are most often used, while wiring techniques are rarely applied. Bony material is used to fuse the occiput to the cervical spine.

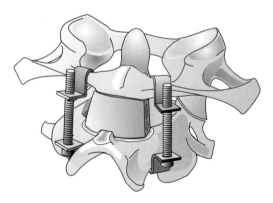

Figure 13.8 Intralaminar hooks according to Halifax.

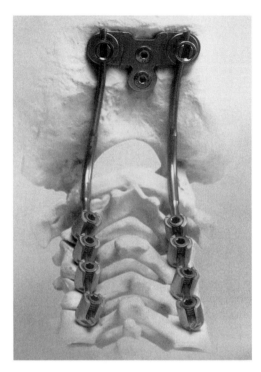

Figure 13.9 Occipitocervical fixation.

Anterior Stabilization

Odontoid Screw Fixation

Odontoid screw insertion is performed for the fixation of odontoid fractures. The compression technique, using one or two screws, to stabilize fractures of the odontoid process equals that of transarticular screw fixation (Fig. 13.10A,B). This technique is not suitable for oblique fractures, and posterior internal instrumentation is required in those cases. Access to odontoid screw fixation is achieved through an anterior approach, described later.

LOWER CERVICAL SPINE

Anterior Approach to the Cervical Spine

The anterior approach has several advantages as compared to the posterior exposure. The patient is operated on in a supine position, thus eliminating the risk of increased compression of the spinal cord during the turn to the prone position. The anterior approach is less

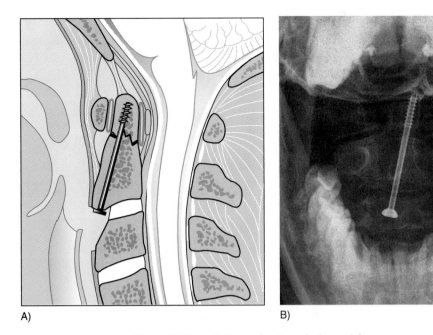

A)   B)

Figure 13.10 A,B: Screw fixation of odontoid fracture.

traumatic and provides better control over the disk space. The incidence of postoperative kyphosis and secondary neck pain is reduced. The anterior plate is considered a simpler device to handle, compared to posterior fixation instrumentation, and the fusion rate is higher with this technique.

The patient is placed in a supine position and the neck is stabilized in extension using either Gardner-Wells traction with 2–3 kg or a horseshoe-shaped support. The cervical spine adopts a natural lordosis as a result of this positioning. The position of the shoulders is corrected to maximize the C-arm view. The skin incision is either performed transversally through a skin crease at the level of approximately C5 or parallel and anteriorly to the sternocleidomastoid muscle (Fig. 13.11A–H; also see same figure in the Color Plate section). The platysma muscle is divided, and the fascia of the sternocleidomastoid muscle is opened. The carotid artery is now identified, and blunt dissection passes medial to the carotid sheath, the jugular vein, and the vagus nerve and lateral to esophagus and trachea. The longus colli muscle, covered by the prevertebral

fascia, is identified. The fascia and the anterior longitudinal ligament are divided. The longus colli muscles are elevated laterally using self-retaining retractors, after which the anterior aspects of the vertebral bodies and intervertebral disks are accessible to decompression, fusion, and internal fixation.

Internal Instrumentation Techniques

Traditionally, internal fixation of the lower cervical spine was obtained by a posterior approach if the injury was localized to the posterior column using the two-column classification. The anterior approach and corresponding fixation were used if the injury was localized predominantly to the anterior column. However, numerous recent studies shows that anterior fixation is sufficient even if the posterior column is damaged, and presently most injuries to the lower cervical spine are fixed via an anterior approach. A combination of both anterior and posterior approaches is used if instability is severe, for instance, in cases with bilateral facet joint dislocation (see Fig. 13.11A–H; also see same figure in Color Plate Section).

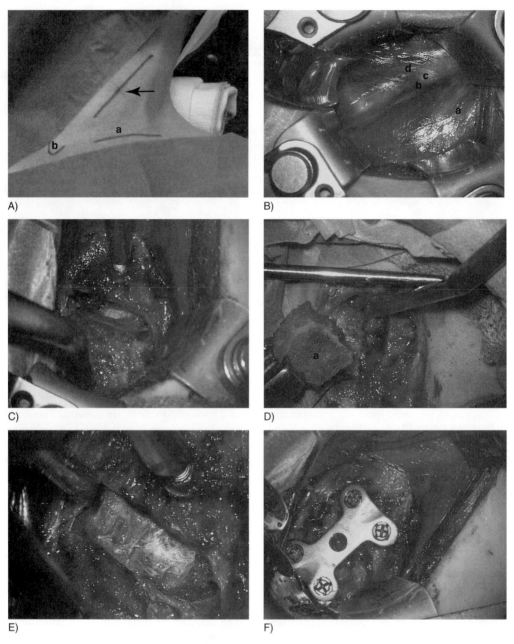

Figure 13.11 Guidelines for anterior and posterior decompression, fixation and fusion (A–H) of bilateral facet dislocation. A: The arrow indicates direction of skin incision along the left medial border of the sternocleidomastoid muscle. *a*, collar bone; *b*, incisura jugularis sternalis (the V-shaped notch at the top of sternum). B: *a*, sternocleidomastoid muscle; *b*, carotic sheath; *c*, disk; *d*, medial attachment of the longus colli muscle. C: The dural sac is exposed following removal of the disk (decompression of the dural sac). D: Tricortical bone (a) is harvested from the left iliac crest. E: The adjusted graft replaces the removed disk. F: Anterior cervical plate fixation. G: Intraoperative photo showing a posterior exposure of the dural sac. The screws and rods are in place. H: Postoperative plain radiography illustrating the location of the anterior cervical plate and posterior instrumentation. See also Color Plates Fig. 13.11A–H.

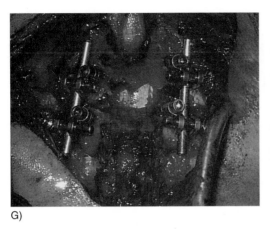
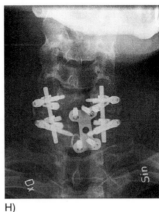

G)   H)

Figure 13.11 (continued)

Anterior Instrumentation

Bone Grafting and Ventral Plate Fixation

Bone grafting (fusion) with ventral plate fixation is the most frequent technique to stabilize the lower cervical spine. The first step in this procedure is to visualize the damaged area using an anterior approach, after which the intervertebral disk(s) and fractured vertebrae are removed (Fig. 13.12; also see same figure in the Color Plate Section).

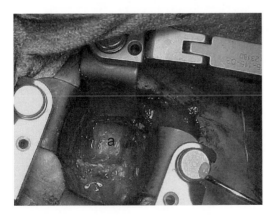

Figure 13.12 Single-level cervical corpectomy. Image shows the decompressed dural sac (*a*). The compression caused by the fractured bone is now removed. See also Color Plate Fig. 13.12.

Fusion using tricortical bone grafts harvested from the iliac crest and fixation with a ventral plate completes the procedure. Modern titanium plates do not significantly interfere with imaging procedures and the most important postoperative questions are obtained by MRI. The most frequently used screws are unicortical and 14 or 16 mm long. The screws pierce only the anterior cortical bone and do not reach beyond the posterior cortical bone, which minimizes the risk of penetrating into the spinal canal and spinal cord. Locking washers or nuts are applied to prevent back-out of the screws.

Posterior Instrumentation

The Gallie wire technique is still used in some trauma centers to fix fractures of the lower cervical spine. However, newer techniques avoid the use of one-point fixation techniques. Figure 13.13 illustrates one-, two-, and three-point fixation techniques, showing an anterior fusion using bone grafting and ventral plate (one-point fixation) and the same technique together with a wire procedure (two-point fixation). The wire technique has been replaced by pedicle screws (Fig.13.13C), resulting in a three-point fixation. The motion segment will thus be prevented to move in any direction.

The posterior instrumentation applied to the lower cervical spine resembles those used in

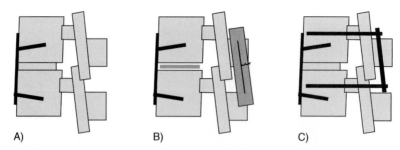

Figure 13.13 One-, two- and three-point fixation corresponding to figure A, B, and C, respectively. (Courtesy of T. Henriques, M.D.)

the upper cervical spine. A few examples are presented here.

Wire Techniques

Various wire techniques are available to stabilize the lower cervical spinal following injury. However, the use of wire techniques resulting in one- and two-point fixation is considered insufficient to stabilize the lower cervical spine. A Halo-vest or other rigid orthotic device is recommended as additional treatment if wire techniques are used. The use of wire techniques have been largely replaced by other methods.

Intralaminar Clamps (Hooks)

The use of intralaminar hooks is similar in both the upper and lower cervical spine.

Screw Selection

Different types of screws can be used together with lateral mass plates (see next section) or rods as alternative to those treatments mentioned earlier. Screws may be fastened either into the lateral masses or into the pedicles. The latter provides three-point stabilization according to Denis and total stability of the motion segment (Fig. 13.14).

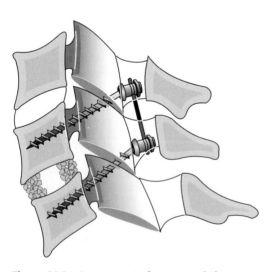

Figure 13.14 Lower cervical spine pedicle screw fixation.

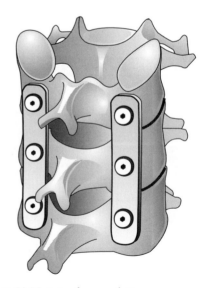

Figure 13.15 Lateral mass plating.

Plating of the Lateral Masses

Various straight plates can be bent and adjusted to fit the configuration of the cervical spine. The posterior plating techniques do not need intact lamina and can therefore be used in patients with multiple fractures to the posterior columns, in addition to injuries of the facet joints and vertebral body fractures (Fig. 13.15). The length of the plates depends on the severity of the injury.

Rod Fixation

Various types of rods have lately been introduced. These rods are adjustable to the configuration of the cervical column. The fixation system comprises either bone screws or hooks that are implanted into the cervical vertebrae of the spine. A rod can be applied across the cervical column to counteract rotational movement in the motion segment (see Fig. 13.11G,H; also see same figure in Color Plate section).

14 | Thoracolumbar Fractures and Ligament Injuries

Stability of the thoracic and lumbar spine is, as in the lower cervical spine, maintained by the intervertebral disks, vertebrae (vertebral bodies and arches), and ligamentous structures. Stability in the thoracolumbar region is much more pronounced, due to the stronger posteriorly located ligamentous structures and larger facet joints. The articulating surfaces of the facet joints have an increased concavity and convexity, resulting in increased contact between these components (Fig. 14.1). The ribs, sternum, ligaments, and large vertebrae also contribute to the greater stability of this part of the spinal column. This results in a different injury profile in the thoracolumbar region as compared to the cervical spine. As a rule, fractures rather than dislocations are seen.

Most of the body weight is carried by the intervertebral disks and vertebral bodies. The ability of the vertebral bodies to bear weight decreases with age as a result of diminished water content in the disks and osteoporosis in the vertebrae. This results in an increased vulnerability to trauma, and fractures as a result of low-energy trauma are seen quite commonly among patients with osteoporosis. The most important task of the intervertebral disks is to absorb and distribute loads as equally as possible between adjacent vertebral bodies. The facet joints have no weight-bearing capacity except in the middle and lower lumbar spine; because of the physiological lumbar lordosis, the center of load is located more posteriorly in that region, giving the facet joints there some weight-bearing ability. The construction and dimension of the lumbar facet joints contribute to their stability. The joints function as bony barriers is to prevent translational and rotational displacement (see Chapter 10).

The anterior longitudinal ligament is one of the strongest ligaments in the body, playing an important role in providing stability to the thoracic spine by preventing hyperextension movements in the motion segments (Fig. 14.1). The posterior ligamentous complex consists of several structures. The posterior longitudinal ligament is much thinner compared to the anterior one, and it thus lacks biomechanical properties of importance. The inter- and supraspinous ligaments and the articular capsule enveloping the facet joint also contribute to stability by minimizing flexion in the motion segment. The combination of flexion bending moments and compression forces is the most common traumatic load to the thoracic spine. For example, in the abrupt transfer of motion that occurs in a motor vehicle accident, the upper part of the body and the head continue to move forward while the lower part of the body comes to a halt. This results in hyperflexion of the thoracic and lumbar spine, with the load concentrated on the anterior part of the vertebral body. A collapse of the vertebral body may occur if the load is severe enough, with the spongiotic bone either compressed or crushed. The posterior ligamentous complex may also be damaged as a result of distraction forces toward these posterior structures. Fractures occur most frequently at the junction of the rigid thoracic spine and the more mobile lumbar spine. Sixty percent of fractures in the thoracolumbar region are located between the levels of T12 and L2. The L1 vertebra is the most affected vertebral body (30%).

THE CONCEPT OF INSTABILITY

The incidence of posttraumatic neurological deterioration, kyphotic deformity, and pain increases in unstable fractures, so classification of these injuries should reflect their relative

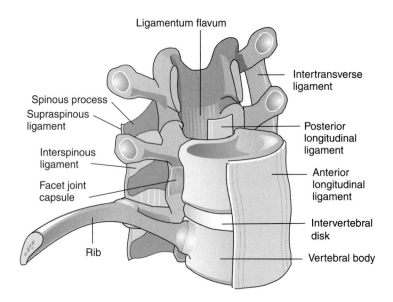

Figure 14.1 Important supporting structures of the thoracic spine.

stability and also help to determine prognosis, especially since the risk of future complications could be decisive in the choice of treatment. Here, we present two frequently used classifications, after which some general principles regarding available treatment options will be discussed.

FRACTURE CLASSIFICATIONS

Various classifications have been presented in the literature. In 1949, Nicoll classified fractures based on morphological changes visualized by radiological examinations. The injury mechanisms were added to the morphological characteristics by Holdsworth in the 1960s, while the classification introduced by Denis in the mid-1980s was based only on morphology observed by computed tomography (CT). These classifications conceptualized the vertebrae into two- (Holdsworth) or three-column models (Denis; Figs. 12.4, 12.5, and 14.2) in order to indicate structures of importance to the stability of the spinal column. Classifications based on the three-column model according to Denis and the two-column model according to Magerl and coworkers (1994) are the most frequently used in clinical practice. These models enable clinicians

to evaluate whether a fracture is stable or unstable and to direct treatment according to this conclusion.

The Three-column Concept of Fracture Classification

In Denis' three-column model, the anterior and middle columns correspond to the anterior

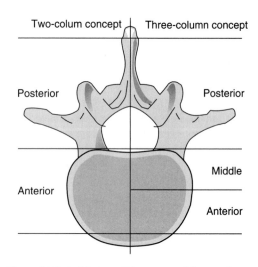

Figure 14.2 Axial view of the two- and three-column spine concept.

TABLE 14.1 Denis three-column classification.

Type of Fracture	Column Failure
1 Compression fracture	Anterior column compression
2 Burst fractures types A–E	Anterior and middle column failure
A – Fracture of both endplates	
B – Fracture of the upper endplate	
C – Fracture of the lower endplate	
D – Burst fracture with rotation	
E – Lateral burst fracture	
3 Seat-belt type of injuries	Middle and posterior column involvement
A – One-level damage	Injury through bone or ligamentous structures
B – Two-level damage	Injury through bone or ligamentous structures engaging two adjacent levels
4 Fracture-dislocation injuries	Posterior, middle and anterior (anterior longitudinal
A – Flexion rotation type	ligament or anterior part of the intervertebral disk)
B – Shear type	column failure
C – Flexion-distraction type	

column in the two-column model, whereas the posterior columns in both models are identical (Fig. 14.2 and Table 14.1).

Compression Fractures

Compression fractures result from a combination of a flexion bending moment and a compressive force. The anterior column is fractured, while the middle column remains uninjured. A wedge is seen in the anterior column, while the posterior part of the vertebral body (i.e., the middle column) is undamaged (Fig. 14.3). Compression fractures neither compromise the size or diameter of the spinal canal (see also Fig. 15.6C).

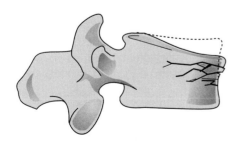

Figure 14.3 Compression fracture.

Burst Fractures

Burst fractures are also seen following a combination of flexion bending moment and compression force, but in these injuries both the anterior as well as the middle columns are fractured (Fig. 14.4). A wedge is also seen following burst fractures since the compression is most severe in the anterior part of the vertebral body. The risk of acquiring neurological symptoms increases in case of damage to the posterior cortical surface of the vertebral body, and bony fragments are often dislocated into the spinal canal (Fig. 14.5). The distance between the pedicles is increased as a result of a lateral dislocation of the pedicle attachment (Fig. 14.6). This is a characteristic sign of burst fractures and occurs following severe compression of the vertebral body.

Burst fractures are subdivided into five types according to Denis (Table 14.1). Types A and B are the most common, engaging both end plates in type A and the upper end plate and vertebral body in type B.

Seat-belt Type Injuries

The term "seat-belt injury" was introduced at a time when cars were equipped with only

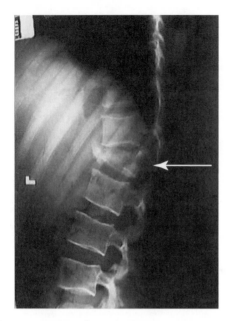

Figure 14.4 Burst fracture (*arrow*).

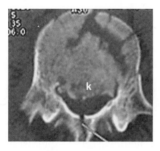

Figure 14.5 Axial view of a burst fracture. Observe the narrowing of the spinal canal caused by the retropulsed bony fragment (*k*).

two-point attachment seat belts. These seat belts lacked a shoulder component, and the load following an accident was absorbed entirely by the horizontally orientated belt. The initial flexion bending moment resulted in a compressive force followed by a distractive force. The load resulted in an impact on the middle and posterior columns. A single-level seat belt type of injury affects the posterior ligament complex, the posterior longitudinal ligament, and intervertebral disk (Fig. 14.7) or bony structures. The most well-known type of this injury, the Chance fracture (Fig. 14.8), extends through the spinous process, pedicles, and vertebral body.

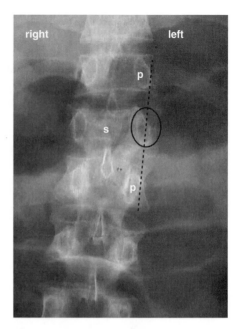

Figure 14.6 Plain radiograph. Frontal view illustrating the increased distance between the pedicles (*p*, pedicle). The *broken line* on the left side marks the outer border of the uninjured pedicles located above and below the injured vertebra. The outer border of the pedicle (*circle*) belonging to the injured vertebrae(s) is located a few millimeters laterally to the broken line, indicating the presence of a burst fracture and a pedicle displacement.

The undamaged anterior longitudinal ligament prevents displacement of vertebrae in the injured motion segment.

An increased distance between the spinous processes of the injured motion segment characterizes both ligamentous and bony single-level injuries. This fracture is quite common among children and is often associated with abdominal injuries.

Fracture–Dislocation Injuries

The fracture-dislocation injury is considered the most dangerous of all thoracolumbar fractures and occurs as a result of high-energy trauma directed toward all three columns (Table 14.1 and Fig. 14.9). Fracture-dislocation injuries are associated with a high percentage of neurological deterioration. They are fortunately uncommon and appear following high-energy loads

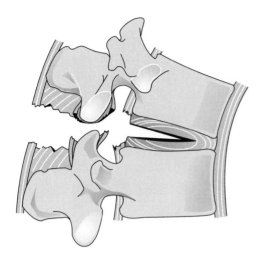

Figure 14.7 One-level type of seat-belt injury with ligamentous failure.

resulting in rotational and translational displacements. All three columns fail as a result of distraction, compression, flexion, rotation, and/or shear loads. Displacement results in a narrowing of the spinal canal and subsequent neurological deterioration.

Stability Assessment Guidelines

It is difficult to translate Denis' fracture classification into corresponding stable and unstable fractures; however, most clinicians agree on the following guidelines regarding stable/unstable fracture classification on the basis of the three-column model.

Compression and Burst Fractures. Compression fractures in general are considered stable. Instability occurs in compression and burst fractures if (a) two or three columns are damaged (fractures are considered unstable if the middle column fails, since damage to this column is always associated with damage to the anterior and/or posterior column as well); (b) the patient has significant loss of neurological function immediately following trauma or exhibits progressive neurological deterioration in close relation to the injury; (c) less than 50% remains of the original vertebral body height; (d) a kyphosis of 25 degrees or more develops after a fracture to a single vertebra or a total kyphosis of more than 30–40 degrees occurs following multiple

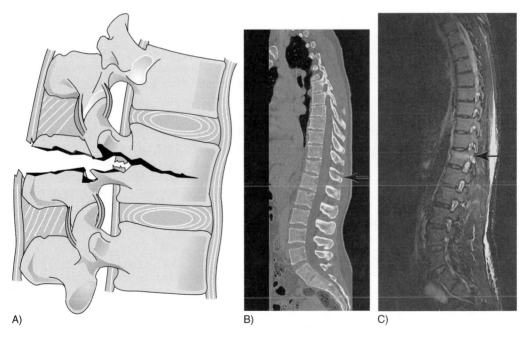

A) B) C)

Figure 14.8 Chance fracture. A: Observe the vertical fracture through the spinous process (*arrow*) demonstrated in a spiral computed tomography (CT) with (B) sagittal reconstruction and (C) the corresponding fracture illustrated using magnetic resonance imaging (MRI).

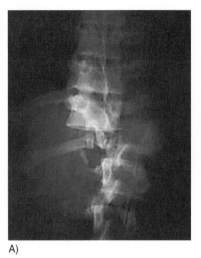
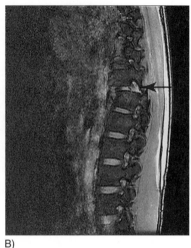

A)   B)

Figure 14.9 Fracture-dislocation type of injury. The plain radiograph shows (A) a lateral and (B) anteroposterior displacement as illustrated by this magnetic resonance image (MRI) obtained sagittal view (*arrow*).

fractures; or (e) the degree of spinal canal compromise is equal to or exceeds 50%.

The presence of three or more individually stable compression or burst fractures in a row is, according to some authors, considered an unstable situation.

Seat-belt and Fracture-Dislocation Injuries. In these types of injuries, failure occurs to at least two columns; thus, these two fracture types are always regarded as unstable.

Guidelines to Determine Stability

Guidelines to determine stability on the basis of Denis' classification are suggested in Table 14.2. These guidelines are based on the assumption that instability occurs if at least two of the three columns are damaged. The table shows which columns are considered stable or unstable following different types of injuries. The table also illustrates which type of further load may increase the risk of additional injury to an already unstable/damaged column.

Compression fractures are typically regarded as stable. The spinal column should, following a compression injury, be protected against flexion bending moment that further increases compressive force. Burst fractures may be either stable or unstable under compressive forces, resulting in the same restriction toward flexion bending moments. Seat-belt and fracture-dislocation injuries are always unstable under distractive forces and all types of loads.

TABLE 14.2 Stability/instability guideline.

Fracture	Column Failure		
	Anterior	*Middle*	*Posterior*
Compression	Compression	*Stable*	*Stable*
Burst	Compression	(Compression)	*Stable*
Seat-belt	Stable	Distraction	Distraction
Fracture-dislocation	Compression		Dislocation
	Rotation		Rotation
	Shear		Shear

Magerl's Two-column Concept of Fracture Classification

The goal of finding a fracture classification that is easy to apply on the basis of radiological and clinical findings has led to several new classification proposals. Nicoll's classification emphasizes the importance of posterior ligamentous structures. The focus on posterior ligamentous structures is lacking in the classification according to Denis, which is based on skeletal CT findings and is, in some respects, regarded as incomplete. In their classification scheme, Magerl and coworkers have once again pointed out the importance of posterior structure integrity as assessed by magnetic resonance imaging (MRI). This classification is based on morphological findings, as well as on the mechanical impact at the time of the accident, with the aim of initially categorizing injuries according to type of trauma, then grouping and subgrouping the injuries with regard to pathomorphological findings discovered by radiological investigation. Magerl's classification is based on the A0 (Arbeitsgemeinschaft für Osteosyntesfragen) fracture concept, and thoracolumbar fractures are thus classified according to a 3-3-3 system. The first number corresponds to injury types A–C, based on the injury mechanisms compression, distraction, and rotation, respectively. The injury severity increases from A to C. Each type of injury is divided into three groups and these groups are further subdivided in a similar manner. A3 is, according to this classification, a more severe injury compared to A1 in the A group and the subgroup A1.1 is a milder form of injury compared to A1.3 in the A1 group (see Tables 14.2 through 14.5). The transition between stable and unstable fractures is not always easy to define, and this type of progressive classification may provide additional information pertaining to treatment decisions. The classifications according to Denis and Magerl are currently used especially when fractures are associated with SCI. We have therefore also chosen to briefly present this classification. Magerl and coworkers' categorization is based on the two-column model, in which the anterior column fails in type A injuries, and both columns are damaged in type B and C injuries.

TABLE 14.3 Type A. Compression fractures of the vertebral body.

A1 Impaction fractures

    A1.1 End-plate impaction

    A1.2 Vertebral body impaction resulting in a wedge formation.

    A1.3 Vertebral body collapse.

A2 Split fractures

    A2.1 Sagittally oriented

    A2.2 Coronally oriented

    A2.3 Pincer fracture

A3 Burst fractures

    A3.1 Incomplete burst fracture

    A3.2 Burst-split fracture

    A3.3 Complete burst fracture

TABLE 14.4 Type B injuries: anterior and posterior element injury with distraction.

B1 Posterior disruption predominantly ligamentous (flexion-distraction injury)

    B1.1 With transverse disruption of the intervertebral disk

    B1.2 With type A fracture of the vertebral body

B2 Posterior disruption predominantly osseous (flexion-distraction injury)

    B2.1 Involving both columns (Chance fracture)

    B2.2 With disruption of the intervertebral disk

    B2.3 With type A fracture of the vertebral body

B3 Anterior disruption of the intervertebral disk

    B3.1 Hyperextension-subluxation

    B3.2 Hyperextension-spondylolysis

    B3.3 Posterior dislocation

Type A, Compression Fractures

Type A injuries comprise fractures on the vertebral body caused by compressive forces. These are seen as a result of flexion bending moments or axial forces. The compression fractures are divided into groups A1–A3 and further into three subgroups.

A1 or Impaction Fractures. A1.1 denotes a compression of the vertebral body (Fig. 14.3). A1.1 fractures

TABLE 14.5 Type C injuries: anterior and posterior element injury with rotation.

C1 Type A injuries with rotation (compression injuries with rotation)

    C1.1 Rotational wedge fracture

    C1.2 Rotational split fracture

C2 Type B injuries with rotation

    C2.1 B1 injuries with rotation (flexion-distraction injuries with rotation)

    C2.2 B2 injuries with rotation (flexion-distraction injuries with rotation)

    C2.3 injuries with rotation (hyperextension-shear injuries with rotation)

C3 Rotational shear injuries

    C3.1 Slice fracture

    C3.2 Oblique fracture

---

are not associated with spinal canal compromise caused by retropulsed fracture fragments.

A1.2 corresponds with Denis' compression group. The transition between A1.1 to A1.2 (Fig. 14.10) occurs if the reduced vertebral body height (wedge shape) results in an angle to the spinal column of more than 5 degrees (Cobb angle >5 degrees; Fig. 14.11).

A1.3 occurs most often among patients with osteoporosis. The fracture is called "fish vertebra" if the compression is seen predominantly in the central part (Fig. 14.12).

A2 or Split Fractures. A2 fractures denote cases in which compression results in a splitting of the entire vertebral body. This splitting may occur in three different fashions (A2.1–A2.3). The so-called *pincer fractures* are characterized by a centrally located splitting, and the defect is filled with intervertebral disk material (Fig. 14.13). Both the end plates and the anterior wall are damaged, but the posterior wall is intact. This type of fracture is typically located in the lumbar region but is usually not associated with the development of kyphosis.

A3 or Burst Fractures. A3 or burst fractures (fragmentation of bone) correspond to burst fractures in Denis' classification and constitute the most severe type of compression fractures. The spinal canal is, as a rule, narrowed by retropulsed fragments. The A3 fractures range in

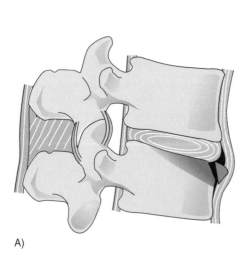
A)

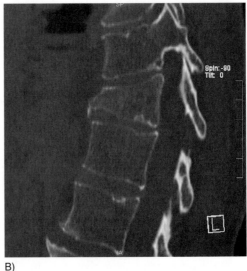
B)

Figure 14.10 A,B: Vertebral body impaction with a clear wedge formation. The degree of impaction is calculated by comparing the vertebral body height of the damaged vertebra to the corresponding height of the adjacent vertebral bodies.

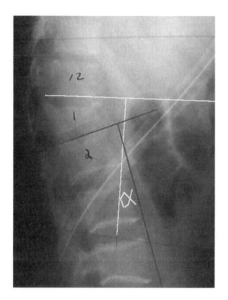

Figure 14.11 Cobb angle = a.

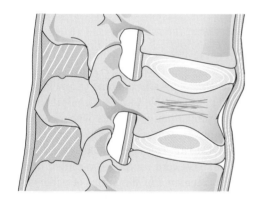

Figure 14.12 Fish vertebra.

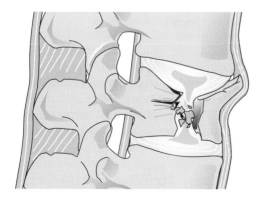

Figure 14.13 Pincer fracture.

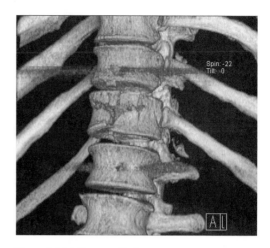

Figure 14.14 Burst-split fracture.

severity from partial (failure of either the upper or lower end plate via burst-split involving fragmentation of one end plate while the rest of the vertebra is split sagittally [Fig. 14.14]) to complete burst fractures, in which the entire vertebral body has been fragmented. An increased distance between the pedicles and fractures of the vertebral lamina is, identically with Denis' burst fractures, seen in the A3 group.

Type B, Anterior and Posterior Element Injuries with Distraction

The B-type fracture, with the exception of B3, is characterized by a transverse disruption of the posterior column. The following division into subgroups is based on the extent and appearance of the anterior column failure.

B1 and B2, Posterior Disruption Predominantly Ligamentous and Osseous, Respectively. Both the anterior and posterior columns are injured in the B1 and B2 groups as a result of a flexion-distraction load. Denis seat-belt injuries affecting the ligamentous (Fig. 14.7; B1.1 injury) or the bony structures (Chance fracture; Fig. 14.8A, B2.1 injury) are included in these groups. Distraction is the dominating force affecting the posterior structures. The combination of the posteriorly locating distraction force and compressive forces acting anteriorly typically results in a type-A vertebral fracture in addition to the type-B injury.

B3, Anterior Disruption Through the Intervertebral Disk. The B3 injury predominantly occurs among patients with Bechterew disease.

Type C, Anterior and Posterior Element Injuries with Rotation. Type C injuries arise following axial rotation forces that are added to forces such as those acting in the type A or B injuries. Type C represents the most severe injuries. Here, both columns fail. Type C injuries are associated with a high incidence of neurological deterioration. The severity of this injury results in displacement in several planes, such as translational and rotational. The C-type injury corresponds to the fracture-dislocation injuries of Denis' classification (Fig. 14.9).

Frequency and Level of Injury

Table 14.6 describes the frequency and distribution of thoracolumbar fractures, according to Magerl and coworkers, among 1,455 patients. The type A fractures comprise two-thirds of all fractures, whereas type B and C fractures, in their many groups and subgroups, comprise only one-third of all injuries. The presence of neurological sequelae, ranging from symptoms

TABLE 14.6 Incidence and level of thoracolumbar fractures according to Magerl and co-workers. n = 1455.

Type and Groups	Incidence (%) of Total Number of Patients	Percent (%) of Fracture Type
A	66.16	
A1		53.51
A2		5.23
A3		42.25
B	14.46	
B1		60.29
B2		38.28
B3		1.44
C	19.38	
C1		55.71
C2		38.57
C3		5.71

TABLE 14.7 Incidence of neurological deterioration in the material of Magerl and co-workers.

Type and Groups	Number	Neurological Deterioration (%)
A	890	14
A1	501	2
A2	45	4
A3	344	32
B	145	32
B1	61	30
B2	82	33
B3	2	50
C	177	55
C1	99	53
C2	62	60
C3	16	50

originating from one nerve root to a complete SCI, were reported in 1,212 patients in this study. Neurological symptoms of any kind were found in 22% (Table 14.7). A significant increase in the proportion of patients with neurological deterioration was seen in the transition from group A2 to A3. This is explained by the increased risk of spinal cord compression caused by retropulsed fragments in the group of patients with burst fractures. The proportion of patients with neurological impairment in group A3 is equal to the number in groups B2 and B3.

Stability Assessment Guidelines

Instability, as illustrated by morphological changes at radiological examination, is only of value after being related to the original type of trauma or load. Three types of load are recognized in the A0 classification: compression, distraction, and rotation. Every degree of reduced resistance toward these loads may be defined as instability. Fractures gradually increase in severity from type A to C, as is also the case within groups and subgroups 1 to 3. An impaction fracture of one end plate (A1.1) is thus considered stable, whereas rotational-shear injuries

TABLE 14.8 Scale of instability from the AO-perspective.

Type	Stable	Unstable
A	A1/A2	A2/A3
B	(B1/B2)	B1/B2
		B3
C		All

with severe displacement in several planes is regarded as unstable (C3.3).

Stable type-A fractures (A1/A2) transform gradually into unstable fractures (A2/A3) (Table 14.8). Increased vertebral body compression is seen at radiological examination, and resistance against compressive forces is likewise gradually decreased. The fracture becomes gradually unstable against additional compressive forces. The B1 and B2 fractures are considered unstable under additional flexion bending moment and, naturally, under compression in the presence of a significant vertebral body injury. C-type fractures are always considered unstable under all types of load.

Treatment. Both Denis' and Magerl's classifications are used in the choice of management following thoracolumbar fractures. The choice of treatment, irrespective of the presence of SCI, is still under debate, although the number of patients receiving surgical management gradually increases, a result of rapid developments in the field of instrumentation and the wish to reduce the length of hospital stay.

Unproblematic compression fractures involving only the anterior column are treated conservatively, whereas burst fractures with an increased distance between the pedicles and with posteriorly dislocated fragments resulting in a narrowing of the spinal canal are treated surgically, since these fractures are assessed as being stable and unstable, respectively. Deciding on surgical versus conservative management in both these fractures is usually easily made. The remaining fractures, however, are treated on the basis of a more complicated assessment as regards stability or instability.

Particular difficulties regarding choice of treatment arise when the patient exhibits a fracture classified as unstable, but the necessity of surgical management may still be questionable because conservative treatment constitutes an equally good alternative.

The type B injuries serve as an example. Conservative treatment is proposed principally if the bony structures are injured, whereas surgical management is suggested if the damage involves the intervertebral disk and ligamentous structures, since conservative treatment usually fails to heal soft-tissue injuries. The importance in these cases of clinical investigation must be emphasized. The clinician must not forget to palpate the spinal processes if a burst fracture (according to Denis) or an A3 group injury (according to Magerl) is discovered at the initial radiological investigation. Soreness, pain, or a suspected defect during palpation of the spinous processes indicates failure of the posterior ligament complex. MRI should then be performed to confirm or exclude such an injury. The mode of treatment may change if the MRI reveals an injury to the posterior ligamentous structures. A fracture that initially was considered for conservative treatment (some A3 fractures) may now, due to clinical and MRI findings, be reclassified as a B-type of injury, because both the anterior and posterior columns are engaged and the patient should receive surgical treatment. This approach is in accordance with the modern view of fracture classifications, which emphasizes the importance of posterior ligamentous structures.

The next sections briefly review some aspects of conservative treatment, followed by the most common surgical interventions for thoracolumbar fractures. Conservative alternatives are presented in more detail in the next chapter. We have deliberately chosen to describe treatment options in general terms, considering how difficult it is to evaluate the relative stability or instability of a fracture and in light of varying regional traditions of management for these types of injuries.

CONSERVATIVE TREATMENT

Conservative (nonsurgical) treatment encompasses three components: bedrest, pain management, and orthotic devices. Varying guidelines exist regarding the length of conservative treatment; most authors suggest bedrest between 4–12 weeks, but long periods of bedrest are usually regarded unnecessary. The trend in modern conservative management is to shorten the period of rest to a minimum and instead, by means of physiotherapy, to mobilize the patient as soon as possible. In most cases, the patient is equipped with an orthotic device to hold the spine in hyperextension as soon as the acute (and often extremely painful) period has passed. In addition to relieving pain, the orthotic serves to correct, stabilize, and support the spinal column until fracture healing is completed and the risk of developing local spine deformities is minimized. Patients are encouraged, during the treatment period, to be as active as their pain allows, but should avoid lifting heavy objects. The severity of pain is thus the deciding factor for the degree of activity and the length of the orthotic treatment period, and is usually estimated at 12 weeks. Plain radiographs are performed during and at the end of the treatment period (see also Chapter 15).

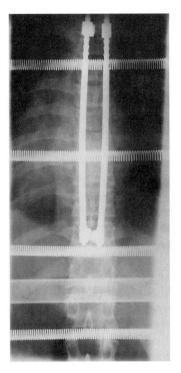

Figure 14.15 Harrington fixation device.

SURGICAL MANAGEMENT

The main goals of surgical management of fractures to the thoracolumbar region are to:

- Decompress nervous tissue to allow restitution of lost nervous function and counteract future neurological deterioration
- Correct anatomical misalignment and prevent future kyphosis development in the injured area
- Fuse unstable spine segments
- Offer rapid mobilization
- Reduce pain
- Minimize length of hospital stay

That the preservation of an acceptable anatomical alignment by rigid fixation prevents future kyphosis in the fracture area has been a strong argument for surgical intervention, since a posttraumatic kyphosis increases secondary pain problems and neurological impairment. The era of fixation began with the introduction of long Harrington rods and similar instruments; distraction or compression of the injured motion segment, achieved through lengthening or shortening the instrument, presented, at that time, the only possibility to correct a posttraumatic deformity (Fig. 14.15). Several motion segments above and below the level of injury were included in the fixation, resulting in an unnecessarily extended exposure in relation to the extent of injury. Since those early efforts, tremendous improvements to both operative technique and instrumentation have been made, and most of the problems and complications associated with the Harrington fixation devices have been overcome. For example, the technique of pedicle fixation, involving only one motion segment above and below the level of injury, has solved many of the previous problems and complications. Many potential solutions exist to problems related to surgical management; three important issues to consider when choosing a surgical approach are:

1. Should the exposure of the fractured area be accomplished through an anterior or posterior approach?
2. How, and to what extent, should decompression and repair of the dural sac be performed?

3. Which internal fixation devices should be used to achieve an immediate, rigid immobilization of the spinal column?

Various points of view regarding the answers to these questions will be presented in the upcoming sections, and some surgical principles related to injury classification will also be illustrated.

Anterior Approach

The anterior approach is preferred if the purpose of exploration is to access the anterior and lateral aspects of the spine. This is achieved either trans-peritoneally (i.e., straight in from the front), or using an anterolateral approach. The latter method is performed through a retroperitoneal approach to the lumbar and thoracic spine at the level of T11 or below, or through a transthoracic access above the level of T11 (Fig. 14.16). The anterior approach may appear attractive because it allows good exposure of the spine, and the technical conditions to perform the decompression and subsequent fusion and fixation are

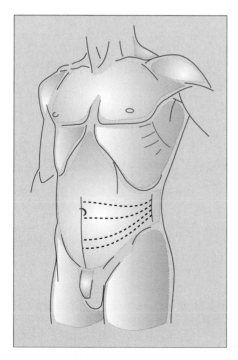

Figure 14.16 Skin incision alternatives used during the anterior approach.

excellent. However, this method requires more surgical skill, and the complication rate exceeds that of the posterior approach. The anterior approach can be especially troublesome at the thoracolumbar junction. Symptoms associated with irritation of the sympathetic nervous system are difficult to avoid since this method includes manipulation of the diaphragm. An insufficient posterior decompression, involving a situation in which a significant and unacceptable compression of the spinal cord remains following the initial procedure, may constitute an absolute indication to perform this procedure. An anterior approach and subsequent fusion and fixation may also be indicated following severe intervertebral disk and vertebral body damage if posterior fusion is regarded as insufficient to prevent the future development of kyphosis.

Fusion and Instrumentation

Tricortical bone harvested from the anterior superior iliac crest replaces the damaged bone removed during the decompression procedure. The purpose of the transplant is to reconstruct the stabilizing and weight-bearing functions of the vertebral body. Artificial transplants filled with spongiotic bone have been used in a similar fashion (Fig. 14.17). The aim of the fusion is to create a long-lasting, stable homogenous bony block involving the replaced vertebra, as well as the vertebral body above and below the level of injury. The Kaneda device can serve as an example of an instrumentation used subsequent to an anterior approach. The very thin plate reaches from the level above to the level below the injury, and the thinness of the plate counteracts pressure on the vessels located adjacent to the vertebral body. The instrumentation provides a rigid fixation of the spinal column, allowing the patients unrestricted mobilization.

POSTERIOR APPROACH

Posterior approaches are the most frequently used techniques for exposing fractures in the thoracolumbar region. The patient is placed in a prone position and access to the posterior structures of the spinal column is routinely achieved

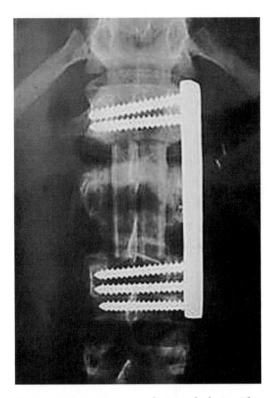

Figure 14.17 Fixation using the Kaneda device. The removed vertebral body is replaced by an artificial cage and the Kaneda device consisting of two threaded rods secured by staples. Vertebral screws are finally placed in the vertebral bodies above and below the injury level.

through a dorsal midline incision (for illustrations, see Chapter 13). The incision is extended a few levels above and below the level of injury, after which the fascia and muscles are elevated through subperiosteal dissection, exposing the spinous processes and lamina of the vertebrae. This exposure is usually sufficient to visualize the injured structures and to perform an adequate decompression of the dura and foramina by removing material compressing the spinal cord and nerve roots, respectively. The dura must be repaired (Fig. 13.4; also see same figure in Color Plate Section, dural tear) when a dural tear is discovered and neural elements are located extradurally.

Posterior fusion and internal fixation then follow decompression and repair of the dura. The disadvantage of midline exposure is the limited exposure of the anterior part of the

spinal canal (i.e., the posterior border of the vertebral body). The removal of bony and/or disk components extruding posteriorly from the vertebral body is hampered by this limited exposure. It is usually difficult to be sure that the anterior part of the spinal cord is decompressed using this technique. Access to the anterior part of the spinal canal and the protruding components may be solved by adding a transpedicular exposure to the initial posterior approach.

However, the midline exposure is used as a standard procedure. Relief of pressure on the dura, spinal cord, and nerve roots caused by bony fragments and disk material is performed via laminectomy, foraminotomy, and various techniques to remove retropulsed components from the anterior part of the spinal canal. Ligamentotaxis is the indirect repositioning of intraspinally located retropulsed bony fragments by the application of lordosis and a distraction force (i.e., an instrumentation technique is used to achieve the repositioning; Fig. 14.18). The

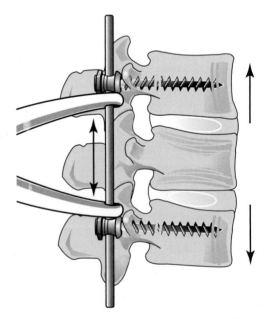

Figure 14.18 Ligamentotaxis by application of distraction forces. A distractor separates the vertebral bodies above and below the injured level. This enables the damaged vertebral body to regain its lost height. The compression of the vertebral body may thus be partially or completely remedied.

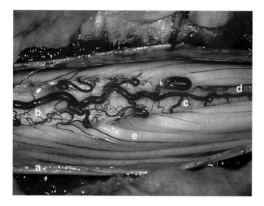

Figure 3.1 Spinal cord topography. Exposed spinal cord. *a*, dural sac; *b*, spinal cord; *c*, conus medullaris; *d*, filum terminale; *e*, dorsal nerve root.

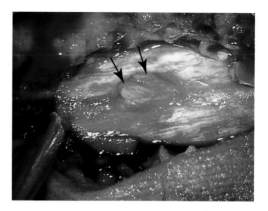

Figure 13.4 Dural tear in the lumbar region showing extradurally located nerve roots (*black arrows*).

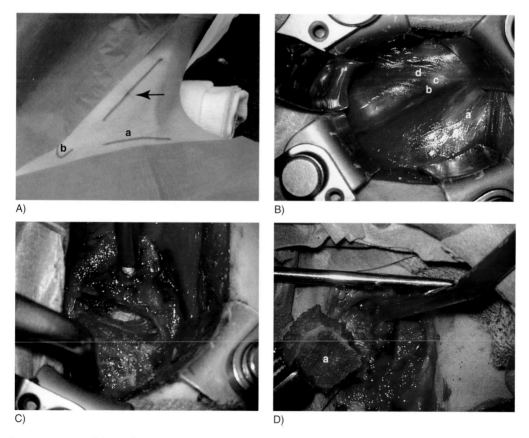

Figure 13.11 Guidelines for anterior and posterior decompression, fixation and fusion (A–H) of bilateral facet dislocation. A: The arrow indicates direction of skin incision along the left medial border of the sternocleidomastoid muscle. *a*, collar bone; *b*, incisura jugularis sternalis (the V-shaped notch at the top of sternum). B: *a*, sternocleidomastoid muscle; *b*, carotic sheath; *c*, disk; *d*, medial attachment of the longus colli muscle. C: The dural sac is exposed following removal of the disk (decompression of the dural sac). D: Tricortical bone (a) is harvested from the left iliac crest.

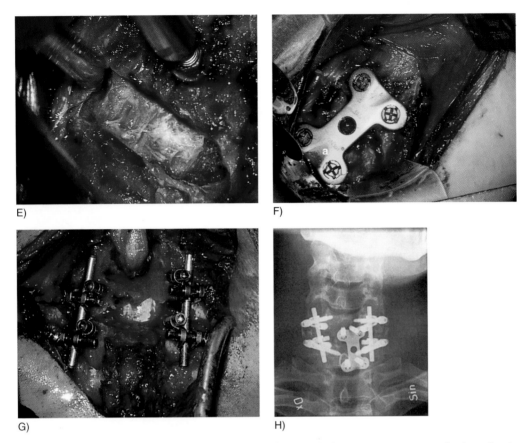

E) F)

G) H)

Figure 13.11 E: The adjusted graft replaces the removed disk. F: Anterior cervical plate fixation. G: Intraoperative photo showing a posterior exposure of the dural sac. The screws and rods are in place. H: Postoperative plain radiography illustrating the location of the anterior cervical plate and posterior instrumentation.

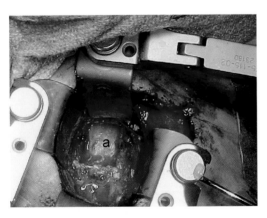

Figure 13.12 Single-level cervical corpectomy. Image shows the decompressed dural sac (*a*). The compression caused by the fractured bone is now removed.

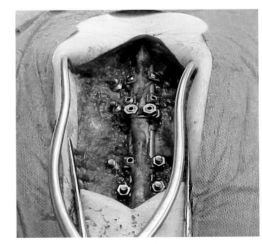

Figure 14.20 Instrumentation. Posterior instrumentation using pedicle screws and rods.

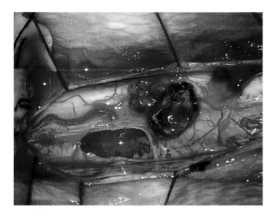

Figure 19.4 Intramedullary vascular malformation. Intraoperative photo showing a vascular abnormality (cavernoma) located in the spinal cord.

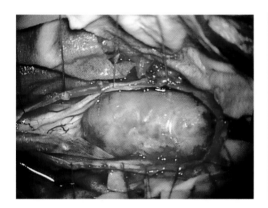 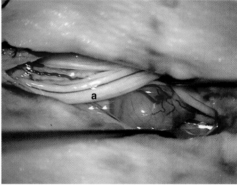

Figure 19.9 Intradural tumor. Intraoperative image showing meningioma at the level of the foramen magnum. In second photo, neurinoma is located adjacent to the conus medullaris. The nerve roots (*a*) are subjected to compression.

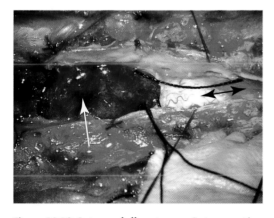 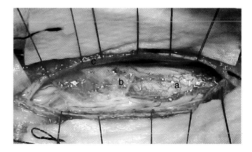

Figure 19.10 Intramedullary tumor. Intraoperative image showing an intramedullary spinal cord tumor (*arrow*, tumor; *double arrow*, spinal cord).

Figure 30.1 Spinal cord tethering and intramedullary cyst formation. Intraoperative illustration of scar formation surrounding the spinal cord. *a*, spinal cord; *b*, scar tissue; *c*, dural sac.

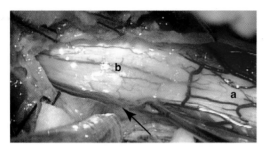

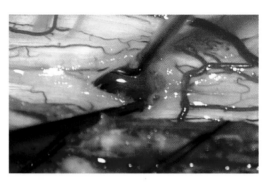

Figure 30.3 Scar formation. Intraoperative photo showing scar formation between the spinal cord and dural sac (*arrow*). *a*, uninjured spinal cord; *b*, lesion level is characterized by its grayish color.

Figure 30.5 The spinal cord is exposed (midline myelotomy).

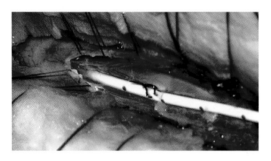

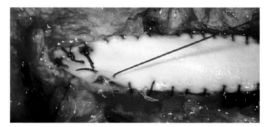

Figure 30.6 Insertion of a shunt catheter through the midline myelotomy.

Figure 30.7 Duraplasty.

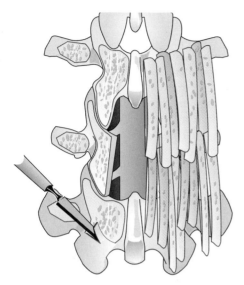

Figure 14.19 The decortication procedure. Using a chisel (to the left) and the placement of autologous bone (to the right).

bony component compressing the dura and spinal cord will partially be removed from the spinal cord vicinity as a result of the restoration of vertebral body height, and pressure on the spinal cord is consequently diminished.

Fusion and Instrumentation

Bone harvested from fractured vertebral arches and spinous processes during the laminectomy, together with bone from the posterior part of the iliac crest, is used as graft material for fusions. The bone grafting takes place after decompression. The most frequent method of fusion is a posterolateral procedure. The harvested bone, containing mainly spongiotic but also cortical bone, is laid over the decorticated surfaces. *Decortication* is the procedure (Fig. 14.19) by which the spongiotic bone is exposed, using a chisel, in the motion segments that must be fused. The exposure of spongiotic bone by the decortication procedure facilitates fusion.

The posterior instrumentation currently used is based on pedicle screw- or hook-rod systems, allowing different possibilities of attachments (Fig. 14.20A,B; also see same figures in the Color Plate Section). These systems, especially the pedicle-rod systems, allow fixation in all directions and prevent translational as well as rotational displacements. The pedicle screws are placed in all columns, thus allowing fixation of the entire injured motion segment. This method is therefore regarded as a possible

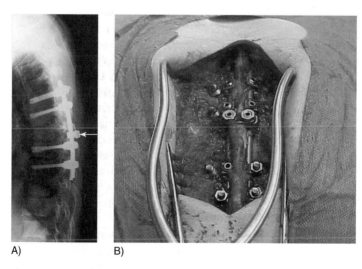

A)   B)

Figure 14.20 Instrumentation. A: Using pedicle screws, longitudinally directed rods, and rods directed at a right angle in relation to the longitudinal rods (*arrow*). B: Posterior instrumentation using pedicle screws and rods. See also Color Plate Fig. 14.20B.

solution to all types of injury in this region. The adjacent levels, historically fixed by Harrington rods, are not involved in the instrumentation. Pedicle screws do not require intact vertebral lamina, as do hooks and wires. As an example, these screws are normally placed in the pedicles belonging to T12 and L2 if the fracture is located at the level of L1. It is important to emphasize that the stability of the damaged spinal column in the long term is accomplished by bony fusion as such, while the immediate and short-term stability is achieved by the instruments applied.

GUIDELINES RELATED TO VARIOUS TYPES OF FRACTURES

Type A, Compression Fractures

Instability in type A fractures is principally related to compressive forces (Table 14.2). Distraction of the anterior part of vertebral body (the posterior wall is uninjured) is therefore the most important maneuvre to correct and restore vertebral height and minimize kyphosis, by restricting the mobility of the vertebral body. The correction of a vertebral body using fixation instruments is called *ligamentotaxis* (see discussion in the preceding section). The restoration of the vertebral body to an anatomically acceptable appearance usually results in normal vertebral body height, and the pressure of retropulsed bony fragments toward the anterior part of the dura is reduced. The fixation device relieves pressure from the restored fracture and protects the injured motion segment from displacement movements during the healing period, since it guaranties stability of the injured motion segment until fusion is accomplished. The weight-bearing duties of the vertebral body are shifted from the spinal column to the instrument as a result of the pedicle screw placement. This also counteracts additional compressive forces on the fractured area and further development of kyphosis.

Type B, Distraction Fractures

The spinal column is partially or totally unstable against flexion (B1 and B2 injuries) or extension forces (B3 injuries) if the patient sustains a type B, distraction fracture. A transverse disruption of the posterior column is seen in the B1 and B2 groups, and the spinal column is consequently always unstable under flexion forces. Stability under extension remains, since the anterior longitudinal ligament is intact. This is of great importance in planning surgical procedures: Increased flexion must be avoided if instrumentation is used to stabilize the motion segment, in order to avoid future kyphosis. The B3 group is unstable under extension since the anterior longitudinal ligament is damaged, whereas this group of fractures is stable under flexion. Pedicle screws or hooks are currently the most widely used fixation devices; their purpose is to replace the function of posterior structures. Pedicle screws are used in a manner similar to that used during the fixation of compression fractures, and hooks placed in a claw position (i.e., bilaterally) have the same properties as pedicle screws. Both techniques enable repositioning of the fracture and a rigid stabilization of the posterior structures, which is of greatest importance in the treatment of distraction fractures. The tendency to use hooks increases the higher up the thoracic spine the fracture is located, due to the gradual decrease in pedicle diameter in the upper thoracic spine.

Type C, Rotation Injuries

Instability under axial rotation always occurs following type C injuries, in addition to the those types of instability associated with type A and B injuries. Type C represents the most unstable type of injuries, with an increased risk for horizontal displacement in all directions (anteroposterior and lateral). (All three columns have failed according to Denis classification; and both columns have failed under the A0 classification scheme.) All type C injuries are, as a rule, treated surgically due to the high risk of instability. This type of injury shares the poor healing properties of other injuries involving disks and other soft tissues such as ligaments. A posterior approach is considered sufficient, since the instrumentation techniques previously presented in this chapter enable sufficient stabilization of the injured motion segment(s). Rods positioned at a right angle in relation to cranio-caudally located rods are used to prevent type C injuries from rotational displacement (Fig. 14.20A,B).

ACKNOWLEDGMENTS

The authors wish to express their gratitude to Associate Professor Lennart Sjögren, Department of Orthopedic Surgery, Södersjukhuset Stockholm, Sweden, for his valuable contribution and support in the creation of this chapter.

Conservative Treatment Following Injuries to the Spinal Column

Orthoses are devices applied externally to support weakened parts of the body. Following an injury to the spinal column, the aim of spinal orthoses is to minimize movements in the injured motion segment, restore spinal alignment, and contribute to trunk stability. The efficacy of spinal bracing is inversely proportional to the volume of tissue that separates the brace from the spine. The use of longer orthoses is usually preferable compared to shorter ones. This circumstance is of importance, especially in the treatment of lumbar fractures (see later in this chapter). As an example, four to five levels above and below the level of injury is included in bracing of thoracolumbar fractures. The so-called three-point supporting devices fulfill these demands when used in the thoracolumbar region, because they offer biomechanical stability despite the localization of injury in this region. Braces that are equipped with several points of contact with the torso and/or those providing a "longer" contact surface are thus more efficacious. Most stable and some unstable fractures may be successfully treated by an external splinting technique (i.e., spinal bracing), but there are several alternatives in the conservative treatment of spinal fractures. Here, we review the most frequently used orthotic models. We have chosen to describe their application only briefly, since local traditions and other factors finally decide the indications (fracture type and injury level) for each individual orthosis.

CRANIOTHORACIC STABILIZING TECHNIQUES

The Halo-vest (Fig. 15.1) remains the most frequently used device for external splinting of the cervical spine. This device offers significant restriction of movement, since both the neck and the head are fixed to the chest. Thus, the Halo device is a suitable option in the treatment of unstable fractures, preferably of the upper cervical spine (see treatment guidelines in Chapter 11).

Contraindications to the Halo-vest are infections in the scalp and skull bone, and skull fractures that may hamper screw fixation, as well as some patient-related factors (age, abuse). The device consists of a crown or ring (available in different sizes) with adherent screws that are attached to the skull bone, a vest, and connecting rods. The single frontal and diagonally located dorsal pins are tightened simultaneously using a torque screw, after which the two remaining screws are applied in the same manner. Injury to the supraorbital nerve must be avoided when applying the frontal screws (see references and Fig. 15.2). The use of the device reduces head flexion and the extension-bending moment significantly, and the extension of the fixation to the chest results in a three-point supporting device. Misalignments, as a result of fractures and/or ligamentous injuries, can be corrected by adjusting the tilt of the ring prior to the fixation of the chest part of the device.

Although the device is the most frequently used external fixation device and provides the best available external stability, it does not provide 100% fixation. Bengt Lind and coworkers showed that significant flexion and extension is seen in every motion segment in the cervical spine despite the use of a Halo device. They also found that the motion is most extensive in the upper cervical spine, but decreases further down. The position of the body and the type of patient-related movements causes great variability of load to the cervical spine. Despite these findings, craniothoracic external fixation

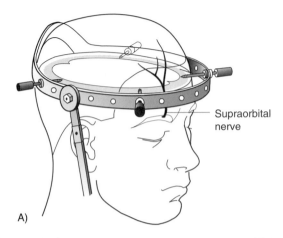

Supraorbital
nerve

A)

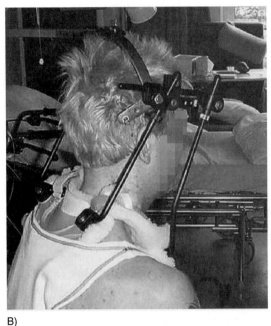

B)

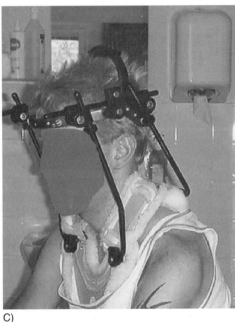

C)

Figure 15.1 Halo-vest. Illustrated version (A). Patient application (B,C). It is of great importance to avoid penetrating the supraorbital nerve and frontal sinus medially, as well as the thin temporal bone and the temporal muscles located laterally.

remains an attractive option following some injuries, especially those to the upper cervical spine. The treatment period is most often around 12 weeks, and radiological examinations are performed repeatedly during and after treatment.

CERVICAL ORTHOSIS

External fixation using orthoses offers acceptable stability to the cervical spine because of the smaller tissue volume separating the cervical spine from the brace and the possibility of using the skull and chest as contact areas.

Cervical orthoses (COs) provide limited restriction of rotation and lateral bending; luckily, these motions are of less importance than sagittal movement (i.e., from maximal flexion to maximal extension), and flexion-extension movement is well prevented by COs.

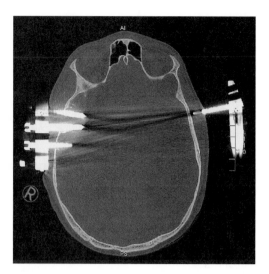

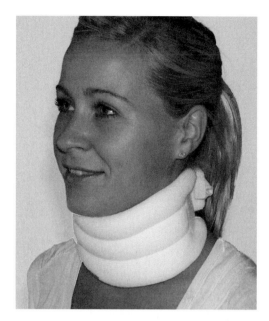

Figure 15.2 Halo-vest. Halo treatment commonly results in local infection at the screw fixation points. Furthermore, penetration of the screws (see figure to the left) through the temporal bone poses another potential risk for the patient.

Figure 15.3 Soft cervical collar.

The possibility of monitoring the treatment effect of CO in each motion segment is questionable, and the use of COs has, therefore, been restricted to fractures considered stable.

COs are subdivided into two groups. The first group offers no contact with the skull or shoulder area (Fig. 15.3). This results in unrestricted sagittal movement, rendering the stabilizing properties of the cervical orthosis practically negligible. The other group is the cervical-shoulder-supporting orthoses. Prefabricated Aspen and Philadelphia hard collars (Fig. 15.4) are examples of cervical-shoulder stabilizing orthoses that provide contact between the mandible and the neck base/shoulder. These collars mainly restrict flexion-extension

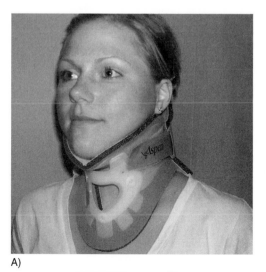

A)

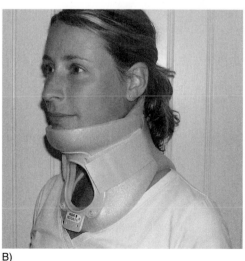

B)

Figure 15.4 Hard cervical collars. Aspen model (A). Philadelphia type (B).

movement in the C1–C7 region. However, the achieved restriction of sagittal motion may be clinically insufficient. These collars are used in the treatment of certain fractures considered as stable, and in some cases as a complementary treatment following surgery.

CERVICOTHORACIC ORTHOSIS

A three-point bending support is achieved by lengthening the cervical orthosis in a caudal direction and by including the chest (Fig. 15.5A,B). The aim of the prefabricated cervicothoracic orthosis (CTO) is to prevent flexion and rotational motion following injuries ranging from C1 to T7. These braces include the sternal-occipital-mandibular immobilizer (SOMI) brace, and they offer substantial limitation of movement in lower parts of the cervical spine.

LUMBOTHORACIC ORTHOSES

Scarce data are available regarding the efficacy of attempts to externally stabilize the thoracic and lumbar spine. Lumbar bracing offers most problems, since four or five levels above and below the fracture must be splinted in order to achieve acceptable stability. The use of orthoses that immobilize one leg is one solution to this problem. However, this extension of the bracing results in an inability to sit, and this type of orthoses is seldom accepted by patients. Many lumbar fractures are, as a consequence of such difficulties, managed surgically. A variety of orthoses to be used for thoracolumbar external splinting are available. The lid-and-box and the three-point corset are two examples of techniques used to splint the thoracolumbar region.

Lid-and-Box

This model is suitable in the treatment of fractures located between T7 and L5. The aim is to prevent flexion, local bending, and rotation. The term "lid-and-box" is used to describe a solid torso corset produced and adapted for individual purposes. The first step in this procedure is to make a plaster cast of the torso. This "plaster-cast

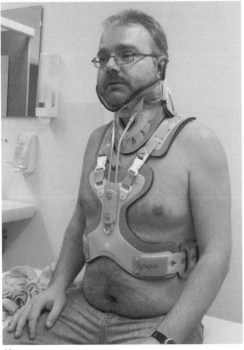
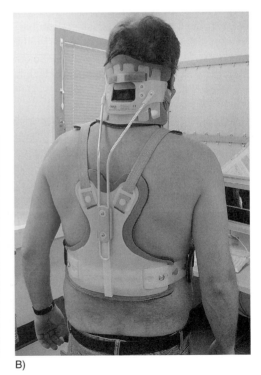

A)   B)

Figure 15.5 Cervicothoracic orthosis (A,B).

positive" is used as a model to produce the final thermoplastic corset. Polyethylene, a high-temperature thermoplastic, is the most frequently used material in the lid-and-box brace. The polyethylene thermoplastic layer is thicker in this model compared to other braces and thus offers a more rigid stabilization of the thoracolumbar region. The lid-and-box model encases the entire torso, with openings located on each side and the anterior part fashioned as a removable "lid." This model has been developed to facilitate the treatment of painful fractures, and it may also be used in the initial period following injury, when assisted rotation in the bed is the only movement that is allowed without the use of a corset. The lid-and-box is removed while the patient in a side-lying position and, thus, the braces are removed only when the patient is lying down. This brace is also used in the treatment of fractures above the level of T7, since the lid can be extended cranially. A cervical orthosis can be attached to the lid-and-box, which further extends the possibility of treating more cranially located fractures. Such a model is called a cervicothoracicolumbar orthosis (CTLO).

Three-point Corset

Three-point corsets are used to treat fractures located between the levels of T8 and L5. They are either prefabricated/customized or hand-made to adapt to individual requirements.

Prefabricated Models

The supporting areas of the three-point corset are located in front of the sternum and pubic regions, while the posterior plate is aligned with the fracture (Fig. 15.6A–C). The sternal-symphyseal distance, as well as the location of the posterior plate, is adjustable, which allows the three-point corset (with some limits), to be adapted to each individual.

Individually Adapted Plaster-cast Models

The plaster-cast model of the three-point corset is used in the treatment of fractures when a high risk of posttraumatic kyphosis is anticipated. The aim of this model is to more sufficiently prevent flexion in the fractured area, as compared to that achievable with prefabricated models. The contact area in this model is broader and larger, and this model also prevents strong lateral bending moment in addition to its antiflexion properties.

LUMBAR ORTHOSIS

The Boston overlap brace (BOB) is the most frequently used model of lumbar orthosis

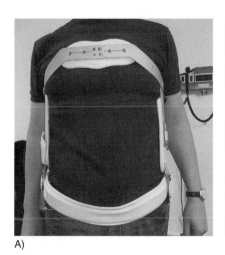
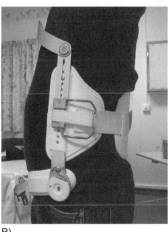
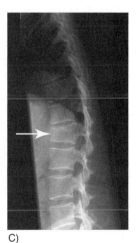

A)   B)   C)

Figure 15.6 Corsets. Customized three-point corset (A,B). A fracture treated conservatively using this type of corset (C).

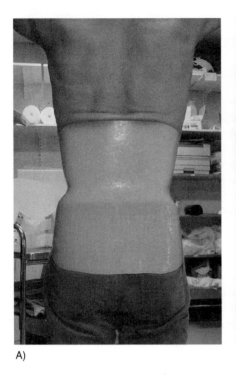
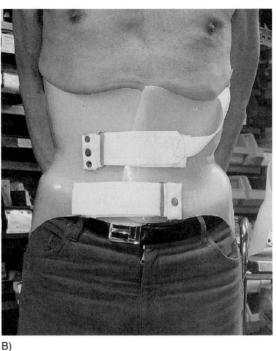

A)   B)

Figure 15.7 Lumbar orthosis (BOB) (A,B).

(Fig. 15.7A,B). The purpose of the BOB is, as with all other corsets, to prevent flexion, lateral bending, and rotational moments. This model is used in the treatment of fractures located between the levels of L1 and L5. Both standard and customized BOBs consist of a 3-mm polyethylene layer over interior cell thermofoam, which is added to improve patient comfort. Customized lumbar orthoses are available in 0, 15, or 30 degrees of lordosis in order to fixate the pelvis and prevent flexion. The BOB normally reaches T10 anteriorly and is opened and closed from the front. Because its purpose is to prevent hyperflexion, and the impact on the posterior part of the BOB in considerably less compared to the front side, the model does not need to reach very far below the level of L1.

ACKNOWLEDGMENT

The authors would like to express their warm gratitude to orthotic engineering technician Charlotta Hübner for introducing us, with a cautious hand, into the world of orthotics.

16 | Children with Spinal Cord Injury

This chapter addresses only those conditions relating to pediatric traumatic SCI that differ significantly from those of adults with traumatic SCI. In addition to certain differences in anatomy and biomechanics, we present certain types of fractures and ligamentous injuries seen solely or predominantly in children. Generally speaking, pediatric SCI is typically more severe. Parents and family obviously become more involved in both the acute and long-term care of children with SCI than in adults in a similar situation; and special medical and psychosocial considerations must be addressed to help children with SCI mature into adulthood in a way that is as normal and harmonious as possible.

There are no universally accepted guidelines for the acute medical care of children with SCI. In part this may be due to the fact that older children (8–10 years of age) begin to demonstrate a spectrum of injuries similar to that of adults. Among young children the differences in injury patterns are significant, but SCI in that age group is extremely rare. However, several articles provide excellent summaries of current medical guidelines (see the section "Suggested Reading").

EPIDEMIOLOGY

It is very uncommon for young children to sustain a SCI; the incidence increases dramatically, however, from the mid-teen years onward. According to current statistics the overall incidence of pediatric SCI in the United States is approximately 2 cases per 100,000 children. The incidence of SCI among children younger than 5 years is extremely low. Among children with SCI who are age 2 or younger, the C1–C2 segment is involved in almost 80% of cases. Although the likelihood of sustaining an SCI in early childhood is low, the injuries are typically more severe than those seen in adults. Traumatic brain injury occurs in about 40% of children with SCI and, as in adults, constitutes the most commonly associated injury.

Table 16.1 presents data from a study of 179 children (110 boys and 69 girls) with spinal *column* injuries (Osenbach & Menezes 1992). Young children, especially infants, show an increased propensity for injuries to the upper cervical spine, due to a disproportionately large head in relation to the body, as well as to undeveloped neck muscles (Fig. 16.1). Among teenagers, the mechanisms of injury are mainly related to risk-taking behaviors such as motor vehicle-, fall-, and sports-related accidents. A trend seems to indicate that the younger the patient, the higher the level of injury on the spinal column.

The Osenbach and Menezes' study also shows that 93 of the 179 patients had complete (42) or incomplete (51) SCI. Children with Down's syndrome, rheumatoid arthritis, and skeletal dysplasias are at increased risk of sustaining spinal cord lesions.

PROGNOSIS

In a study involving 20 children with complete injury, Wang and colleagues showed that neurological improvement was recorded in 30% of the patient group, which is significantly better than in adults. The neurological improvement occurred over a long period of time post injury. However, cervical dislocations with severe neurological deficit were associated with a low rate of neurological improvement, and atlantooccipital injuries were often associated with early death.

Table 16.1 The causes and localizations of skeletal injuries[*] presented with the percentage of patients with neurological involvement in relation to level of injury[**]

	Children 0–8 years	Children 9–16 years	Percentage of patients with SCI in relation to level of injury
Cause			
Motor vehicle accidents	28 (45%)	72 (61%)	
Falls	15 (24%)	15 (13%)	
Sports	1 (2%)	23 (20%)	
Birth injuries	10 (16%)	—	
Other	8 (13%)	7 (6%)	
Total	62 (100%)	117 (100%)	
Distribution			
C0–C3	33 (53%)	31 (26%)	36%
C4–C7	16 (26%)	32 (27%)	73%
Th + ThL	9 (14%)	33 (29%)	67%
Lumbar	4 (7%)	21 (18%)	28%
Total	62 (100%)	117 (100%)	

[*] Expressed in absolute numbers, with percentages in brackets.
[**] C = cervical, Th = thoracic, ThL = thoracolumbar.

UNIQUE PRESENTATIONS

The types and localizations of spinal column injuries differ between adults and children/adolescents due to the unique anatomical and biomechanical characteristics present in children:

- The center of load for cervical mobility is at the C2–C3 level in children, whereas the greatest load centers around the C5–C6 level in adults. This increases vulnerability among children to injuries in the upper cervical spine and in the transition between occiput and cervical spine with extreme flexion and extension.
- The facet joints are more horizontal in children than in adults, especially in the upper cervical spine, and the vertebral bodies are more wedge-shaped, which predisposes children to sliding movements in a forward–backward direction.
- Mobility is exaggerated due to flaccid ligaments and inadequately developed paraspinous muscles, which compromises support for the spinal column. Although this may protect against injury to the vertebral body, it also increases the risk of ligamentous injuries

and the so-called *SCI without radiological abnormalities* (SCIWORA).

Because of these factors, and because the youngest children in particular have a disproportionately large head and weak neck muscles, injury often occurs in the upper cervical region (Fig. 16.1).

ACUTE CARE

Before we discuss the specific injuries that afflict children, we will first present a general overview of the care of children and adolescents with SCI in the acute phase and general principles for workup and treatment.

Care at the Accident Scene

As in adults, the purpose of care at the accident scene is to prevent further deterioration of the neurological deficit and other injuries. The procedures are the same as for adults with one exception: Because of the size of the child's head in relation to the body, the cervical spine will be *flexed* when the child is placed in

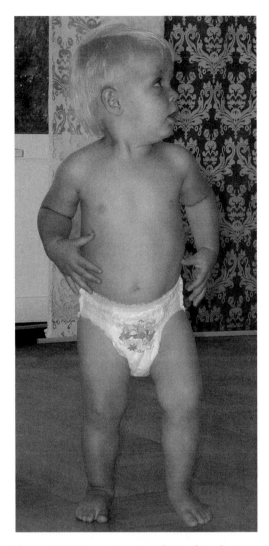

Figure 16.1 Proportionate relationship between head and body of young child.

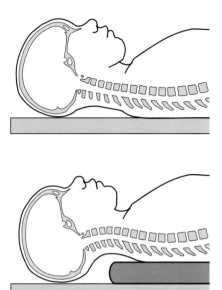

Figure 16.2 Moving the injured child. Placing the child on a mattress counteracts flexion, making it easier to achieve a neutral position for the cervical spine.

Removal of helmets from adolescents involved in moped or bicycle accidents is guided by the same principles as in adults.

Care at the Hospital

Care of children and adolescents in the hospital also follows the same general principles that guide the care of adult patients, with certain exceptions (Table 16.2). For example, children are at higher risk for abdominal complications following flexion-distraction injuries of the lumbar spine (seat belt injuries), and children should be extubated as soon as possible to avoid the risk of long-term ventilator dependence.

Radiologic Workup

Radiologic workup is indicated following a trauma if the child:

- Is uncommunicative because of young age and/or head injury
- Has neurological deficits

a supine position on a spineboard (Fig. 16.2). To achieve a neutral position in the cervical spine, some authors recommend that the body be elevated about 25 mm in children between the ages of 4 and 8, and somewhat more for children younger than 4 years. Ideally, a child should be immobilized using a combination of a rigid cervical collar and taping of the body against the spineboard after the child is placed on a mattress. However, there may be reason to avoid taping since this significantly reduces vital capacity.

TABLE 16.2 Differences between principles of care of children and adults in the hospital.

Children	Adults
Head large and difficult to control, in part due to un-developed neck muscles	Head smaller, fully developed neck muscles
Skeletal structures still growing and developing	Mature skeleton
Thin skull, sutures open	Thick skull, sutures closed
Use of steroids untested	Steroid treatment is an option in adults
Respiratory problems indicated by hypercapnia	Respiratory problems indicated by hypoxia
Crying may camouflage respiratory problems	
Fluid balance highly sensitive	Fluid balance usually easier to regulate
Calorie requirements high	Calorie requirements essentially follow normal metabolic demands
Rapid metabolism	Slow metabolism
Rehabilitation focus – to teach the child various steps of development	Rehabilitation focus – relearning
Latex allergy: greatly increased risk	Latex allergy: moderately increased risk

- Complains about neck pain
- Is assessed to have other painful injuries that may distract attention from a neck injury
- Shows signs of intoxication

Radiologic workup is *not* indicated if the child has undergone trauma but remains alert, has a normal neurological examination, has no neck pain or stiffness, has no distracting injury, and shows no signs of intoxication. Recommendations for the radiologic workup of children follow.

Conventional X-ray. If an isolated cervical spine injury is suspected, radiologic workup begins with a conventional radiograph of the cervical spine. If the child is unable to open the mouth, a rubber tongue blade may be inserted to facilitate imaging of the dens in the frontal projection.

Plain films may show indirect signs of ligamentous injury. If conventional x-rays are normal, but the child's clinical status raises suspicion of ligamentous injury, flexion-extension radiographs should be carried out about 1 week post injury.

Considerable difficulties may be associated with the interpretation of plain films in children. For example, in adult patients, the distance between the posterior arch of the atlas and the

dens (the atlas-dens interval, ADI; Fig. 16.4) may be up to 2.5 mm, according to some authors. In children, the ADI changes with age, and various distances are specified in the literature. The ADI may be up to 4.5 mm, especially in young children, due to loose ligaments and incomplete ossification. Consequently, variations in ADI occur that that may complicate assessment of problems such as atlantoaxial instability.

Computed Tomography Scan. Computed tomography (CT) is always the diagnostic procedure of choice for the workup of high-energy trauma, since CT is the superior method for imaging the skeleton. Modern CT scanners create imaging slices less than 1 mm thick through the entire cervical spine, with an acceptable radiation dose, and then convert the images into three-dimensional reconstructions.

Magnetic Resonance Imaging. Only magnetic resonance imaging (MRI) provides direct information about ligamentous injury, disk herniation, and hemorrhages in and around the spinal cord. MRI can also provide guidance for how long immobilization should continue, when return to activity is acceptable, and aid in prognostication in the presence of spinal cord changes.

CONSERVATIVE TREATMENT

Traction, for the purpose of restoring normal spinal column anatomy or reducing pressure on the spinal cord, is not well documented in the literature. In children, treatment with traction is complicated by several factors, such as the child's thinner cranium, lower body weight, more elastic ligaments, and less developed musculature, all of which may lead to excessive traction, with its attendant risk of SCI. The literature contains no definite evidence that traction is superior to surgical treatment. However, Halo-vest treatment has been successfully used in children as young as 7 months of age. In such cases, 10–12 pins have been used, and the Halo-vest was applied in the conventional manner (see Chapter 15).

SURGICAL TREATMENT

The literature contains no studies that conclusively determine whether early or late surgical decompression of the spinal cord is preferable after acute SCI in children. The primary indication for early surgical intervention is progressive neurological deficit in patients with incomplete injuries. According to reports, surgical treatment of children is now more common than in the past. This observation applies to severe dislocation, unstable injuries, and in cases where the spinal cord is exposed to mechanical pressure.

Laminectomy at multiple levels should be avoided in growing children, especially if the anterior portion of the spinal column is injured, since this increases the risk of progressive instability and further neurological damage. Therefore, a posterior fusion should be carried out in conjunction with any unavoidable laminectomies.

Early surgery is more common than external immobilization for stabilization of the thoracic and lumbar spine, not for the purpose of improving neurological recovery, but to prevent future spinal deformity and to accelerate the rehabilitation process.

SPECIFIC INJURIES

Five conditions are considered more or less unique to or specific in children. These conditions and the treatment of pediatric fractures in general have been thoroughly reviewed by Roger M. Lyon. The conditions are SCIWORA, atlantooccipital dislocation, SCI related to childbirth, epiphysiolysis of the axis, and C1–C2 dislocations. In addition, this overview also describes injuries to the lower cervical spine and to the thoracolumbar spine.

SCIWORA

SCIWORA deserves particular mention among traumatic injuries in children and adolescents. In 1982, Pang and Wilberger defined SCIWORA as objective signs of posttraumatic myelopathy without concurrent signs of fracture or ligamentous instability either on plain films or CT. Consequently, this condition involves traumatic SCI without any radiographic signs of damage to the spinal column. This paradox is mainly explained by the highly elastic ligamentous structures in children. The ligamentous hypermobility and elasticity of the immature spinal column allows the spinal column and spinal cord to be stretched to different lengths during trauma. The spinal cord is estimated to be able to tolerate a stretch of 5 mm, whereas the spinal column can be lengthened by up to 2 cm without sustaining injury. This difference in elasticity probably explains the high incidence of SCIWORA among children.

Incidence

The incidence of SCIWORA in pediatric traumatic SCI is estimated to be 20–50%. The majority of cases occur among children under the age of 8. In 70% of cases, SCIWORA entails a complete injury with an unfavorable prognosis (Pang & Wilberger 1982). In children over the age of 12, SCIWORA occurred in only 12% of cases and was less often associated with complete injury; the prognosis was better for this group. About 80% of injuries afflict the cervical spine, and about half of the children demonstrate neurological deficit with a delay of up to 4 days post-trauma.

More recent studies show that "true" SCIWORA is a rare occurrence. This is indicated by MRI, which can visualize injuries to the spinal column that do not appear on plain film or CT.

MRI findings include injuries to the anterior longitudinal ligament, C2–C3 disk herniation, and posterior ligament injuries. Changes seen in the spinal cord include hemorrhages and edema.

Radiologic Workup

If pain, muscular spasm, or other factors prevent obtaining flexion-extension views at the time of the injury, the child should be immobilized until such examination can be carried out. However, flexion-extension views are difficult to interpret, especially early on, and therefore all children with SCIWORA should have an MRI examination. For this reason, flexion-extension views are rarely done by many trauma centers.

SCIWORA is associated with an increased risk for recurrence of neurological deficits among patients who have had transient spinal cord manifestations. Deficits may reappear without any further traumatization at all or if a new low-energy trauma occurs. Such neurological deficits are often more severe than those caused by the initial injury. In the case of recurrent trauma, even minor injury may cause the patient renewed and severe spinal cord symptoms.

Treatment

Medical treatment of pediatric SCI is essentially consistent with the general guidelines that apply to adults. Should early transient symptoms of spinal cord involvement arise, these children should be treated to prevent recurrent spinal cord problems.

It is not unusual for children with incomplete neurological injury to experience a recurrence of symptoms a few weeks after the initial injury. This fact is the rationale behind the indication for treatment with fixed cervical collar. Since no dislocation or displacement is present, treatment focuses on immobilization and avoidance of activity. Although there is insufficient evidence to issue guidelines, the recommendation is for external immobilization for the suspected level of injury for up to 12 weeks and to have the child avoid high-risk activities for an additional 12 weeks. The purpose of this treatment is to allow the soft tissues to heal and to prevent progression or recurrence of spinal cord symptoms.

Atlantooccipital Dislocation

Atlantooccipital instability occurs in about 8% of fatal motor vehicle accidents, and this injury is twice as common in children as in adults. The diagnosis is extremely uncommon from a treatment standpoint, because this injury usually severs the spinal cord at the cervicomedullary junction, which is usually immediately fatal. Children and adolescents who manage to survive this injury typically have severe neurological deficits. Cervical traction should not be used in suspected atlantooccipital instability because of the risk of stretching the spinal cord further. For additional information, see the section on atlantooccipital dislocation in Chapter 11.

Neonatal Spinal Cord Injury

The incidence of birth-related SCI is estimated at 1 in 60,000 deliveries; 70% of these injuries occur with breech presentation. The spinal column and ligaments of a newborn infant can stretch about 5 cm without sustaining injury, but the spinal cord can stretch only about 5 mm. The most common levels of SCI in newborns occur at the upper cervical spine and the cervicothoracic junction. Excessive longitudinal traction afflicts the lower cervical spine and cervicothoracic junction, especially in cases of breech delivery, and the risk of injury increases if the cervical spine is simultaneously hyperextended. A SCI that afflicts the upper cervical spinal cord is associated with conventional delivery and the use of instruments to rotate the child.

Birth-related SCI is associated with high mortality. The diagnosis is made based on clinical findings during the child's first day of life and through radiological or neurophysiological examinations. Spinal shock and respiratory problems are common symptoms. Signs of spinal shock comprise flaccidity and absence of spontaneous movement of the extremities. Deep tendon reflexes are absent on clinical examination. Apnea and flaccid tetraparesis after breech delivery with manipulation are characteristic of an upper cervical spine injury. The absence of independent breathing during the first 24 hours of life is associated with the need for long-term assisted ventilation.

Epiphysiolysis of the Odontoid Process

The epiphysis between the C2 vertebral body and the odontoid process does not fuse until the age of 7 and remains vulnerable to cervical spine trauma up to that point (Fig. 16.3). The hangman's fracture is unusual in children. Instead, avulsions of the epiphyseal plate may occur up to the age of 10 (Fig. 16.4). Ligamentous laxity and incomplete closure of the epiphyseal area are factors that make the transition between the dens and the C2 vertebral body particularly

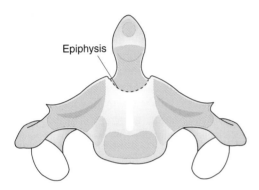

Figure 16.3 The C2 vertebral body in a young child. The areas marked in pink correspond with ossified portions of the vertebral body. The epiphysis (growth zone) between the C2 vertebral body and the odontoid process are labeled in the figure.

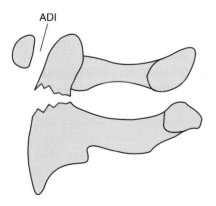

Figure 16.4 Fracture through the odontoid process. The odontoid process is easily bent backwards in relation to the C2 vertebral body. The atlas-dens interval (ADI) increases with this displacement.

vulnerable in young children. The most common cervical spine injury in children under 7 years is a dens fracture or epiphysiolysis. Such disruption of the growth zone can result even from low-energy trauma. A conventional lateral radiograph shows this epiphysiolysis; the odontoid process is shifted in relation to the vertebral body of the axis. This injury usually occurs in preschool-aged children and, as a rule, treatment is conservative. Since the injury only affects the epiphysis, the potential for healing is good with immobilization.

Closed reduction and external fixation for about 10 weeks are recommended, and about 80% of such injuries heal with this treatment. Halo-vest treatment for 6 weeks followed by a soft cervical collar for an additional few weeks is usually sufficient. Surgical treatment may be appropriate when an initially successful reduction of epiphysiolysis combined with external fixation reverts to a new displacement, or if the initial displacement is pronounced and cannot be corrected through closed (nonsurgical) reduction. The most common surgical measure on such occasions is a posterior fusion of C1 and C2.

Atlantoaxial Instability

An anterior dislocation of the atlas in relation to the axis of 4.5 mm or more is required in order for rupture of the transverse ligament to occur, since a normal ADI may be up to 4.5 mm. An ADI greater than 4.5 mm indicates a ruptured ligament, whereas a displacement of greater than 5 mm between C1 and C2 in a child is an indication of greater instability, in which all ligaments have ruptured. If the ADI is greater than 10 mm or if the patient has symptoms of spinal cord compression at the C1–C2 level, posterior fusion is recommended (see Chapter 13).

Atlantoaxial Rotary Fixation

A combination of rotary dislocation between the occiput and atlas together with a subluxation between the atlas and axis is not unique to children, but is proportionately more common in this group. Such dislocation may arise with minor trauma, resulting in the head being rotated to one side while simultaneously tilting

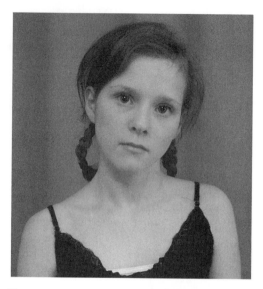

Figure 16.5 Cock-Robin appearance.

to the other side, referred to as the "Cock-Robin appearance" (Fig. 16.5). The child is unable to turn the head back across the midline. Neurological examination is typically normal, and attempts at passive movement of the head are painful. The patient experiences spasm of the sternocleidomastoid muscle on the same side to which the head is rotated and usually presents with a complaint of torticollis. Reduction followed by immobilization is the standard therapy for this rotary subluxation. Surgical treatment may be required if the dislocation cannot be reduced, the subluxation recurs following reduction, or if the original displacement lasts more than 3 weeks.

Lower Cervical Spine Injury

Lower cervical spine injuries are relatively uncommon in children under the age of 8. The pattern of injury for children over the age of 8 is similar to that of adults. Compression fractures dominate, and dislocations do not occur until the late teens. Flexion is the most common mechanism of injury.

Surgical treatment is seldom necessary in children with lower cervical spine fractures, even when ligamentous injury causes instability. Halo-vest treatment after reduction and traction is the most common treatment option. Surgical stabilization becomes necessary in case of progressive neurological deterioration, severe displacement cannot be reduced, or if instability that develops over time. Surgical treatment usually involves some type of posterior fusion of the injured segment followed by orthotic treatment.

Thoracolumbar Injuries

Thoracolumbar fractures are often located at the juncture between the rigid thoracic segments and the more mobile lumbar segments. Teenagers are more likely to sustain vertebral body fractures and injuries of the posterior structures, while younger children tend to sustain only ligamentous injuries. Pediatric fractures often involve active growth zones. When a fracture involves the end plates, growth of the vertebral bodies is affected, with the consequent risk of developing spinal deformity. The occurrence of neurological deficits follows the same principles as for adults.

Major trauma is needed to cause fractures and dislocations of the thoracic spine. Because of limited rotational capacity in the upper thorax, most injuries occur after flexion and axial compression. The profile of injuries and the treatment of fractures in teenagers resembles that of adults. Immobilization is a common form of treatment since most of these injuries do not typically cause instability or neurological involvement.

Conservative treatment is indicated for compression fractures that result in a less than 50% reduction of height in the vertebral body. Severe compression fractures (i.e., >50% loss of height in the anterior portion of the vertebral body) and minor multiple vertebral compression fractures that together result in unacceptable kyphosis, as well as herniated disks, bone fragments, or hematomas that compromise the spinal cord are indications for surgery. Multiple small wedge-shaped vertebral fractures of the thoracic spine are particularly characteristic in children. It is often necessary to stabilize pediatric patients more extensively than adults (more levels involved) since the purpose of the procedure is to prevent future deformity of the spinal column (see the section "Progressive Back Deformities").

Burst fractures tend to occur in the lower thoracic and lumbar spine, where axial forces are large. Many burst fractures may be treated conservatively, but severe dislocation requires surgical treatment. The principles for stabilizing these fractures are similar to those for compression fractures.

Treatment of seat-belt injuries and fracture-dislocation injuries follows essentially the same guidelines as those for the adult population.

SUMMARY OF EMERGENCY CARE

Although a review of the literature on the treatment of children with acute cervical SCI presented in *Neurosurgery* (Apuzzo 2002) concluded that the available literature only offers diagnostic guidelines and treatment options, but no conclusive treatment protocols, there appears to be consensus regarding certain aspects of workup and treatment:

- It is difficult to achieve a neutral position for the cervical spine during transport on a spineboard.
- It is possible to rule out spinal column and/or SCI solely on clinical grounds (see also Chapter 6).
- Conventional radiographs of the cervical spine should include frontal and lateral views, open mouth (dens frontal), and oblique projections.
- Most pediatric spinal column injuries can be treated conservatively, and Halo-vest treatment is the most effective immobilization method. This treatment is associated with acceptable risks, including some increase of morbidity due to infections and loosening of pins.
- The only specific pediatric injury for which there is solid evidence for choosing a specific treatment is epiphysiolysis of C2 in children under 7 years. First-line treatment for this injury involves closed reduction and immobilization.
- Isolated ligamentous injuries of the upper cervical spine may heal with external fixation alone. If the injury is associated with deformity, surgical treatment may be considered.

- Pharmacological treatment with steroids in children under age 13 lacks sufficient scientific evidence; methylprednisolone thus is usually not given in this age group.

SPINAL CORD INJURY-RELATED SEQUELAE IN THE PEDIATRIC GROUP

Hypercalcemia

Hypercalcemia related to increased bone resorption (as reflected in elevated serum calcium) is particularly common in teenage boys. In typical cases, onset of symptoms is insidious, with abdominal pain, nausea, vomiting, malaise, fatigue, polyuria (i.e., large urine volumes), polydipsia (i.e., large fluid intake), and dehydration. In some cases, behavioral changes are also present, and psychotic symptoms can occur. The condition may also be asymptomatic. Hypercalcemia may lead to conditions such as renal failure and stone formation in the urinary tract. Treatment includes intravenous fluid administration, diuretics, and bisphosphonates.

Autonomic Dysreflexia

Autonomic dysreflexia in small children often presents atypically as vague malaise, rather than the classic description with severe pulsating headache. An increase in blood pressure of 20 mmHg or more above baseline should arouse suspicion of this condition.

Disturbance of Temperature Regulation

Poikilothermia—the tendency for body temperature to passively adjust to ambient temperature—is particularly pronounced among young children with SCI, in part due to a disproportionately large surface area in relation to body weight, and in part because the youngest children cannot adequately communicate that they feel too cold or too hot.

Children typically react more readily with fever than do adults, and this also applies to children with SCI. Common causes of fever include respiratory infections, deep vein thrombosis, heterotopic ossification, fractures, pressure ulcers, wound infections, and various intraabdominal disorders. In some cases, no underlying pathology can be demonstrated as the cause of the fever, which leads to the assumption that the fever is due to a SCI-related disruption of temperature regulation.

Pain

Pain often occurs in children with SCI, as is the case in adults with SCI. However, assessment of pain is more difficult in children. One pain-related phenomenon reported to be more common among children is *autophagia*, mainly in the form of nibbling on the fingertips, which in turn may be related to dysesthesia (i.e., unpleasant sensations).

Latex Allergy

Latex allergy has been reported to occur in 6–18% of children with SCI. The reason is likely increased latex exposure, since it has been shown that the risk of developing latex allergies increases with prolonged exposure to latex-containing products at a young age. Allergic manifestations may include rash, urticaria, angioedema (i.e., swelling of lips, tongue, or throat) and/or anaphylaxis (i.e., allergic shock). Latex allergy is particularly common among persons who are allergic to kiwis, bananas, avocados, and chestnuts. Diagnosis is confirmed by history, in vitro tests, and skin testing. Given the risk of allergy, children with SCI should avoid exposure to latex.

Urogenital Sequelae

Intermittent catheterization is currently the standard method for emptying the bladder in children with SCI. This bladder-emptying regimen can usually be initiated from the age of 3, and self-catheterization can typically be started at the age of 5–7.

Gastrointestinal Problems

A bowel-emptying regimen on a regular daily or every-other-day schedule using a microenema and/or manual removal can typically be initiated at the age of 2–4 years. Prior to that age, diapers are used for fecal incontinence.

Musculoskeletal Problems

Progressive Spinal Deformity

The risk of developing progressive deformity of the spinal column is great for patients who sustain SCI in childhood. It has been reported that almost 100% of patients who sustain injury before growth plate closure develop secondary spinal deformity, while more than 50% of patients who are injured after epiphyseal closure are similarly affected. Contributing factors to the development of spinal deformities such as scoliosis and kyphosis include injuries to the epiphyseal plates and paralysis of the supporting trunk muscles below the level of injury. So-called paralytic scoliosis may lead to secondary pelvic tilting, difficulties in sitting, pressure ulcers, and pain. An angulation of 60 degrees or more increases the risk of both impaired cardiopulmonary function and urinary and bowel problems.

Young age at the time of injury is the most important factor for the development of scoliosis. Preteens in particular must therefore be monitored with frequent radiographic checkups. Orthotic treatment initiated early on can reduce the development of scoliosis, but surgical correction often becomes necessary. There is consensus that children with unstable thoracolumbar fractures and concurrent SCI should have a fusion procedure if scoliosis continues to progress. In young individuals with complete SCI, fusion should encompass several levels above and below the injured segment.

Hip Deformities

Hip deformities related to subluxation, dislocation, and contracture are common in young children and often require prophylactic orthotic treatment, and sometimes even surgical intervention. Hip contractures combined with subluxation occur in almost one-quarter of patients who sustain SCI in childhood.

Heterotopic Ossification

Heterotopic ossification is less common in children with SCI than in adults and characteristically has a later onset (on average more than 1 year after the injury, compared with only a few months in adults).

Fractures

As in adults, children with SCI are at increased risk of sustaining fractures in paralyzed limbs. Fractures, often seen in conjunction with osteoporosis, should be suspected if local swelling is present in an extremity, especially swelling of the supracondylar portion of the femur and the proximal tibia. Fractures may also manifest as fever of unknown origin.

ACKNOWLEDGMENTS

The authors would like to warmly thank Associate Professor Peter Pech, Radiology Unit, Uppsala University, for his assistance in the creation of this chapter.

Suggested Reading

Bosch PP, Vogt MT, Ward WT. Pediatric spinal cord injury without radiographic abnormality (SCIWORA): the absence of occult instability and lack of indication for bracing. *Spine* 2002;27(24):2788–2800.

Bilston LE, Brown J. Pediatric spinal injury type and severity are age and mechanism dependent. *Spine (Phila Pa 1976)* 2007;1;32(21):2339–2347.

Cirak B, Ziegfeld S, Knight VM, et al. Spinal injuries in children. *J Pediatr Surg* 2004;39(4):607–612.

Goetz E. Neonatal spinal cord injury after an uncomplicated vaginal delivery. *Pediatr Neurol* 2010;42(1):69–71.

Hadley MN, ed. Management of pediatric cervical spine and spinal cord injuries. *Neurorsurgery* 2002;50(3):S85–S99.

Hadley MN, ed. Spinal cord injury without radiographic abnormality. *Neurosurgery* 2002;50(3):S100–S104.

Kochanek PM, Tasker RC. Pediatric neurointensive care: 2008 update for the rogers' textbook of pediatric intensive care. *Pediatr Crit Care Med* 2009;10(4):517–523.

Lennarson PJ, Menezes AH. Pediatric spinal cord injury. In: Tator CH, Benzel CH, eds., *Contemporary Management of Spinal Cord Injury: From Impact to Rehabilitation*. Park Ridge, IL: American Association of Neurological Surgeons, 2000:209–229.

Lyon RM. Pediatric spine injuries. In: Frymoyer JW, Wiesel SW, eds., *The Adult and Pediatric Spine*, 3rd ed. Philadelphia: Lippincott, Williams & Wilkins, 2004:425–444.

Osenbach RK, Menezes AH. Pediatric spinal cord and vertebral column injury. *Neurosurgery* 1992;30(3):385–390.

Pang D, Wilberger JE Jr. Spinal cord injury without radiological abnormalities in children. *J Neurosurg* 1982;57(1):114–129.

Puisto V, Kääriäinen S, Impinen A, et al. Incidence of spinal and spinal cord injuries and their surgical treatment in children and adolescents: a population-based study. *Spine (Phila Pa 1976)* 2010;1;35(1):104–107.

Vogel LC, Anderson CJ. Spinal cord injuries in children and adolescents: a review. *J Spinal Cord Med* 2003;26(3):193–203.

Vogel LC, Krajci KA, Anderson CJ. Adults with pediatric-onset spinal cord injuries: part 3: impact of medical complications. *J Spinal Cord Med* 2002;25(4):297–305.

Wang MY, Hoh DJ, Leary SP, Griffith P, McComb JG. High rates of neurological improvement following severe traumatic pediatric spinal cord injury. *Spine* 2004;29(13):1493–1497.

Yucesoy K, Yuksel KZ. SCIWORA in MRI era. *Clin Neurol Neurosurg* 2008;110(5):429–433. Epub 2008 March 19.

17 | Cervical Spinal Column and Spinal Cord Injuries in Athletes

Injuries to the spinal column, with or without spinal cord involvement, account for 2–3% of all sports-related injuries. Fracture-dislocation injuries are seen in one-third of all cases, mainly in conjunction with American football, rugby, wrestling, ice hockey, and diving accidents. C5 is the most common level of injury, probably because mobility is greatest at this level, and these activities involve axial compression with a component of flexion at the time of the injury. Although few injured individuals sustain severe fractures and SCI, those who do so in conjunction with elite-level sports receive considerable publicity. This chapter describes injuries related to a number of sports, as well as various forms of spinal cord involvement resulting from athletic activity. Finally, we present two algorithms on the various aspects to consider when deciding whether to allow players to return to contact sports following serious injury to the spinal column, with or without spinal cord involvement.

HIGH-RISK ATHLETIC ACTIVITIES

Diving

Diving accidents account for 75% of patients who sustain a SCI during athletic activities (Fig. 17.1), although they only account for about 10% of all SCI. Those individuals who sustain a SCI are usually males diving into lakes or the open sea, and injury to the spinal column and/or spinal cord is usually the sole high-energy injury found. Diving accidents that entail a fracture of the fifth vertebra are in 70% of cases associated with a simultaneous SCI, and it is not uncommon for more than one vertebra to be fractured. The mechanism of injury is a combination of axial compression and flexion to which the individual is exposed when the depth of the water is misjudged and the head hits a rock, the ocean floor, or the bottom of a pool. By providing information to avoid diving into water of unknown depth (shallow water), avoiding alcohol in conjunction with diving, and being certain about pool depth, the number of diving accidents with this tragic outcome could be reduced.

Skiing

Trauma resulting in SCI, for obvious reasons, is more common in downhill than in cross-country skiing. The helmets that many people wear today reduce the risk of head injury, but not of SCI, and information on the slopes should point out the importance of always skiing in groomed areas.

American Football

This sport is associated with a relatively high risk of incurring SCI, compared with other contact sports. The incidence of tetraplegia in organized American football is estimated at about 1 case per 100,000 registered athletes, which corresponds with about 10–15 new cases annually among 1.5 million active football players. Most of these SCI occur in high school athletes. The explanation may lie in differences in size, age, strength, and maturity among players in this age group. Most injuries are related to tackling; players with long slender necks appear to be most vulnerable. Most SCI occur to the tackler when he hits his opponent with the crown of his head while his neck is bent slightly forward, producing axial compression in combination with mild flexion at the moment of impact (Fig. 17.2).

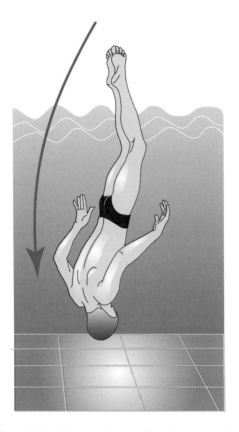

Figure 17.1 Diving accident with axial compression and flexion as the mechanism of injury.

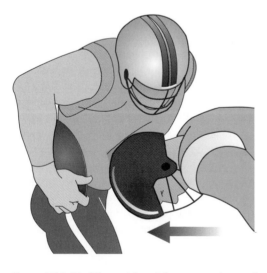

Figure 17.2 Tackling with axial compression and flexion.

Neck muscles are extremely strong when extended, but significantly weaker when flexed. When the player drops his head slightly forward and unleashes the axial trauma with the tackle, his ability to absorb the opponent's energy is compromised and he is therefore at greater risk of sustaining injury to the cervical spine.

Torg and colleagues (1993) introduced the term *spear tackler's spine*, a condition defined as including (a) narrowing of the cervical spinal canal (cervical spinal stenosis), (b) straightening of normal cervical lordosis, (c) a medical history that includes episodes of plexus neurapraxia (see *burning hands syndrome*) or transient SCI, (d) the presence of preexisting or posttraumatic radiographic abnormalities of the cervical spine, and (e) regular use of "spear tackling," in which, at high speed, the player uses his body as a spear by throwing himself against the opponent and tackling head first while his body is still airborne, or when an opponent is shoved head-first to the ground, like a spear.

Rugby

Rugby is the most common sport related to SCI in some countries, such as South Africa. Certain phases of play are deemed particularly dangerous. Players are particularly vulnerable to trauma when forming a "scrum"(the formation players make when they group in a cluster at the start of play). The player who gets the ball and has the misfortune to have the cluster pile on top of him after falling with his head against the surface could then be exposed to hyperflexion trauma combined with a rotational component, and the injury that usually arises is a unilateral facet dislocation. Tackling in rugby is also dangerous, especially when the tackler uses his outstretched arms to fell the opponent with a headlock-like grip, which subjects the tackled player to hyperextension, often combined with a rotational component. In a *sandwich tackle*, a player is hit by two tacklers, one of whom tackles the legs and the other the upper body. A particularly dangerous type of tackle is similar to that seen in American football, with flexion and axial compression.

Wrestling

Fortunately, neck injuries and SCI in wrestling are extremely uncommon. Unless a wrestler is forced down with the neck extensor muscles in hyperextension, SCI is almost always avoided.

Martial Arts

SCI is also extremely uncommon in the martial arts sports, although SCI with lethal outcome have occurred in connection with cervical fracture-dislocation injuries. For example, a dangerous situation may arise with the *sweeping ankle* throw, in which the feet are kicked out from under an individual, causing the head to hit the ground without allowing the falling person time to break the fall with body or arms.

Gymnastics

The use of trampolines has been a matter of concern. SCI has occurred when mistakes are made when jumping on a trampoline, especially with jumps involving rotation, causing a risk for neck injuries.

Ice Hockey

SCI usually affects ice hockey players who are about 20 years of age. As in other sports, the C5 level appears to be the most vulnerable. The usual mechanism of injury involves shoving, tackling, or cross-checking with a club, either against the boards or in the middle of the rink. Axial compression is probably also involved here, when the head hits the ice or the wall of the rink, although flexion is also a factor.

SPECTRUM OF INJURIES

Four patterns may be described among individuals with SCI:

Permanent Spinal Cord Injury (Type 1)

In cases of permanent SCI (type 1), clinical and/ or radiological signs of SCI are present. The clinical picture is characterized by symptoms of spinal cord involvement of varying severity, and magnetic resonance imaging (MRI) reveals intramedullary changes such as swelling, bleeding, or contusion.

Transient Neurologic Deficit with Radiological Findings (Type 2)

Symptoms of transient spinal cord involvement are uncommon, but have been well described in athletes. Torg and colleagues introduced the term *neurapraxia* in sports medicine to describe these types of transient symptoms, usually involving bilateral impairment of sensation in the upper extremities, but sometimes also motor deficits. Neurapraxia involving the cervical spinal cord is caused by sudden mechanical deformation of the spinal cord. Sensory symptoms manifest as burning pain or loss of sensation. These symptoms are transient and disappear within 15 minutes to 48 hours. The prevalence of neurapraxia has been estimated at over 30%, which means that one in three participants at the high school level suffered some form of spinal cord trauma during their athletic career.

Burning hands syndrome is an example of neurapraxia that may have its cause in a disturbance at the spinal cord level or the nerve roots and brachial plexus. Burning hands syndrome at the spinal cord level is a variant of *central cord syndrome*, and the spinothalamic tract is probably exposed to some type of transient vascular involvement. The syndrome consists of a burning dysesthesia and paresthesia in the hands. Muscle weakness may occur, but is uncommon. No other signs of SCI are present, and the entire spectrum of symptoms resolves in about 24 hours. Cervical spinal stenosis is the predominant radiological finding, as this condition predisposes to this syndrome.

Transient Neurologic Deficits Without Radiological Findings (Type 3)

This category includes individuals afflicted with transient symptoms of nerve root or spinal cord involvement, but without any radiological findings. It has been speculated that the spinal cord is compressed at the moment of the injury. The pincer mechanism, as described by Penning, is considered to be an accurate descriptive model. According to this theory, the spinal cord is compressed between the lower posterior corner of the upper vertebral body and the base of the spinous process of the lower vertebra (Fig. 17.3). Given these circumstances, a differential diagnostic cause of burning hands syndrome should also be considered.

"Burners" or "stingers" correspond to brief episodes of paresthesias or motor weakness in the upper extremities. This spectrum of symptoms is caused by a traction or compression injury to the brachial plexus or to the 5th or 6th cervical nerve roots (Fig. 17.4).

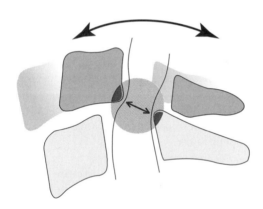

Figure 17.3 Penning's pincer mechanism.

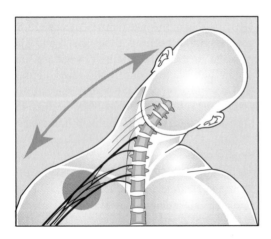

Figure 17.4 Traction on the cervical nerve roots and/or brachial plexus.

Isolated Radiographic Signs of Spinal Column Injury (Type 4)

Type 4 injuries includes posttraumatic cases that only demonstrate radiographic changes such as fractures, herniated disks, or ligamentous injury at the cervical spine level, but demonstrate no neurological involvement (Table 17.2).

GUIDELINES FOR RETURN TO ATHLETIC ACTIVITY

Tables 17.1 and 17.2 present guidelines for returning to or termination of athletic activity after the various types of injuries just described.

Type 1, 2, and 3 Injuries

The recommendation for individuals afflicted with permanent SCI (type 1) or with repeated transient episodes of spinal cord involvement (type 2 and 3), such as central cord neurapraxia, is not to return to physically demanding athletic activity (Table 17.1). The number of episodes of transient spinal cord involvement required to recommend refraining from returning to contact sports varies in the literature. An athlete may return to activity after one episode, but after three such episodes it is recommended that the individual refrain from the activity. The controversy stems from how to handle a return to sports for athletes who have sustained two type 2 or 3 injuries.

Type 4 Injuries

Despite extremely scanty data on fractures, it is generally accepted that unstable fractures or ligamentous injuries assessed as unstable contraindicate returning to contact sports, regardless of whether the fracture heals after treatment (Table 17.2). Another generally accepted principle is that athletes with a fracture or dislocation requiring Halo-vest treatment or surgical stabilization must not or should not return to contact sports. Even when such injuries heal, mobility may remain somewhat impaired, and the loads above and below the level of injury are greater following a fracture or dislocation that has stabilized.

TABLE 17.1 Algorithm for return to athletic activity after various types of neurological involvement.

Neurological Injury (Type 1, 2, 3)	Number of Injury Incidents	Return to Activity
Type 1	One or more	No
Type 2 and 3	One episode	Yes
	Two episodes	Recommendations vary/no consensus
	Three or more episodes	No

TABLE 17.2 Algorithm for return to athletic activity following type 4 injury and cervical spinal stenosis.

Radiological injury (Type 4)	Stability Aspects	Return to Activity
Fracture, ligamentous injury	Unstable	No
	Injury treated with either Halo-vest or surgery	No
	Stable under load	Yes
	Spear tacklers' spine	No
Cervical spinal stenosis	Clinical assessment more important than radiological finding	Recommendations based on injury type 1, 2, and 3

Athletes who sustained a fracture deemed stable under load, that did not require Halo-vest treatment or surgical stabilization, and who have a normal neurological examination may return to athletic activity. Laminar fractures, spinous process fractures, and minor vertebral compression fractures are examples of fractures in which the athlete may resume activity.

Athletes meeting Torg's definition of *spear tackler's spine* may not return to activity.

Recommendations are difficult to make in cases of cervical spinal stenosis, and there are no truly effective screening methods for assessing the risk of active participation in sports in cervical spinal stenosis (defined as an anteroposterior diameter of less than 12 mm). The recommendations for cervical spinal stenosis mainly take into account the presence of neurologic symptoms and essentially follow the recommendations for type 1–3 injuries. An incidental finding of cervical spinal stenosis probably poses very little risk for athletes who engage in contact sports.

Suggested Reading

Bailes JE. Spinal injuries in athletes. In: Menezes AH, Sonnntag VK, eds. *Principles of Spinal Surgery.* New York: McGraw-Hill Companies, 1996:465–492.

Boden BP, Jarvis CG. Spinal injuries in sports. *Neurol Clin* 2008;26(1):63–78; viii. Review.

Chao S, Pacella MJ, Torg JS. The pathomechanics, pathophysiology and prevention of cervical spinal cord and brachial plexus injuries in athletics. *Sports Med* 2010;40(1):59–75.

Giovanini MA, Day AL. Spinal injuries in athletes with cervical stenosis. *Techniques Neurosurg* 1999;5(2): 185–193.

Kuhlman GS, McKeag DB. The "burner": a common nerve injury in contact sports. *Am Fam Physician* 1999;60:2035–2042.

Maroon JC, Bailes JE. Athletes with cervical spine injury. *Spine* 1996;21(19):2294–2299.

Rihn JA, Anderson DT, Lamb K, et al. Cervical spine injuries in American football. *Sports Med* 2009;39(9):697–708.

Tator CH. Recognition and management of spinal cord injuries in sports and recreation. *Neurol Clin* 2008;26 (1):79–88; viii. Review.

Torg JS, Sennett B, Pavlov H, Leventhal MR, Glasgow SG. Spear tackler's spine. An entity precluding participation in tackle football and collision activities that expose the cervical spine to axial energy inputs. *Am J Sports Med* 1993; 21(5):640–649.

Torg JS, Ramsey-Emrheim JA. Management guidelines for participation in collision activities with congenital, developmental, or post-injury lesions involving the cervical spine. *Clin Sports Med* 1997;16(3): 501–530.

Wilberger JE Jr. Athletic spinal cord and spine injuries. Guidelines for initial management. *Clin Sports Med* 1998;17(1):111–120.

Spinal cord injuries caused by projectiles (e.g., bullets) are among the severest types of injury an individual can endure (Fig. 18.1). One of the great pioneers in neurosurgery, Dr. Harvey Cushing, who was active during World War I, was of the opinion that only patients with incomplete injuries could survive. He estimated mortality at about 80% among soldiers who sustained any type of SCI. The general rule of thumb at that time was that surgery was not indicated for patients with a complete injury unless that injury was below the level of the spinal cord; that is, caudal to L1, in which case this patient group was treated with superficial wound debridement, just as those with incomplete SCI. During the interval between the world wars, treatment strategy was to carry out debridement of only the entry and exit wounds. A relatively dramatic improvement of medical care for bullet wounds with spinal cord involvement occurred during World War II with the introduction of sulfa drugs and penicillin, improved transportation from the scene of injury, and because appropriate rehabilitation row could be offered. Modern principles of war surgery were first employed on a large scale during the Vietnam War, including those principles that apply today with respect to debridement and closure of dural defects.

EPIDEMIOLOGY

In contemporary civilian life, low-caliber pistols and rifles with bullet speeds of less than 700 m/s give rise to most SCI. Few epidemiological studies are available, but one frequently cited report from Rancho Los Amigos Hospital in California reflects the spectrum of injuries in that state, where bullet wounds are second only to motor vehicle accidents as the most common cause of trauma-induced paraplegia. Of cases caused by shooting, 40% were due to shots entering from behind and about 20% were caused by shots that entered from the front. Half of these SCI involve the thoracic spine and, not surprisingly, young men were typical victims. Many of those persons have substance abuse problems, which may be a contributing factor to their often poor rehabilitation outcomes. In all, bullet wounds account for about 15% of all SCI in the United States (data from 1980s), and 1 in 20 bullet wounds involves an SCI. Knife wounds, the other type of penetrating injury, appear to be particularly common in South Africa, possibly because firearms are not yet commonly available.

BULLET WOUNDS

Ballistic Aspects

Ballistics is the study of the motion of unguided projectiles. The wound caused by a bullet is a function of its shape, mass, and velocity. The kinetic energy (energy of motion) of a bullet, E_k, can be calculated from the formula $E_k = 1/2\ mv^2$, where m is bullet mass (kg) and v is bullet velocity (m/s). Factors such as the bullet's shape (round, pointed, or flat) and consistency (solid or hollow) also influence the effect of the energy. In addition to kinetic energy, the path of the projectile to the tissue is also of significance. The appearance of the tissue wound is dependent on whether the bullet has a straight track, an element of torque, or if a tumbling effect influenced the path of the bullet toward the body. The severity of a wound can also vary at the same velocity depending on

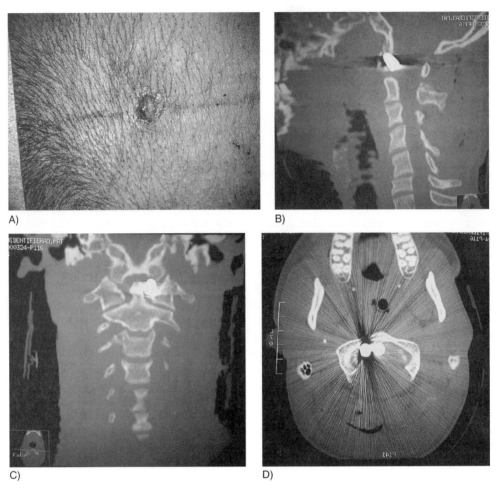

A)

B)

C)

D)

Figure 18.1 Gunshot wound. Illustration of (A) skin entry wound and a computed tomography (CT) collage of a bullet located at the C1 and C2 level. Lateral view (B). Frontal view (C). Axial projection (D).

the type of tissue hit. Thicker and thus more resistant bone slows the kinetic energy of the bullet, although secondary missiles in the form of bone fragments may cause significant tissue damage. In summary, the severity of the wound varies with the velocity of the projectile, the density of the tissue, and the characteristics of the projectile, such as shape, mass, and pattern of movement.

Each bullet creates a path through the tissue and, in conjunction with this path, a cavity is formed. The size of the cavity is directly proportional to the kinetic energy. The spinal cord may become injured by the projectile itself, but the shock wave or pressure wave generated is the most common mechanism of injury, combined with secondary projectiles such as bone fragments that may penetrate the spinal cord. It is indeed entirely conceivable that contusion injuries to the spinal cord and nerve roots may occur without penetration of these tissues by the bullet.

Local and Systemic Pathophysiology

Acute Phase

Bullet wounds in the thoracic spine between T1 and T10 thus often result in complete injuries, probably because of the narrow diameter of the spinal canal, which amplifies the effect of the shock wave. It is uncommon for bullet wounds at the lumbar level to cause complete injuries, since injuries at the L1 and L2 level and further caudally involve peripheral nerves that belong to cauda equina rather than central nervous system tissue.

Twenty-five percent of all bullet wounds at the thoracic level have at least one associated systemic injury. The most common thoracic injuries include hemopneumothorax, as well as pleural and parenchymal hemorrhage.

The severity of the SCI thus is related to the kinetic energy of the bullet and on the other factors mentioned earlier. Additional factors that may influence the pathophysiologic processes are whether or not a direct mechanical trauma (direct hit by the bullet) afflicts the spinal cord, whether the trauma was caused by the recoil effect of fragments, or if a contusion wound occurred because of a shock wave. Epidural and subdural hematomas are relatively rare compared with intramedullary hemorrhage. The pathophysiologic chain of events, with a primary and secondary phase followed by a chronic phase, is similar to that of other contusion and crush wounds. Penetrating injuries below the conus are not infrequently associated with injury to the lumbosacral plexus. Fragments from clothing, skin, and other debris that accompany the bullet in its track constitute a special pathophysiologic process. Bullets may also be mobile and shift around in the spinal canal, which entails a dynamic pathophysiologic process over time.

The material of which the bullet is made also appears to be significant. For example, bullets made of lead are not as toxic to the local tissues as are copper bullets.

The presence of a foreign body may also entail a rejection process around the bullet. If the bullet is located near the spinal cord, a compression of the spinal cord may arise, but there is also an increased risk of various infectious processes, such as meningitis, epidural and intramedullary abscesses, and osteomyelitis.

In the abdominal region, colonic injuries in particular are associated with osteomyelitis and meningitis. Penetrating wounds through the ventricle and small intestine are far less likely to cause infection.

Fistulae occur late in the course of events after a bullet wound, and may extend from the spinal column to the intestines, bladder, or pleura. Arteriovenous fistulae may form adjacent to injuries involving the vertebral artery.

Chronic Phase

Among the complications arising after penetrating bullet wounds is the development of cysts in the spinal cord. These cysts are usually multilobular. The unique pathophysiologic pattern following bullet wounds is for these cysts to assume the form of microcysts, rather than forming one single cyst centrally located in the spinal cord. Arachnoiditis, causing scar tissue formation and tethering of the spinal cord, may often precede cyst formation.

Pain is very common after bullet wounds. Pain is usually dysesthetic and amplified by light touch. According to some authors, this pain is worse at night, but otherwise remains relatively constant.

Patients with SCI caused by penetrating trauma demonstrate a higher incidence of neurological deterioration in late stages than do those with other types of SCI, especially if the bullet is allowed to remain in the spinal canal. Development of pain may indicate neurological deterioration as a result of inflammatory processes. Otherwise, patients with penetrating wounds manifest similar late complications as those with SCI of nonpenetrating etiology (see Chapter 30).

Management

General Guidelines During the Acute Phase. Treatment of any systemic effects resulting from the trauma (thorax, abdomen, etc.) must be given priority before addressing the actual injury to the spinal cord and its consequences. Immobilization, attention to breathing and circulation, neurological assessment, and transport to the hospital follow the same principles that govern management of patients with SCI in general.

Particular note should be given to the fact that a patient with SCI and simultaneous injury to the thorax and/or abdomen often cannot experience infralesional pain, which may mask serious conditions such as active intraabdominal bleeding. The ability to distinguish between neurogenic shock and hypovolemic shock due to bleeding is very important (Table 6.6). It is also important to initiate treatment with antibiotics as soon as possible post trauma.

For radiologic workup, conventional x-ray and computed tomography (CT) are most commonly employed. Workup of penetrating trauma should include the probable trajectory of the bullet with a good margin if only the entry wound is detected. Magnetic resonance imaging (MRI) has its limitations, especially if the bullet contains iron, in which case there is a risk that the bullet may move in response to the magnetic field, which may enlarge the area of tissue damage. The risk of MRI workup should therefore be avoided.

Vascular injury to the carotid artery or jugular vein must be suspected if hematoma is palpable around entry wounds in the cervical spine. Some authors suggest radiographic assessment of the cervical vessels in order to diagnose possible fistulae. Injuries to the throat and esophagus can be evaluated through the use of contrast x-ray imaging; this is important, since an injury to the esophagus that remains undiagnosed after 24 hours is associated with high mortality. In the presence of visceral damage within the abdomen, neurosurgical procedures are associated with a high risk of complications. Therefore, repair of visceral damage combined with initiation of antibiotics should precede neurosurgery aimed at decompressing the spinal cord and stabilizing the spinal column. In summary, exploration of injuries to the skull, cervical region, chest, and abdomen, as well as other fractures outside the spinal column, should be given higher priority than the radiologic diagnosis of SCI and neurosurgical intervention in patients with multisystem trauma and SCI after a penetrating trauma.

Surgical Treatment

Indications for Surgery. Indications for surgical intervention following penetrating trauma are subject to endless discussion, but only a few scientific studies have addressed the prognosis in penetrating injuries. The authors conclude that the prognosis is probably not as dire as previously believed and is comparable to the prognosis after motor vehicle accidents. Consequently, surgical intervention for such injuries has increased.

In cases of progressive neurological deterioration caused by fragments that put pressure on the spinal cord, surgical treatment with decompression is typically recommended. Such surgery entails relieving the pressure on the spinal cord by removing the bullet or other tissue that presses against the spinal cord. Penetrating wounds to the spinal cord that cause an immediate complete injury are not, per se, an indication for surgical exploration. The risks of infection, development of fistulae, and anesthesia-related complications are too high in relation to the marginal potential for improvement of neurologic function through surgical intervention. Surgery is usually done for incomplete myelopathy with persistent significant spinal cord compression, and complete cervical injuries may be explored if surgical decompression may improve function in one or two nerve roots; in other words, if surgical intervention focuses on the nerve roots, rather than the spinal cord.

Cauda equina injuries with small intraspinal metal or bone fragments are not usually operated. However, if a largely intact bullet or large bone fragment compresses the spinal cord or nerve root, surgical exploration is generally carried out, since large fragments remaining in this region cause an increased incidence of posttraumatic pain.

Most surgeons agree that surgical intervention to close cerebrospinal fluid fistulae is indicated. In highly unusual cases where spinal fluid leakage occurs and the point is to prevent infection, patients with both complete and incomplete injuries may be explored. Initially, however, a 5–7-day trial of lumbar drainage may be tried in combination with 1 week of antibiotic treatment. These measures are typically sufficient to close fistulae.

Research presented by colleagues at Louisiana State University Medical Center reflects generally accepted opinion regarding indications for surgical intervention for such injuries. Their study, encompassing 15 cases, including 10 involving the thoracic level and 5 at the lumbar level, shows that none of the patients with complete injury demonstrated any meaningful neurological recovery, regardless of whether bullets or bone fragments compressing the spinal cord were removed or not. By contrast, all patients with incomplete cauda equina injury improved after decompression of the spinal cord. None of the patients in this material suffered from complications such as fistulae, spinal fluid leakage, infection, or progressive neurologic dysfunction. All patients who experienced hyperesthesia prior to surgery showed significant improvement after removal of the bullet or bone fragment.

Goals for Surgical Intervention. The goal of surgical treatment is to:

- Prevent progressive neurologic dysfunction
- Prevent cerebrospinal fluid fistulae
- Debride devitalized tissue to minimize the risk of infection
- Remove projectiles that contain lead or copper to reduce the inflammatory response
- Relieve the spinal cord and nerve roots from pressure resulting from hematoma, bone, and bullet fragments

Special Technical Aspects. Decompressive laminectomy should be carried out extending at least one arch above and below the actual level of injury in order to achieve a good overview of the field of injury. The procedure is initiated by loosening the muscles from each arch, followed by identification of as much of the devitalized tissue as possible, which is then debrided and rinsed with a liberal amount of saline mixed with antibiotics. Fragmented bone and metal fragments in the extradural space may be removed. The use of ultrasound is recommended to find remaining fragments or hematoma located intradurally or in front of the dural membrane. Devitalized dura should be removed, followed by thorough irrigation with warm -saline. The dural defect is replaced with artificial dural tissue. The entire wound should be rinsed repeatedly, after which the wound is closed in several layers, to avoid postoperative fistula formation.

Instability. Instability is extremely uncommon after a bullet wound. However, if instability should be present, the stabilizing procedure is not carried out during the acute phase. Instead, the patient is treated with traction or orthosis until such time that surgery is appropriate.

Conclusion

The prognosis for recovery of neurological function is very poor for complete acute SCI following gunshot wounds. Management is essentially similar as for other high-energy trauma in which SCI has occurred. However, SCI is given low priority if the trauma has given rise to systemic effects such as in injuries to the thorax and abdomen.

Surgical measures for bullet wounds of the spinal column and the spinal cord play a limited role. Surgical treatment is indicated for progressive neurological deficits and to close cerebrospinal fluid fistulae. In patients with preserved neurological function who have a significant simultaneous residual compression of the conus and cauda region, surgery may be considered to counter the increased risk of posttraumatic pain. Late complications such as pain are common after penetrating trauma.

KNIFE WOUNDS

In the few studies at hand, the cervical spine appears to be the area most vulnerable to stab wounds. In cases in which the spinal cord is injured, the path of the stab wound goes between the vertebral arches, which usually are not injured (Fig. 18.2). In two-thirds of cases, the resulting SCI presents as a Brown-Séquard syndrome. At the time of the injury, the knife penetrates between the spinous process and transverse process. As the knife penetrates between these structures, the blade crosses the midline on in its trajectory into the spinal canal/ spinal cord. Treatment of these injuries essentially follows the same principles described for penetrating projectiles, although there are some differences, mainly with respect to systemic effects, since knife wounds do not have the same high-energy consequences.

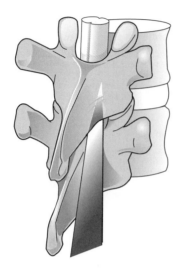

Figure 18.2 Knife wound. Direction of knife where a SCI may arise.

Suggested Reading

Al-Habib AF, Attabib N, Ball JR, et al. Clinical predictors of recovery following blunt spinal cord trauma: systematic review. *J Neurotrauma* 2009;15 (Epub ahead of print).

Bhatoe HS, Singh P. Missile injuries of the spine. *Neurol India* 2003;51(4):507–511.

Couture D, Branch Jr. CL. Spinal pseudomeningoceles and cerebrospinal fluid fistulas. *Neurosurg Focus* 2003;15(6):1–5.

Hanigan WC, Sloffer C. Nelson's wound: treatment of spinal cord injury in 19th and early 20th century military conflicts. *Neurosurg Focus* 2004;16(1):E4.

Jallo GI. Neurosurgical management of penetrating spinal injury. *Surg Neurol* 1997;47(4):328–330.

Jallo GI, Cooper PR. Penetrating injuries of spine and spinal cord. In: Menezes AH, Sonnntag VK, eds., *Principles of Spinal Surgery*. New York: McGraw-Hill, 1996:807–815.

Kendall JL, Anglin D, Demetriades D. Penetrating neck trauma. *Emerg Med Clin North Am* 1998;16(1):85–105.

Kitchel SH. Current treatment of gunshot wounds to the spine. *Clin Orthop* 2003;(408):115–119.

Landy HJ, Arias J, Green BA. Penetrating injuries. In: Tator CH, Benzel CH, eds., *Contemporary Management of Spinal Cord Injury: From Impact to Rehabilitation*. Park Ridge, IL: American Association of Neurological Surgeons, 2000:199–207.

McKinley WO, Johns JS, Musgrove JJ. Clinical presentations, medical complications, and functional outcome of individuals with gunshot wound-induced spinal cord injury. *Am J Phys Med Rehabil* 1999;78(2):102–107.

Medzon R, Rothenhaus T, Bono CM, et al. Stability of cervical spine fractures after gunshot wounds to the head and neck. *Spine (Phila Pa 1976)* 2005;15;30(20):2274–2279.

Mirovsky Y, Shalmon E, Blankstein A, Halperin N. Complete paraplegia following gunshot injury without direct trauma to the cord. *Spine (Phila Pa 1976)* 2005;1;30(21):2436–2438.

Putzke JD, Richards JS, Devivo MJ. Gunshot versus nongunshot spinal cord injury: Acute care and rehabilitation outcomes. *Am J Phys Med Rehabil* 2001;80(5):366–370.

Rivkind AI, Zvulunov A, Schwartz AJ, Reissman P, Belzberg H. Penetrating neck trauma: hidden injuries-oesophagospinal traumatic fistula. *J R Coll Surg Edinb* 2001;46(2):113–116.

Waters RL, Sie IH. Spinal cord injuries from gunshot wounds to the spine. *Clin Orthop* 2003;(408): 120–125.

Wortmann GW, Valadka AB, Moores LE. Prevention and management of infections associated with combat-related central nervous system injuries. *J Trauma* 2008;64(3 Suppl):S252–S256. Review.

Nontraumatic myelopathies refer to spinal cord disorders that are not caused by external trauma. However, from a rehabilitation standpoint, certain nontraumatic myelopathies bear close resemblance to trauma cases, especially those characterized by focal involvement (i.e., in which the lesion affects only a limited portion of the spinal cord) and in those where disease progression after onset of illness is essentially stationary. Even patients with progressive myelopathy (i.e., conditions in which underlying disease entails progressive worsening) may in some cases benefit from treatment at spinal centers. An overview of the most important nontraumatic myelopathies is presented in this chapter. For details please refer to general neurology textbooks.

INFLAMMATORY CONDITIONS

Multiple Sclerosis

In Europe and North America, multiple sclerosis (MS) is the most common cause of nontraumatic neurological impairment among persons between the ages of 15 and 50. Spinal cord–related symptoms are the first manifestation in 10–30% of cases. The disease can be relapsing-remitting or chronically progressive (primary-progressive). It is not uncommon for a disease course that is initially relapsing-remitting to become chronically progressive after a number of years. This is referred to as secondary-progressive MS. The disease is characterized by autoimmune inflammatory lesions in the white substance of the brain and spinal cord. These lesions lead to demyelinization and the subsequent formation of scar tissue, known as *plaques*. Spinal plaques in MS are most commonly found in the dorsal half of the spinal cord

and preferentially involve the cervical and upper thoracic levels rather than more caudal segments. MS plaques tend to have a symmetric and bilateral distribution. Diagnosis is confirmed by magnetic resonance imaging (MRI) of the brain and spinal cord, which may demonstrate scattered plaques within the central nervous system (CNS) (Fig. 19.1). During the acute phase, with active inflammatory lesions, MS plaques will enhance with intravenous contrast. Cerebrospinal fluid (CSF) examination may demonstrate oligoclonal banding in electrophoresis and selective γ-globulin elevation.

Three main variants of MS have been described at the spinal cord level: neuropathic, subacute spinal cord compression, and acute transverse myelitis.

In the *neuropathic* variant, sensory symptoms dominate, such as peripheral paresthesias, which may either be spontaneous or provoked by touch. Sensory impairment is minimal, and is often felt as if a thin layer of fabric was located between the skin and the stimulus. Often the patient experiences *Lhermitte's phenomena*, characterized by electric shock-like sensations that radiate down along the spine and sometimes out into the extremities in response to neck flexion. However, this phenomenon is not pathognomonic of MS, as it may occur in several other spinal cord disorders. In general, reflexes are increased, abdominal reflexes may be absent, and Babinski's sign is present.

The *subacute spinal cord compression* variant most closely mimics the medical history of cervical spondylotic myelopathy (see below). MRI workup is here necessary to rule out conditions causing spinal cord compression. However, careful history may reveal that many of these patients have also had previous flare-ups with transient neurological symptoms from other parts of

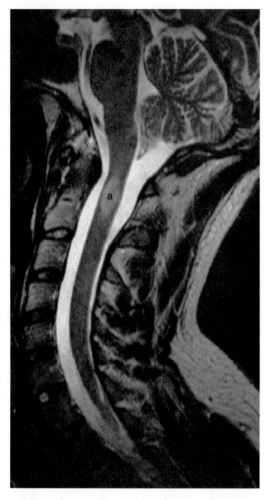

Figure 19.1 Multiple sclerosis. Magnetic resonance image (MRI) shows plaques of multiple sclerosis (MS) in the cervical spinal cord. There is no thickening of the spinal cord and the MS plaque (*a*) is enhanced in this T2-weighted sequence.

the CNS, parallel to the development of a gradually progressive spastic paraparesis.

An MS attack typically develops from the onset of symptoms to the maximum deficit over a period of 1 day to 1 week. Remission from maximum deficit to maximum functional recovery typically occurs over a period of 1–3 months. In many cases, the patient has an attack about every other year. Sensory symptoms completely remit in more than 75% of all cases. The prognosis for motor deficits is poorer. Among patients with motor symptoms, about half with mono- or hemiparesis will achieve complete remission, but less than 20% of patients with tetra- or paraparesis will recover full function. Only 15% of patients with bladder symptoms will recover normal bladder function. Severe flare-ups are often treated with high doses of intravenous or oral steroids, which shorten the time until remission; however, they probably do not affect either the degree of functional recovery or the frequency and intensity of future attacks.

The *Uhthoff phenomenon*, which is characteristic for MS, should be mentioned in this context. Here, an elevation of body temperature leads to a temporary increase in neurological symptoms. Although this phenomenon may appear to be a flare-up, it is in reality a "pseudo-relapse," and is not associated with new plaque formation.

Long-term therapy with subcutaneous interferon β-1b (Betaseron), intramuscular (Avonex), or subcutaneous (Rebif) interferon β-1A as well as subcutaneous glatiramer acetate copolymer-1 (Copaxone) has been shown to slow the course of the disease in MS, mainly by decreasing the frequency of flare-ups. More recently, intravenous infusion of natalizumab has been very promising in preventing neurological deterioration in relapsing-remitting MS. The effect on primary- and secondary-progressive MS is controversial. Cytotoxic drugs and autologous bone marrow transplants are rare treatment options in severe cases.

Acute transverse myelitis is caused by lesions that involve more or less the entire spinal cord cross-section within one or several spinal cord segments. The spectrum of symptoms is identical to that which occurs in other acute causes of transverse lesions of the spinal cord, such as those of a traumatic or vascular nature. Onset of symptoms may be immediate or progress over several days. It is not uncommon for the patient to experience band-like pain at the level of lesion. Initially flaccid paresis, paresthesias, and sensory deficits arise below the level of lesion, with urinary retention and a distinct sensory level. In rare cases, acute transverse myelitis is associated with bilateral retrobulbar neuritis, a condition known as *Devic disease* (neuromyelitis optica).

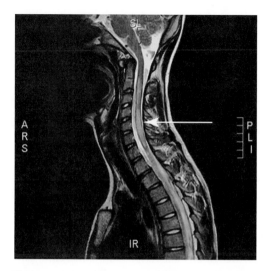

Figure 19.2 Myelitis. T2-weighted image in which diffuse myelitis has been diagnosed (*arrow* indicates area of maximum involvement). In transverse myelitis, craniocaudal involvement is not typically as widespread as in this case.

The condition is often precipitated by an immunological reaction, in which disease onset is preceded by immunization or viral infection. In rare cases, transverse myelitis may be due to direct infection of the spinal cord by agents such as herpes simplex, varicella zoster, cytomegalovirus, or Epstein-Barr virus. In some cases, no precipitating event can be identified. In the acute phase, MRI shows either normal findings or nonspecific spinal cord swelling (Fig. 19.2). CSF examination may be normal or show lymphocytic pleocytosis and elevated proteins.

In about 5% of cases, symptoms of transverse myelitis signal the onset of MS. In certain of these cases, MRI of the brain may demonstrate clinically "silent" plaques, lending credence to the diagnosis of MS. MS is also to be suspected by detection of specific CSF findings, as described earlier.

About one-third of patients with acute transverse myelitis achieve complete functional recovery, one-third improve but experience some degree of neurological sequelae, and one-third remain paraplegic.

Arachnoiditis

Arachnoiditis is characterized by inflammation of the spinal cord meninges, giving rise to scar tissue formation and adhesions (tethering) between the arachnoid and the spinal cord and/or spinal nerve roots. Etiology may be infection, trauma, chemical irritation from intrathecal (i.e., in the spinal canal) injections of x-ray contrast medium, back surgery, or other insults to the spine. The adhesions may cause symptoms through traction or strangulation of neural tissue or its blood supply and/or through blockage of CSF circulation. Symptoms may include back pain or rhizopathy, as well as sensorimotor symptoms associated with the development of arachnoid or intramedullary cysts. MRI confirms the diagnosis. The treatment is usually conservative (analgesics, intrathecal steroids). If symptomatic intramedullary cysts develop, surgical drainage and spinal cord untethering may become necessary.

VASCULAR CONDITIONS

Spinal Cord Infarction

Spinal cord infarction may be caused by insufficient blood flow in the aorta, segmental arteries, and/or arteries within the spinal cord itself, such as the anterior or posterior spinal arteries. The condition known as *anterior spinal artery syndrome*, with infarction of the anterior portion of the spinal cord cross-section, causes paralysis and loss of pain sensitivity below the level of the lesion, with preservation of proprioception and vibration sense (see Chapter 5). Control over bladder function is usually lost as well. In typical cases, onset is acute and associated with back pain over the infarcted area. However, frank occlusion of the anterior spinal artery can rarely be demonstrated. Causes of spinal cord infarction may include dissecting aortic aneurysm, surgical procedures involving the aorta, embolic or arteriosclerotic vascular occlusion, and/or stenosis of a segmental or spinal cord artery, especially in conjunction with an episode of severe systemic hypotension and/or cardiac arrest. Most infarctions involve the bulk of gray matter. Infarction is particularly common in the thoracic spinal cord, where blood supply is more limited. In occlusion of the major anterior segmental medullary artery, also known as the great radicular artery of Adamkiewicz (Fig. 3.10), which is typically located in the lower thoracic or upper lumbar spine, a massive infarction often occurs that is equivalent to an anterior cord syndrome at the spinal cord level. About half of patients with spinal cord infarction achieve significant motor functional recovery after the injury. Typically, these are young patients with incomplete paresis.

Intraspinal Bleeding

Hemorrhage within the spinal canal may be epidural (Fig. 19.3), subdural, subarachnoid, or intramedullary, involving the substance of the spinal cord itself (hematomyelia). About 25% of hemorrhages occur in patients with ongoing anticoagulant therapy or coagulopathy (i.e., diseases with increased bleeding diathesis); trauma accounts for 10% of cases, and hemorrhage from vascular malformations or tumor account for another 5%. No demonstrable cause can be found in the remaining 60% of cases. The spectrum of symptoms is characterized by acute back pain, rapidly followed by progressive paresis and sensory deficits below the level of the lesion.

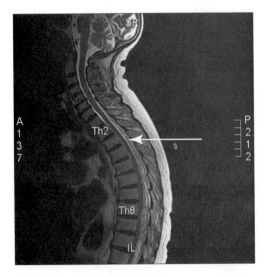

Figure 19.3 Spinal epidural hematoma. Lesion extends proximally to the level of the T2 vertebral body. Hematoma located posterior to the subarachnoid space and the dura (*arrow*).

Treatment is surgical for circumscribed spinal hematomas that compress the spinal cord, and comprises removal of the hematoma.

About half of patients with total sensorimotor deficit at the time of surgery will achieve some degree of functional recovery, and about 10% will experience total functional recovery.

Intraspinal Vascular Malformations

Extramedullary vascular malformations within the spinal cord are typically caused by a fistula between the feeding artery and the draining vein. The resultant increase in pressure within the venous system leads to a serpentine dilatation of the vessels. The cause of the spinal cord symptoms may be either compression from a mass effect from these vascular tangles, or due to shunting of the blood past spinal cord tissue, resulting in local hypoxia. A vascular malformation may also become manifest, with acute onset of clinical symptoms due to hemorrhage or infarction in the spinal cord (see earlier discussion). Most of these patients are middle-aged or older men who experience slowly progressive symptoms.

Intramedullary vascular malformations typically have their onset earlier than those that are extramedullary, usually in childhood or in early adulthood.

Diagnosis of intraspinal vascular malformation is confirmed by MRI (Fig. 19.4A), MR angiography, and/or spinal angiography. Treatment is determined on a case-by-case basis and consists either of some type of surgical intervention and/or embolization (Fig. 19.4B; also see same figure in Color Plate section).

INFECTIOUS CONDITIONS

Spinal Epidural Abscess

This condition is characterized by an abscess (i.e., focal accumulation of pus) in the spinal canal, which can damage the spinal cord either through a direct-acting mass effect and/or through secondary infarction caused by infectious thrombophlebitis (i.e., occlusion of spinal cord vessels caused by infection). The abscess arises as a result of spread from a nearby focal

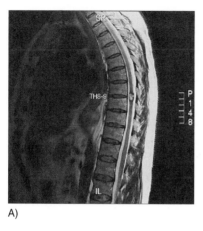
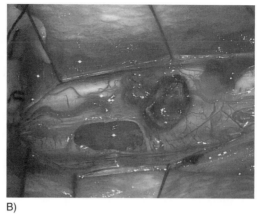

A) B)

Figure 19.4 Intramedullary vascular malformation. A: Intramedullary vascular malformation at the level of the T8–T9 disk. B: Intraoperative photo showing a vascular abnormality (cavernoma) located in the spinal cord. See also Color Plate Fig. 19.4B.

infection (e.g., a vertebral body), or may result from hematogenous spread from a focus of infection elsewhere in the body, such as the lungs or urinary tract. The most common causal organism is *Staphylococcus aureus*. Risk factors include diabetes, intravenous drug abuse, subacute bacterial endocarditis, septicemia, and immuno-deficiency conditions. Yet another infectious cause is tuberculosis, either in the form of skeletal tuberculosis (Potts disease) or involving direct infection of the spinal cord (Fig. 19.5).

Epidural abscesses are most commonly located in the thoracic spine, where the loose dural attachment permits rapid spread of the abscess. Initial symptoms include localized back pain and fever. As the abscess grows, the nerve roots become compressed, leading to radiating pain. In the final phase, the spinal cord and/or cauda equina will be compressed, producing cross-sectional symptoms. Typically, symptoms progress over a period of several days. Leukocytosis (increased white blood cell [WBC] count) is noted on laboratory studies. Initially, MRI usually demonstrates a *phlegmon* (a diffuse area of infection) and subsequently a circumscribed abscess develops. Note that lumbar puncture may cause acute neurological deterioration due to pressure gradients, and should thus be avoided. Patients treated at an early stage—before paraparesis becomes manifest—as a rule

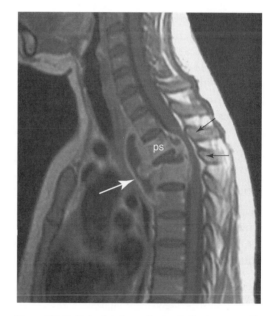

Figure 19.5 Spinal tuberculosis. Infectious condition caused by the tubercle bacillus. Note the abscess on the anterior (*white arrow*) and posterior side of the spinal column. One of the vertebral bodies is involved by the disease (Potts disease; ps in the figure). Moreover, one of the vertebral bodies is resorbed (there is one spinous process "too many" in relation to the number of vertebral bodies in the picture). The spinous process from the missing vertebral body corresponds with the lower of the two *red arrows*.

recover completely, in contrast to patients who have become paraplegic more than a day or so before initiation of treatment, who will typically suffer permanent paralysis. The treatment consists of urgent surgical decompression and antibiotics. Intraoperatively, abscesses are often found to be relatively firm in consistency rather than in a liquefied state.

Epidemic Poliomyelitis and Post-polio Syndrome

Immunization has essentially eradicated this disease in the developed world, but many persons who have survived the disease still live with the sequelae. The neurotrophic polio virus attacks the anterior horn motor neurons in the spinal cord, leading to more or less widespread and pronounced paresis and muscle atrophy.

Some persons previously afflicted with polio have experienced progressive symptoms after a stable period of 25–30 years. This condition is sometimes referred to as *post-polio syndrome*. The cause of this condition has not been established. The fact that patients with a past history of polio have spent some of their neuronal "reserve capacity" may lead to disproportionate progressive functional deficits when additional neuronal death, as part of physiological aging, occurs. Immunological mechanisms have also been proposed. This diagnosis should be considered in patients with a past history of poliomyelitis, although other possible causes must also be ruled out.

Tabes Dorsalis (Tertiary Syphilis)

Syphilis (lues) is a sexually transmitted infection with a shifting spectrum of symptoms during the protracted course of the untreated disease. During what is known as the tertiary stage of syphilis, which is usually reached 10–20 years after primary infection, the spinal cord may become involved. At this point, progressive scar tissue formation of the spinal meninges may secondarily impact the dorsal columns and other neural structures. Typical symptoms include attacks of sudden electric shock-like pains, known as *tabetic crises*. Interruption of the sensory reflex arc causes loss of deep pain sensation, areflexia, and muscular hypotonia. Moreover, there is loss of proprioception leading to a positive Romberg test (i.e., patients lose their balance when asked to stand up with their eyes closed). In addition, neurological examination may reveal Argyll-Robertson pupils (i.e., pupils are unequal in size, irregular, and react to convergence but not to light), optic nerve atrophy with peripheral visual field loss, and sometimes also signs of upper motor neuron injury including the presence of a bilateral Babinski sign.

AIDS-related Myelopathy

Myelopathy may signal the onset of acquired immune deficiency syndrome (AIDS), with spastic paraplegia, often in combination with peripheral neuropathy. The condition may also appear in the late stages of the course of the disease.

HTLV-1–associated Myelopathy

This condition, also known as *tropical spastic paraplegia*, is caused by infection with the human T-lymphotropic virus type 1 (HTLV-1) and mainly occurs in the West Indies, equatorial regions of Africa, and in Japan. The virus is transferred sexually or by blood. Clinically and on MRI, the condition may resemble the findings of MS, but it occurs in an Afro-Asian population where MS is rare. The condition is characterized by chronic inflammation of the spinal meninges and perivascular regions of the spinal cord. Severe demyelination of the corticospinal tract, and in the thoracic spinal cord in particular, may be noted. Lymphocytic pleocytosis and elevated proteins may be seen in the cerebrospinal fluid. HTLV-1 antibody serology is positive.

DEGENERATIVE CONDITIONS

Herniated Disk

Disk herniation of the cervical and thoracic spine may lead to compressive myelopathy (Fig. 19.6). The herniation may arise suddenly or gradually. Usually, some local pain is present, combined

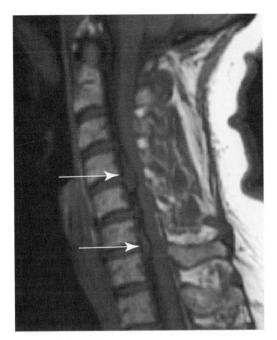

Figure 19.6 Herniated disk. Lateral magnetic resonance image (MRI) illustrating multiple herniated disks in the cervical spine. (*white arrows*)

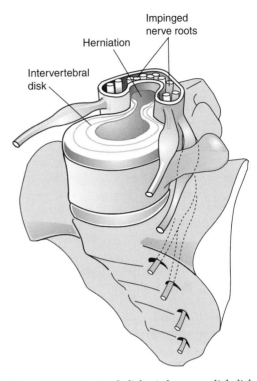

Figure 19.7 Herniated disk. A large medial disk herniation in the lumbar spine may compress several nerve roots below the spinal cord level.

with radiating pain within the affected dermatome. The herniated disk usually projects posterolaterally or laterally, thereby compressing nerve roots, but not the spinal cord. However, in medial (i.e., posterior) herniation the spinal cord may be compressed, resulting in paresis and sensory loss below the level of the lesion. In addition, bladder symptoms such as urgency, incontinence, and/or urinary retention may arise.

Medial herniation within the lumbar spine—below the termination of the spinal cord—may compress the cauda equina (Fig. 19.7). In these cases, motor and sensory loss affects the "saddle" area—the perineum, medial, and posterior thighs; voiding may also be affected, with urinary retention (i.e., paralysis of the bladder muscles with inability to empty the bladder) and overflow incontinence (i.e., passive urine leakage once bladder capacity is exceeded).

MRI will typically demonstrate the herniated disk and the resultant spinal cord or carda equina compression (Fig. 19.8). Patients with acute onset of spinal cord compression due to disk herniation should be referred for acute neurosurgical assessment.

Spondylotic Myelopathy

Spondylosis is a degenerative condition of the spinal column that occurs in about 50% of all 45-year-olds and 90% of all 60-year-olds. The primary pathology involves disk degeneration (with decreased elasticity and water content in the disks, which results in shrinkage) that secondarily leads to reactive deposition of bone on the vertebral bodies and narrowing of the spinal canal (spinal stenosis). The resultant encroachment of the spinal canal may give rise to neurological symptoms of a myelopathic nature.

In *cervical spinal stenosis* (Fig. 12.18), myelopathy usually has an insidious onset with progressive paresis, without significant sensory symptoms or bladder involvement in the early stages. The spectrum of symptoms may, in such cases, resemble that of amyotrophic lateral sclerosis (ALS; see later discussion). Cervical spinal stenosis is reported to be the most common cause of gait disorders among persons

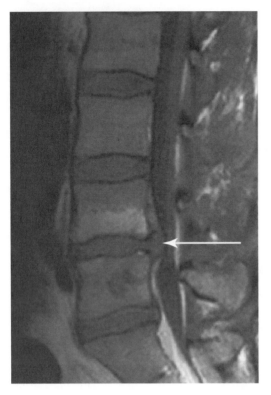

Figure 19.8 Herniated lumbar disk (*arrow*).

over 50 years of age. Local neck pain occurs in about half of these patients. In some cases, vibration sense in the distal lower extremities may become impaired early in the course. Clinical examination demonstrates hyperreflexia in the lower extremities and presence of a bilateral Babinski sign. At the levels of stenosis, segmental lower motor neuron lesions may develop, with muscle atrophy and areflexia in the hands and forearms. Over a period of several years, paresis and sensory deficits increase, and ultimately bladder, bowel, and/or sexual functions may become impaired. A sudden forceful hyperextension of the neck in patients with cervical spinal stenosis may result in acute SCI, as found in central cord syndrome (see Chapter 5).

In *lumbar spinal stenosis* of the upper lumbar spine, compression of the conus and/or cauda equina may occur, as may neurogenic intermittent claudication (also referred to as *pseudoclaudication*). This condition is characterized by pain, numbness, and/or weakness of the lower extremities when standing or walking. Clinically, this condition displays similarities with "true" intermittent claudication due to arterial insufficiency, but peripheral circulation is normal in neurogenic claudication; moreover, true vascular intermittent claudication does not cause symptoms when the patient is simply standing still, whereas the neurogenic variety may do so.

MRI will demonstrate reduction in disk height, disk protrusion/prolapse, facet hypertrophy, and foraminal stenosis. Computed tomography (CT) and CT myelography also provide good depiction of the anatomical conditions. However, the clinical manifestations determine whether surgery is appropriate, as many asymptomatic individuals have severe degenerative changes on radiologic examination. Patients with pronounced subjective symptoms, mainly involving pain and neurological deficit, are usually offered surgical decompression.

Spinal Manifestations in Rheumatoid Arthritis

Rheumatoid arthritis (RA) may involve the spinal column and indirectly also its neural elements. The atlantoaxial ligament keeps the C2 odontoid process fixated toward the anterior arch of the atlas. This ligament can become involved in RA, which leads to atlantoaxial subluxation, which in its turn can lead to compressive myelopathy. MRI may show inflammatory changes in the ligament, any instability, and sometimes the occurrence of granulomatous soft tissue thickening, known as *pannus* formation.

TUMORS

Epidural

Spinal *epidural* tumors are typically metastases from a carcinoma, myeloma, or lymphoma. The mother tumor is often in the kidney, prostate, lungs, or breast. It is not unusual for metastasis-related symptoms to be the first sign of disease. Symptoms include local and/or radicular pain and later signs of progressive myelopathy. Treatment usually involves partial removal of the tumor mass combined with fusion if necessary, high-dose corticosteroids, chemotherapy, and/or radiation therapy. The prognosis as

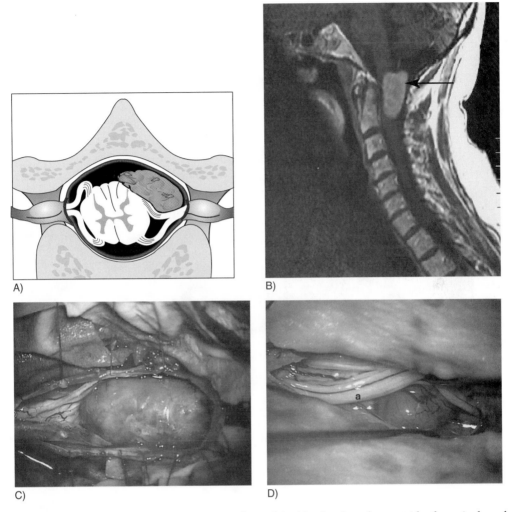

Figure 19.9 Intradural tumor. A: The tumor is located inside the dura but outside the spinal cord. B: Magnetic resonance image (MRI) showing a spinal meningioma at the level of the foramen magnum. C,D: Intradural tumor. C: Intraoperative image corresponding to B. D: Neurinoma located adjacent to the conus medullaris. The nerve roots (*a*) are subjected to compression. See also Color Plate Fig. 19.9C,D.

regards neurological deficits depends on how soon treatment is initiated after onset of symptoms. In cases of rapidly progressive paraparesis, surgery should be performed immediately if there is to be any chance of neurological recovery. Prognosis for survival depends on the biological properties of the tumor and the degree of spread.

Intradural Extramedullary

Intradural extramedullary tumors are usually benign, with very slow growth, and can often be cured by surgical removal. Common types of tumors include meningioma and neurinoma (Fig. 19.9A–D; also see Fig. 19.9C,D in Color Plate section). Symptoms are similar to those produced by spinal epidural tumors, but the course of disease is usually longer.

Intramedullary

Intramedullary tumors typically comprise ependymomas and astrocytomas (Fig. 19.10A–C). An ependymoma is often localized in the lower

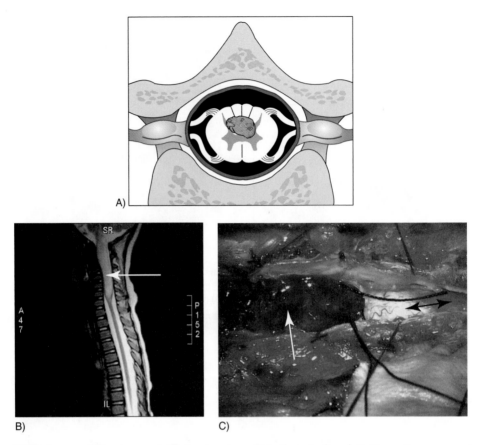

Figure 19.10 Intramedullary tumor. A: Tumor location within the spinal cord. B: Magnetic resonance image (MRI) showing a tumor in the upper spinal cord (*arrow*). C: Intraoperative image showing an intramedullary spinal cord tumor (*arrow*, tumor; *double arrow*, spinal cord). See also Color Plate Fig. 19.10C.

portion of the spinal cord and the cauda equina, whereas an astrocytoma arises mainly in the upper spinal cord. Ependymomas and "benign" (i.e., low grade of malignancy) astrocytomas are associated with a postoperative 10-year survival of about 80%, whereas the corresponding figure for malignant astrocytomas is 15%.

Intramedullary tumors are often associated with a clinical course with initial neuronal irritation and subsequently a breakdown of crossing pain and temperature fibers within the affected segment. As the tumor expands laterally, the segmental reflex arcs will be interrupted. Disease affecting the sympathetic pathways of the cervical spinal cord may produce a unilateral or bilateral Horner syndrome (i.e., ptosis, miosis, and enophthalmos). If the lesion extends toward the anterior horn cells, segmental muscle atrophy and paresis will also arise. Only at a

later stage, when the tumor has expanded far out into the periphery of the spinal cord, will the long pathways be affected. In these cases, bilateral signs of injury to the pyramidal tracts with progressive spastic paraparesis are noted. The dorsal columns appear to be relatively resistant to infiltration or distortion, and any manifestations from these pathways are late signs in intramedullary lesions. In the final stages of this process, only the most peripheral fibers that conduct sacral sensory nerve impulses will function (sacral sparing).

MYELOMENINGOCELE

Myelomeningocele (MMC) is caused by a defective closure of the neural tube and occurs in about 3/10,000 births (Fig. 19.11). Etiologically, the condition is associated with hereditary factors,

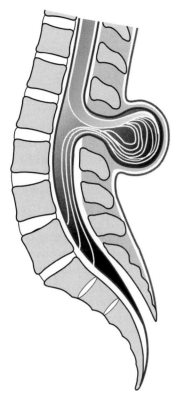

Figure 19.11 Myelomeningocele. The hernial sac contains both spinal meninges and neural tissue.

obesity, folic acid deficiency, diabetes mellitus, and treatment of pregnant women with certain antiepileptics. The hernia is usually located at the lumbosacral level, and there is a common association with congenital defects of the brain, especially hydrocephalus (i.e., dilatation of the cerebral ventricular system due to disruption of CSF circulation) and Chiari II malformations. Mortality during childhood is particularly high in this patient group, and has been reported to be about 40% up to the age of 20. The increased mortality is mainly due to shunt–associated CNS infections and to complications associated with the malformations.

Treatment for MMC involves early closure of the defect and ventriculoperitoneal shunting for hydrocephalus (i.e., surgical implantation of a tube to shunt the CSF from the ventricles of the brain to, e.g., the abdominal cavity). The rehabilitation process is complicated by a high rate of cognitive disorders, in part related to more or less extensive concomitant cerebral malformations, in part to hydrocephalus-related complications such as infection and dysfunction within the shunt system. Chiari II malformations are sometimes complicated by the development of *hydrosyringomyelia*.

This condition is neurologically characterized by flaccid paralysis and a predominance of sensory deficits. Neurological function may deteriorate, mainly due to shunt dysfunction, hydrosyringomyelia, and/or tethering of the spinal cord. Tethering may lead to progressive sensorimotor impairment, increased spasticity, pain, progressive scoliosis, orthopedic deformity in the lower extremities, and/or bladder and bowel dysfunction.

Other medical problems may include stunted growth, impaired growth of paralyzed extremities, precocious puberty, and/or growth hormone deficiency. Obesity is common. The risk of pressure ulcers is high given the unfavorable combination of sensorimotor impairment with concurrent cognitive dysfunction. Orthopedic problems may include club foot, hip dislocation, and knee flexion contractures. Kyphoscoliosis is very common, and its incidence increases with age, particularly up to the point of skeletal maturity. Progression of scoliosis must be regularly monitored both clinically and radiologically, and surgical intervention is often indicated.

Considering the rarity and complexity of this condition, children with MMC should be treated in specialized pediatric neurology units. Once these individuals reach adulthood, continued monitoring and management may be transferred to the adult SCI unit.

MOTOR NEURON DISEASE/AMYOTROPHIC LATERAL SCLEROSIS

Motor neuron disease is characterized by progressive degeneration of neurons in the motor cortex and in the anterior horns of the spinal cord. The etiology is unknown. A small number of cases are familial. In 90% of cases, disease onset is after the age of 40. Different clinical variants occur: *primary lateral sclerosis* (dominance of upper motor neuron lesions), *progressive muscular atrophy* (dominance of lower motor neuron lesions), *and progressive bulbar paralysis* (muscles innervated from the brainstem are preferentially affected). The different variants frequently overlap. Clinically, patients often present a mixed picture of upper and lower motor neuron damage. Bladder and bowel function, as well as sensory function, are unaffected. The disease often leads to death due to respiratory insufficiency within 3–5 years. Typically, the hands are involved first with progressive paresis and muscle atrophy, followed by insidiously increasing spastic paraparesis. This clinical syndrome may resemble that seen in cervical spondylotic myelopathy (see earlier discussion), which thus is an important and treatable differential diagnosis. MRI should therefore always be done. Neurophysiological investigations are also often carried out, mainly to rule out treatable motor polyneuropathy, which constitutes another differential diagnosis. Electromyography (EMG) typically demonstrates widespread muscular denervation.

We should also briefly mention some other rare diseases characterized by progressive muscle atrophy due to involvement of the anterior horn motor neurons. *Werdnig-Hoffman disease* (spinal muscular atrophy type I) is usually fatal in early childhood. *Kugelberg-Welander disease* (spinal muscular atrophy type III) is a juvenile and more benign variant of Werdnig-Hoffman disease, and *Duchenne-Aran disease* is an adult form of this condition. Please refer to specialist literature for further details.

OTHER CONDITIONS

Radiation-induced Myelopathy

Radiation-induced myelopathy may arise after radiation therapy especially for larynx, bronchial, and esophageal cancer, as well as Hodgkin disease. The pathogenic process is likely related to radiation-induced vasculitis (inflammation with occlusion of the spinal cord vessels). Spinothalamic sensory symptoms dominate the acute clinical picture. Sensory symptoms appear to be more severe than motor symptoms, in contrast to the clinical picture seen with spinal cord compression due to metastasis, which constitutes an important differential diagnosis. Onset of symptoms is typically within 9–18

months following radiation therapy, in contrast to so-called acute transient radiation myelopathy which has a clinical picture characterized by early onset a prominent Lhermitte sign.

Cystic Myelopathy/Syringomyelia

This condition is characterized by fluid-filled expansive cavities within the spinal cord caused by a disturbance in CSF circulation. This obstruction to the normal flow of CSF may be due to a congenital malformation such as an Arnold-Chiari syndrome (Fig. 19.12). In this condition, the cerebellar tonsils are pulled down to the level of the C2 arch, instead of being at the level of the foramen magnum (Arnold-Chiari type II). An obstruction of CSF circulation may also arise secondary to prior arachnoiditis. Early symptoms include dissociated sensory loss and pain due to damage of the crossing spinothalamic fibers. As the cavity expands in a

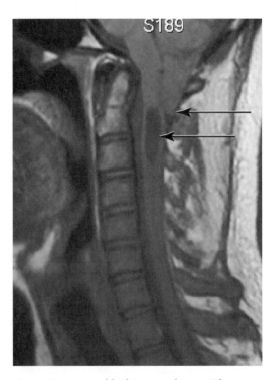

Figure 19.12 Arnold-Chiari syndrome. The cerebellar tonsil (amygdaline nucleus) in this case is pulled down to the C2 arch level, upper arrow, the cerebellar tonsil is positioned at the C2 arch level; lower arrow: intramedullary cyst.

craniocaudal direction, additional spinal cord segments successively become involved. During expansion from the central spinal cord to the periphery, progressive paresis and impairment of other sensory modalities also occur. MRI confirms the diagnosis. The course of this disease is rather unpredictable. Treatment is surgical in cases where syringomyelia produces significant symptoms (see Chapter 30).

Subacute Combined Degeneration

This condition is due to vitamin B_{12} deficiency. Most patients are elderly. Degenerative changes occur in both central and peripheral nervous system myelin. The earliest symptoms are related to peripheral nerve damage and include paresthesias, areflexia, and gait ataxia. Within the spinal cord, the posterior columns become involved first, followed by the lateral columns (thus "combined degeneration"). Neurological examination shows decreased vibration sense and proprioception in the lower extremities. Deep tendon reflexes may be hyperactive (due to pyramidal tract involvement) or weak (due to peripheral nerve involvement). This condition may also be accompanied by dementia and optical nerve atrophy. One-quarter of patients with this condition do not demonstrate the megaloblastic (pernicious) anemia, which otherwise usually accompanies this condition. Most cases involve an underlying deficiency of intrinsic factor, which is required for B_{12} absorption from the small intestine. Further tests may show depressed serum levels of vitamin B_{12} and high levels of homocysteine and methylmalonic acid. Antibodies to intrinsic factor are also present. It is important to diagnose this condition, since vitamin B_{12} substitution may lead to complete cure of symptoms.

Hereditary Spastic Paraplegia

Hereditary spastic paraplegia is a rare condition with variable heredity and a protracted course. The pathology involves the lateral corticospinal tracts, and sometimes the dorsal columns. The course of disease is progressive, and onset is characterized by progressive stiffness of the legs. Involvement of the upper extremities comes later

and may be less pronounced. Significant bladder involvement is uncommon until the late stages of the disease. Spasticity strongly dominates the clinical picture. Deep tendon reflexes are highly increased, and in some patients muscular hypertonia is so pronounced that reflexes cannot be elicited because the muscles are constantly in maximum contraction. Sensory involvement may occur. A recessive hereditary form usually has its onset at age 7–10 and is associated with a poorer prognosis, while a dominant hereditary form usually begins after age 20 years and has a more benign course.

Friedreich Ataxia

Friedreich ataxia is autosomal (i.e., non–sex-linked) recessive (i.e., both parents must carry the trait). Pathologic changes, usually degenerative in nature, involve structures such as the dorsal root ganglia, dorsal columns, lateral corticospinal tract, and the dorsal spinocerebellar tract. Onset of symptoms is usually before age 20. Signs of myelopathy are prominent. Patients demonstrate progressive gait ataxia, decreased deep tendon reflexes in the lower extremities, presence of Babinski sign, diminished proprioception and vibration sense in the lower extremities, and dysarthria. Many patients exhibit cardiomyopathy and 10–20% develop diabetes mellitus. The diagnosis is confirmed through demonstration of a characteristic chromosomal defect.

High-voltage Electric Shock

Electricity, passing through the spinal cord as in lightning strikes or accidents involving high voltage may result in a progressive myelopathy.

Decompression Illness

Decompression illness, also known as "the bends," is caused by rapidly moving from a high atmospheric pressure environment to one with low pressure, and results in the formation of intra- or extravascular bubbles from inert dissolved gases within the blood and tissues. These bubbles may cause symptoms by directly damaging axons, or indirectly via thromboembolism. Treatment involves recompression in a hyperbaric chamber. In 90% of cases, the prognosis is good, provided that treatment is initiated early after onset of symptoms.

Psychogenic Paraplegia

Psychogenic or "functional" paraplegia refers to paraplegia without a demonstrable organic cause. Functional paraplegia poses a major challenge for everyone involved. It is believed that the condition is due to conscious or subconscious psychological factors. It is uncommon for people to consciously feign paraplegia. When the condition is partly or completely thought to be due to subconscious psychological factors, the term *conversion disorder* is applied. In certain cases an obvious precipitating psychological trauma or overt secondary gain is present. Not infrequently, patients appear to be surprisingly emotionally unaffected, given the degree of severity of the functional deficit.

Clinically, the condition often presents with flaccid paraplegia, but with normal deep tendon reflexes, normal bladder and bowel function, and absence of muscle atrophy (other than possibly as secondary to inactivity/immobilization). Sensory loss may involve a stocking or glove distribution, or may in other ways be inconsistent with expected anatomic distribution. The diagnosis is one of exclusion. An experienced examiner often finds support for the diagnosis in the physical examination, but sometimes organic conditions such as MS may present with bizarre symptoms and be associated with psychosocial problems or personality disorders; therefore, such findings do not necessarily exclude concurrent organic disease. Despite extensive neuroradiological, neurophysiological, and clinical laboratory workup, no organic etiology for the clinical picture may be found. The psychological and psychosocial circumstances need to be tactfully addressed. It is rarely appropriate to directly confront the patient, who then risks humiliation, which may result in deterioration of the condition or legal action. Sometimes these patients respond well to regular SCI rehabilitation process at a spinal unit. The prospect of a favorable prognosis should be conveyed to the patient, preferably with some elements of positive psychological suggestion ("your legs will almost certainly be able to support you by next week if you train hard").

ACUTE STRESS REACTIONS AND PSYCHOLOGICAL DEFENSE MECHANISMS

Sustaining an acute SCI always entails a major psychological trauma for victim and family alike. The course of the stress reaction may span many years. During the early stages, both patient and family protect themselves against the scope of the event through several more or less subconscious *defense mechanisms*. Common psychological defense mechanisms include denial, projection, intellectualization, and avoidance.

Denial means that the patient simply does not accept that she is the victim of a severe injury with probably irreversible consequences. As long as denial dominates the psychological picture, it is extremely difficult to convey to the patient information and insight that requires an adequate perception of reality.

Projection may sometimes entail aggressive outbursts toward healthcare staff and others as a reaction to the frustration caused by the injury. In such cases, it is important to understand the underlying cause of the patient's behavior and avoid direct confrontation.

Intellectualization may be expressed as a purely cognitive (intellectual) acceptance of the injury, such as by focusing on all available factual information, but without any emotional reaction.

Avoidance is reflected by various ways of defending oneself from reminders of the disability, for example by avoiding looking in the mirror and/or by avoiding contact with other people with disabilities.

ADAPTATION

To handle the crisis that an SCI entails, the patient's *coping strategies* (i.e., the ways in which the patient handles the situation) will come to play a major role. Usually, it is more difficult for introverts to cope with the situation than for extroverts. Persons with poor self-confidence and/or self-esteem who previously were highly concerned with physical appearance and achievement will experience the injury as particularly frustrating. Persons with an *external locus of control* will consider their chances of affecting their life situation as negligible and will thereby experience problems in the rehabilitation setting. Conversely, an internal locus of control is associated with a feeling of ability to impact personal destiny, something which significantly facilitates the rehabilitation process. Moreover, the presence or absence of a well-developed social network will affect the rehabilitation process. Persons who live in relative isolation will, as a rule, require more support from staff than will those who are more gregarious.

The adaptation process following SCI may last several years. This is particularly important to bear in mind in the current healthcare setting, as hospital stays become successively shorter for economic reasons. A significant portion of the psychological reactions to the injury will often first become manifest *after* the patient has been discharged home, due in part to the short length of stay in the hospital, the early presence of insight-blocking defense mechanisms, and sometimes heavy sedation with drugs during the early rehab phase. This underscores the significance of a well-structured outpatient follow-up post trauma.

MENTAL DISORDERS

Several studies suggest that mental disorders are more common among persons with SCI than in the general population. It has been reported that *depression* or significant depressive symptoms occur in about 25% of men and 50% of women during the post-acute phase. Differentiation from a "normal" grief reaction to trauma is sometimes difficult, and treatment with antidepressants often should be initiated in unclear cases.

Sleep disturbances are common (see later discussion) and may be both a reason for and effect of mental problems. Disturbed sleep results in a number of adverse psychological and physical effects, and a short course of hypnotics is often indicated.

In some cases, a patient may suffer from *posttraumatic stress disorder* (PTSD). Typically, in this condition, a person who has been exposed to a traumatic event continually relives the experience in thoughts or nightmares, avoids stimuli associated with the trauma, and suffers from a decrease in vitality and an increase in irritability. Studies have shown that up to one-third of patients demonstrate this condition.

Other emotional sequelae may relate to clinical or subclinical *traumatic brain injury* sustained at the same time as the SCI. In suspected cases, a neuroradiological and neuropsychological workup may help define the degree of organic brain damage.

Poor mental health has a negative impact on the rehabilitation process. For example, depression increases the risk of urinary tract infections and pressure ulcers, and also contributes to general poor health. The tendency for such patients to engage in substance abuse and other self-destructive behavior increases. All things considered, well-structured psychological management becomes an essential component of both the initial and long-term rehabilitation of persons with SCI. It is important not to view the psychologist or psychiatrist as someone to consult only in the presence of overt psychiatric disease; instead, they should be considered as integral to the rehabilitation team as the physical or occupational therapist.

Many of the psychological challenges of SCI will first manifest after patients are discharged home and confront "a new reality." A few of the many challenges to be met include the ability to clearly communicate need for assistance, an increased dependence on partners and other family members, and coping with sexual dysfunction.

The risk of substance abuse and self-destructive behavior must be considered. *Suicide* is reported to be the most common cause of death in the post-acute phase following discharge from the hospital; the suicide rate among patients with SCI is five to ten times greater than that in the population at large.

When considering long-term satisfaction and quality of life after SCI, the degree of neurological deficits appears to play a lesser role than factors such as presence of pain, incontinence, and spasticity.

MANAGEMENT

All patients with SCI should be met with an open, optimistic, and affirming attitude. They should be encouraged to express their feelings, and time must be allotted to listen to what they have to say. It is essential to be understanding of aggressive behavior and poor compliance, especially during the early post-injury stages. Respect for the patient's personal dignity is paramount. This approach is reflected in how the caregiver handles sensitive issues in the rehabilitative process, such as bladder and bowel management, personal hygiene, and incontinence. Many patients need formal counseling. Such counseling should be part of the rehabilitation plan. It is important for each patient to have the opportunity for assessment by a psychologist or psychiatrist in order to determine whether psychopharmacological treatment, psychotherapy, and/or additional psychiatric and neuropsychological testing are needed. Among psychotherapeutic treatment options, cognitive psychotherapy has made significant inroads in recent years. Not only patients, but also family and friends, need to be made aware of their psychological reactions in conjunction with an injury.

SOCIAL IMPACT

The nuclear family is the social unit most strongly affected by SCI. In many cases, the social roles within the family change radically. With respect to the relationship between man and woman, there is a risk that the caregiver role outcompetes the partner role. The divorce rate is higher in relationships in which one party has a SCI. This is mainly true when the injury afflicts one of the partners in an already established relationship. In cases where the relationship was formed after the SCI occurred, divorce rates are not elevated.

With respect to parenting, several studies have shown that persons with SCI are neither better nor worse in this role than able-bodied parents. Physical disability in and of itself does not preclude being a good parent.

In most cases, the SCI clearly has a negative impact on personal finances. However, on the contrary, in some cases there may actually be a *negative* economic incentive for returning to work. This is unfortunate, since employment, in addition to its financial value, also serves to improve quality of life and promote health. In general, the ability to return to work should command greater attention in the rehabilitation process than what is currently the case. Routine approval of disability retirement is to be avoided, and a majority of patients with SCI regrettably fail to return to the work force.

Thanks to legal reforms involving service support and assistance for people with disabilities, many SCI patients in several countries are now entitled to *personal assistance*. The law contains provisions for monetary compensation to certain people with disabilities, to cover the cost of such assistance. In many cases, such acts have allowed persons with SCI to engage in work, leisure, and community activities to a much greater extent than previously. However, such reforms also entail a risk of becoming a substitute for optimal rehabilitation interventions. The option to become self-sufficient is always preferable to remain being dependent on assistance, even if this will require a greater investment during the initial care period. It is reasonable to assume that a rehabilitation outcome resulting in optimal functional capacity and a high degree of autonomy is preferable to dependence on assistance and subsidies.

Suggested Reading

Several textbooks are available for further study as regards long-term management of SCI. The following selection includes the major "classic" textbooks on the subject (e.g., Guttman, Bedbrook, Rossier), which are perhaps mostly of historic interest. In addition, the list includes some recommended comprehensive current textbooks.

Bedbrook GM. *The Care and Management of Spinal Cord Injuries.* New York: Springer-Verlag, 1981.

Guttmann L. *Spinal Cord Injuries: Comprehensive Management and Research.* Oxford: Blackwell Scientific Publications, 1973, 1976.

Illis LS. *Spinal Cord Dysfunction, Vol. II. Intervention and Treatment.* Oxford: Oxford University Press, 1992.

Kirshblum S, Campagnolo DI, DeLisa JA, eds. *Spinal Cord Medicine.* Philadelphia, Pa.: Lippincott Williams & Wilkins, 2002.

Lee BY, Ostrander LE, Cochran GVB, Shaw WW. *The Spinal Cord Injured Patient: Comprehensive Management.* Philadelphia: W.B. Saunders Company, 1991.

Lin VW, ed. *Spinal Cord Medicine: Principles and Practice.* New York: Demos Publishing Medical, 2003.

Mathias CJ, Bannister R. *Autonomic Failure. A Textbook of Clinical Disorders of the Autonomic Nervous System,* 4th ed. New York: Oxford University Press, 1999:494–513.

Randal R, Betz MJ. *The Child with a Spinal Cord Injury.* Shriners Hospitals for Crippled Children Symposium. American Academy of Orthopaedic Surgeons, 1996.

Randolph W, Evans MD. *Neurology and Trauma.* Philadelphia: W.B. Saunders Company, 1996:276–322.

Rossier AB. *Rehabilitation of the Spinal Cord Injury Patient.* Zurich: University Medical Clinic, Cantonal Hospital Zurich.

Somers MF. *Spinal Cord Injury: Functional Rehabilitation.* New Jersey: Prentice Hall. Inc., 2001.

Zejdlik CP. *Management of Spinal Cord Injury,* 2nd ed. Jones and Bartlett Publishers, Inc. 1992.

21 Pain

Pain receptors, also called nociceptors, are structures that become stimulated when there is a threat of tissue damage. Such receptors consist of free nerve endings, of thin *myelinated* A-δ fibers or *unmyelinated* C fibers (Fig. 21.1).

A-δ and C fibers convey different types of pain sensations. The A-δ fibers have higher conduction velocity and give rise to a fast, distinct, well-localized pain. Pain conveyed through the C fibers is dull, diffuse, more difficult to localize. The pain fibers enter the spinal cord via the *dorsal root entry zone* (DREZ), and usually terminate in Rexed laminae I, II, and V (Fig. 21.2). At the first synapse located in the dorsal column or dorsal horn, the signal is received and modified via interneurons and descending pathways before continuing to the supraspinal levels via the second neuron.

Certain primary afferents branch along the longitudinal axis of the posterior horn in the Lissauer tract (Fig. 21.2), which means that these primary afferents are connected at several levels in the spinal cord. According to convergence theory, an individual neuron within the dorsal horn may communicate with several neurons from one type of tissue and/or with several neurons from different tissues. This complicates the task of the brain to adequately localize the origin of the pain.

The posterior horn of the spinal cord contains various types of nociceptive neurons. In part, there are specific neurons that only receive a small number of primary nociceptive afferents; these neurons only cover a small area of the body, such as one foot. In part, multireceptive or *wide-dynamic-range neurons* (WDR neurons) with large receptor fields receive impulses from different A and C fibers (Fig. 21.3).

When the spinal cord is injured, anatomical and neurochemical changes occur within its tissue, the end result of which is an excitatory condition characterized by hyperactivity (hypersensitivity) within the receptor neurons of the dorsal horn. This hyperactivity may be due to either an increase in C-fiber activity or an increase in demyelination. Intracellular biochemical changes, especially within Rexed lamina II (substantia gelatinosa), also contribute to hyperreactivity. Substances involved in nociceptive transmission include peptides like substance P, excitatory amino acids (e.g., glutamate and aspartate), inhibitory neurotransmitters (e.g., glycine and γ-aminobutyric acid [GABA]), opioids, and nitric oxides. GABA and the opioids are of particular interest in the context of surgical treatment. GABA has been identified as an inhibitory amino acid for impulse transmission in the spinal cord. Animal studies have shown that release of GABA decreases in response to peripheral injury and the presence of neuropathic pain.

Pain is a major problem in the aftermath of SCI. More than two-thirds of all SCI patients suffer from chronic pain, and in about one-third the pain is so severe that it interferes with daily activities and reduces quality of life.

According to the International Association for the Study of Pain (IASP), pain is defined as "an unpleasant sensory and emotional experience associated with actual or potential tissue damage, or described in terms of such damage." This definition emphasizes the subjectivity of pain, and that pain can be both a physiological phenomenon as well as an emotional and cognitive *reaction*.

The pain system encompasses peripheral receptors; afferent neural pathways; connecting and modulating centers in the spinal cord; ascending pathways; centers in the brainstem, thalamus, cerebral cortex, and other areas; and descending pathways.

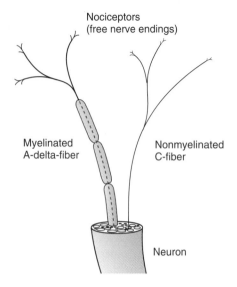

Figure 21.1 Nociceptors.

A person with paraplegia or tetraplegia is of course potentially subject to all painful conditions which can affect the general population. In addition, spinal cord lesions predispose to certain additional painful conditions. In particular, the spinal cord lesions can directly engage pain pathways, creating neuropathic pain (discussed later in this section). Moreover, people with para- and tetraplegia are also forced to use remaining nonparalyzed muscles and joints in a nonphysiologic manner, with musculoskeletal pain as a common result. On the other hand, impaired sensation may *mask* some normally painful conditions: for example, a fracture below the level of injury may manifest itself by malaise, sweating, and spasticity but no pain, and a distended bladder may result in autonomic dysreflexia with severe pulsating headache, but without the otherwise expected local pain.

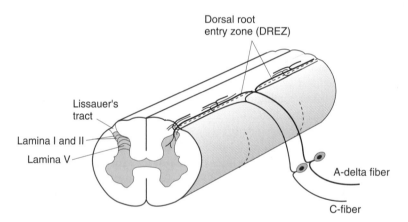

Figure 21.2 Entry of pain fibers into spinal cord tissue.

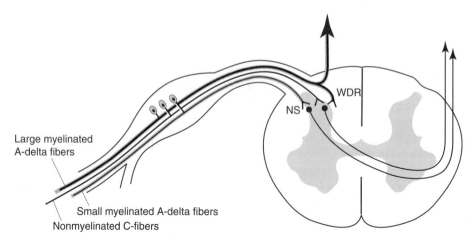

Figure 21.3 Wide-dynamic-range (WDR) neuron.

Pain may be nociceptive or neuropathic in nature. *Nociceptive* pain arises when intact pain pathways are activated by an injury to tissues outside the nervous system, such as the skin, internal organs, or musculoskeletal system. *Neuropathic* pain arises when a direct injury occurs to the neural pathways within the peripheral or central nervous system. Both these types of pain are overrepresented among SCI patients.

Consequently, we must take into consideration not only the "conventional" spectrum of pain-inducing conditions, but also pain as a direct result of SCI, and also the "pain equivalents" unique to persons with SCI (e.g., where pain may manifest by "proxy symptoms" such as spasticity or dysreflexia). These factors combine to make the workup of pain especially challenging in this patient group.

The most problematic type of pain following SCI is the neuropathic kind. Neuropathic pain is accompanied by a variety of symptoms that may occur in isolation or in combination:

- *Allodynia*: Pain elicited by a normally non-painful stimulus, such as light touch
- *Anesthesia dolorosa*: Pain within an anesthetic area
- *Dysesthesia*: An unpleasant and abnormal sensation
- *Hyperalgesia*: An amplified sensation of pain in response to a painful stimulus
- *Hyperesthesia*: Increased sensitivity to both touch and pain stimuli
- *Hyperpathia*: An amplified sensation of pain, especially with repetitive stimulation, with concurrent elevation of the pain threshold
- *Causalgia*: Persistent burning pain, allodynia, and hyperpathia, often combined with vasomotor and sudomotor dysfunction (e.g., altered vascular perfusion and sweating) and trophic changes (e.g., skin atrophy).

The reasons for the frequent occurrence of neuropathic pain after SCI have not yet been fully elucidated. Suggested theories include: (a) "spontaneous" generation of impulses in damaged nerve fibers; (b) "cross-conduction" from one nerve fiber to another via adjacent demyelinated areas that create "false" synapses,

known as *ephapses*; (c) a "release" phenomenon of pain transmission due to interruption of descending pain-inhibiting pathways and/or interruption of afferent pain-inhibiting sensory impulses; and/or (d) chemical hypersensitivity in deafferentated neurons and receptors.

It is important to elucidate both the type and the degree of pain, since these factors govern treatment strategies. Unfortunately, there is no single, generally accepted pain classification system for SCI. Hereafter, we will adhere to the system proposed by Bryce and Ragnarsson, which is based on three cornerstones: *pain distribution* in relation to neurological level of lesion (above, at, below); neuropathic or nociceptive *pain*; and various *etiological subgroups*. This system is not perfect, especially in regard to the concept of neuropathic versus nociceptive pain. Neuropathic-type pain (e.g., burning, cutting, stabbing, electric) sometimes occurs in proven nociceptive conditions, whereas nociceptive-type pain (e.g., dull pain, myalgia, load-induced pain) sometimes occurs in proven neuropathic conditions. There is a risk that the thought process will be led astray if such labels are rigidly applied. This pitfall may be avoided by remembering that in this context, the terms "neuropathic" and "nociceptive" refer to descriptions of *symptoms* rather than of causes. It is therefore preferable to record the patient's actual description of pain and postpone applying the label "neuropathic" or "nociceptive" until the etiology has been confirmed.

PAIN ABOVE THE LEVEL OF INJURY

Nociceptive Pain

The prevalence of *musculoskeletal shoulder pain* among persons with paraplegia is 40–50%. Common underlying causes include chronic impingement, subacromial bursitis, biceps tendinitis, and aseptic necrosis of the humeral head. An imbalance of the shoulder musculature, with relative weakness of the adductors and external rotators, contributes to the development and persistence of rotator cuff impingement. Exercise programs should therefore be aimed at improving strength in the posterior shoulder muscles (external rotators, rhomboids, trapezius, and adductors) and stretching of the anterior shoulder muscles, in order to restore muscular balance in the joint. The sitting position in the wheelchair should be optimized. In addition, the patient should avoid using the arm in positions that provoke impingement, especially abduction/flexion of the arm in excess of 90 degrees in combination with inward rotation. Symptoms may be alleviated by avoiding overuse, by prescription of anti-inflammatory drugs, and/or by corticosteroid injection of the bursa or joint (see also the section "Shoulder Problems" in Chapter 22).

Neuropathic Pain

Carpal tunnel syndrome (with median nerve compression) is common among persons with paraplegia and low-level tetraplegia; prevalence increases with time. Contributing factors to this problem include repetitive trauma from wheelchair propulsion and repetitious increases in pressure within the carpal tunnel, such as during transfers.

Ulnar nerve neuropathy with site of compression in the wrist is also common. Preventive measures include padded gloves to protect the palmar aspect of the wrist and avoidance of weight-bearing on an extended wrist, by instead using a neutral wrist position. For more discussion please refer to Chapter 23.

PAIN AT THE LEVEL OF INJURY

Nociceptive Pain

Spinal posttraumatic instability may cause pain at the level of injury. This pain is often aggravated by movement and weight-bearing.

The prevalence of *musculoskeletal shoulder pain* among persons with tetraplegia (for whom this condition will be classified as being "pain at the level of injury," in contrast to persons with paraplegia where it is classified as "pain above the level of injury") is, as for persons with paraplegia, 40–60%. The causes are similar. In addition, a specific type of shoulder pain in tetraplegics may occur, known as *scapular pain,* located along the medial border of the scapula. Tenderness to palpation can be found over the

rhomboids, levator scapulae, and supra- and infraspinatus muscles. The pain is triggered by an imbalance of the rotator cuff muscles, with disproportionately more power for scapular retraction (pulling back) than for protraction (pushing forward). To avoid shoulder problems, an adequate sitting position in the wheelchair is important; in particular, the arms should be supported by the armrests, so that the weight of the humerus does not pull the humeral head from its socket. When performing range-of-motion exercises, the shoulder joint should not be flexed or abducted more than 90 degrees. Excessive loading of a shoulder joint with weak dynamic stabilizing musculature stresses the capsular ligaments, ultimately resulting in joint instability.

Pain from internal organs located at the level of injury mainly occurs when the neurological level of injury is below the midthoracic spinal cord. Nociceptive stimuli arising from the abdominal and pelvic organs are conveyed rostrally through visceral afferents that follow the sympathetic neural pathways. This kind of pain is often characterized as vague, diffuse, and difficult to localize. In these patients, it is necessary to be vigilant for diseases affecting internal organs, since the clinical presentation will be atypical.

Neuropathic Pain

Pain of this type may be either peripheral or central in origin. The former may be caused by a *segmental nerve root injury.* Such pain is often unilateral and paroxysmal (episodic), and distributed along a single dermatome. The latter, so-called central neuropathic pain, is often bilateral, with a band-shaped distribution and usually persisting. It is denoted as *transitional zone pain,* since it occurs at the border between normal and impaired or absent sensitivity. The cause is usually a direct lesion to the pain pathways in the spinal cord, with onset immediately after injury. Should onset of pain occur more than 6–12 months after injury, underlying *progressive posttraumatic myelopathy* (PPM) have to be ruled out. That condition is believed to be precipitated by scar tissue formation between the spinal cord and the meninges, which impairs cerebrospinal fluid circulation. It occurs in 2–5% of patients with traumatic SCI, and pain is the most

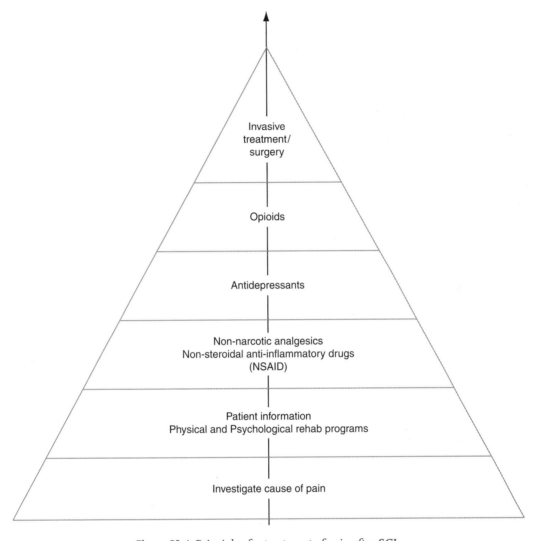

Figure 21.4 Principles for treatment of pain after SCI.

common presenting symptom. If the condition progresses, the pain may sometimes decrease concomitantly with loss of sensation in the affected segment. This corresponds to an ascending sensory level. Progressive paresis and other symptoms may also occur, see Chapter 30. Spinal cord MRI is the study of choice when PPM is suspected.

Patients with tetraplegia may display a *complex regional pain syndrome* (CRPS), producing neuropathic pain involving the upper extremities. This chronic pain is believed to be precipitated by impaired autonomic innervation. The CRPS concept has replaced the earlier terms *sympathetic reflex dystrophy* and *causalgia*. Such

pain is not distributed along a single peripheral nerve or nerve root, but has a more diffuse regional distribution. Frequent signs include local swelling, a change in skin circulation, and increased sweating. Bone scan may show a diffuse increase in uptake.

PAIN BELOW THE LEVEL OF INJURY

Nociceptive Pain

Nociceptive pain below the neurological lesion level may occur persons with incomplete SCI, or in patients with complete injuries but with a *zone of partial preservation* (segments below the level of injury with partially preserved function). Underlying causes include all medical conditions that cause nociceptive pain such as fractures, soft-tissue injuries, and diseases of the internal organs.

Neuropathic Pain

This pain is often of the central type; distribution is diffuse and the character is burning. The pain is continuous, but increases with stress, anxiety, fatigue, smoking, weather changes, and nociceptive stimuli below the level of injury. This type of pain is associated with an increase in electric discharge in the dorsal horns of the spinal cord and in the somatosensory thalamus. It is likely that central sensitization ("hypersensitivity") plays an important role, where an increase in neuronal excitability (irritability) for further nociceptive and non-nociceptive stimuli occurs.

CONSERVATIVE (NONINVASIVE) PAIN MANAGEMENT

Many patients with SCI suffer at least one type of chronic pain and about one in three patients suffers from such intense pain that quality of life is negatively impacted. Treatment for neuropathic pain, in addition to physical therapy and other nonpharmacological modalities, includes a large arsenal of possible medications. Drugs such as acetaminophen, tricyclic antidepressants, tramadol hydrochloride, gabapentin, baclofen, and sedatives may be tried. Unfortunately, the efficacy of drugs for neuropathic pain is often inadequate, and medication side effects create additional problems for these patients. Figure 21.4 provides an overview of treatment options, in stages from the basic to the advanced, for pain following SCI.

For causal treatment of nociceptive pain, see chapters devoted to specific affected organs.

22 | Musculoskeletal Problems

Musculoskeletal problems are very common after SCI and may give rise to added chronic disability. Several studies have shown the prevalence of musculoskeletal pain to be between 50% and 75%, and many factors contribute to this situation. *Osteoporosis* (i.e., loss of bone mass) is extensive below the level of lesion and the risk of fractures is high. Paralysis in itself causes *ergonomic problems,* in part due to poor trunk stability. The load on remaining functioning muscles increases, and normally non–weight-bearing joints are forced to support considerable body weight during transfers, pressure relieving maneuvers, and wheelchair propulsion. The list of factors contributing to musculoskeletal problems is lengthy. In addition to negative impact on the ability to perform activities of daily living (ADL), pain in itself often have a markedly negative effect on quality of life. Chronic pain is probably the major cause of diminished quality of life in the long-term after SCI (see also Chapter 21).

NECK AND BACK PROBLEMS

A number of factors contribute to pain in the neck and back. Individuals with traumatic SCI by default have various degrees of damage to the spinal column. Spinal paralysis typically leads to impaired muscle function in the trunk and thereby frequently to the development of *kyphoscoliosis.*

SHOULDER PROBLEMS

The most common causes of musculoskeletal pain after SCI involves pathology in and around the shoulder joints. The shoulder joint is designed for flexibility, rather than for weight-bearing, but SCI typically necessitates such increased demands on use of the upper extremities in daily life.

Skeletal components of the shoulder (Fig. 22.1) include the scapula, the clavicle, and the humerus. The humeroscapular joint is constructed to allow for movement, and is ill-suited for weight-bearing. The glenoid cavity is small and shallow in relation to the head of the joint. This joint has been likened to a golf ball resting on a peg; consequently the humeroscapular joint is dependent on a well-developed muscular "cuff" for its stability. The tendons of the muscles comprising this cuff—teres minor, subscapularis, infraspinatus, and supraspinatus—are gathered into a shared common tendon aponeurosis. This structure, known as the *rotator cuff*, is readily subject to injury, both from acute trauma and from chronic repetitive overuse. The approach to workup of shoulder problems includes a thorough history and clinical examination. Skeletal changes may be seen on plain x-ray. Soft-tissue changes can be visualized by magnetic resonance imaging (MRI) or with arthroscopy.

Rotator cuff ruptures, aseptic necrosis of the humeral head, and osteolysis of the distal clavicle are more common in persons with SCI than in the general population, especially among wheelchair-bound patients with paraplegia. Repetitive trauma to the upper extremities in conjunction with activities such as transfers and wheelchair propulsion is responsible for the damage. Among persons who manually propel their wheelchair, the space under the "ceiling" formed by the acromion, coracoid process, and ligaments will be narrowed. This situation predisposes to *impingement* of the rotator cuff.

Mild shoulder problems may be alleviated with anti-inflammatory drugs and possibly local corticosteroid injections. It is not settled whether

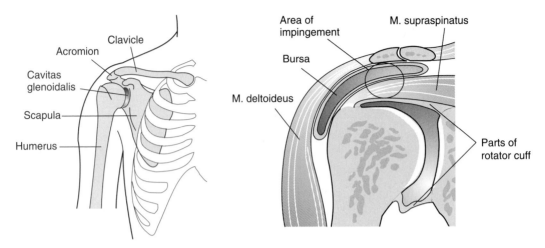

Figure 22.1 Anatomy of the shoulder. The picture illustrates the shallow joint socket, the basic construction of the joint that prioritizes mobility over stability, and the cuff surrounding the joint (rotator cuff). These anatomical conditions predispose the joint to impingement and overuse injuries resulting from the excessive loads placed upon the shoulder joint after SCI.

indications for surgical treatment of shoulder problems among SCI patients should be more liberal than those applied to the general population. However, it is clear that most surgical shoulder interventions in SCI patients require intense postoperative rehabilitation often in an in-patient setting. As long as postoperative immobilization is required for the shoulder joint, many persons with SCI will essentially be completely ADL-dependent.

ARM PROBLEMS

Not only the shoulders, but the entirety of upper extremities will typically be chronically overloaded after SCI, resulting in tendonitis and compression neuropathies. A correlation has been noted between such problems, and obesity and/or poor wheelchair handling technique.

The prevalence of elbow pain has been shown to be about 15%. A common maneuver that provokes such pain is pronation of the forearm, extension of the elbow, and simultaneous wrist extension while grasping grip rings as the person manually propels the wheelchair. The loads incurred during this maneuver put the patient at risk for *lateral epicondylitis* ("tennis elbow"). This condition is characterized by radial pain, especially with activation of the extensor

muscles. Due to chronic inflammation of the extensor muscle attachments, distinct palpatory tenderness may be elicited just distal to the epicondyle. Treatment options include anti-inflammatory medications, support strap, local steroid injection and, in therapy-resistant cases, surgical release of the extensor tendons from the epicondyle.

PREVENTATIVE AND REHABILITATIVE MEASURES

If musculoskeletal problems arise following SCI, the resultant impairment will become disproportionately great. Wheelchair-bound individuals with SCI have no opportunity to rest the upper extremities without becoming completely immobilized and ADL-dependent. Preventative exercises, appropriate trials of assistive devices, and early diagnosis and treatment are thus of great importance. In the shoulder joints, the external rotators are usually weaker than the internal rotators. Since the external rotators also help to hold the shoulder joint down, these muscles are important for preventing impingement. Exercise programs must therefore focus on restoring muscular balance around the shoulder joints. If chronic shoulder problems do arise, it becomes important to motivate the patient to accept an electric wheelchair at least in certain situations early on to relieve the shoulder joints. Recent years have seen the advent of a "hybrid" between manual and electrical wheelchairs, known as *push rim activated power assist wheelchairs* (PAPAWs). These wheelchairs are equipped with an assist motor that facilitates manual propulsion.

Obese patients should receive help with weight loss. Modern SCI units should offer exercise programs, qualified assistance in trying out assistive devices, and a thorough ergonomic analysis of sitting position and propulsion technique in order to counter the growing epidemic of musculoskeletal problems among SCI patients. Rehabilitation clinics should offer postsurgical inpatient care for adequate postoperative immobilization and functional training.

HETEROTOPIC OSSIFICATION

Heterotopic ossification (HO) was first described in 1918. HO is characterized by the formation of bone in tissues adjacent to joints (Fig. 22.2). The newly formed bone tissue is histologically identical to normal bone.

This condition may arise secondary to direct muscle trauma (so-called traumatic myositis ossificans), as a sequel of fracture or surgery in the hip joint, and in response to paralysis after central nervous system (CNS) injuries. HO has been described after both traumatic SCI and brain injuries. In the latter instances, the condition is always localized to a neurologically afflicted area; thus, in SCI, HO occurs *below the level of lesion*. The condition is more common among patients with complete lesions and with pronounced spasticity. The incidence is 20–30%, but only in about half of these patients does the condition pose clinically significant consequences. Large-scale HO may preclude a good sitting position in the wheelchair, contribute to the occurrence of pressure ulcers, and may worsen spasticity. Its cause is unknown. Probably both local and systemic inflammatory factors play a role, the latter referred to as *systemic inflammatory response syndrome* (SIRS).

Ossification is a three-stage process: in the first stage, an extracellular matrix called *osteoid* is formed, next the osteoid is *mineralized,* and finally, *mature bone tissue is formed.*

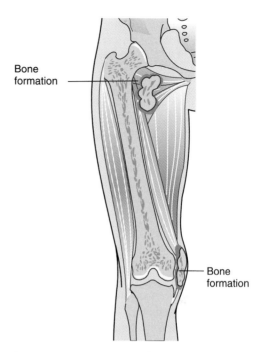

Figure 22.2 Heterotopic ossification. The process is characteristically located around the hip and knee joint.

This process usually begins during the first few weeks following trauma. The earliest symptom is *progressive limitation in the range of motion* within the afflicted joint, followed by *swelling, erythema, increased local tissue temperature,* and *pain*. Differential diagnosis includes deep vein thrombosis, erysipelas, osteomyelitis, and septic arthritis. In 60% of cases, the abnormal ossification occurs around the *hips*, typically anteromedial to the joint, and in 30% of cases around *the knee joints*, especially medially. In individuals with tetraplegia, bone may form around the shoulder or elbow joint in rare cases.

The Brooker classification divides HO into four groups:

- Class 1: Isolated islands of bone
- Class 2: More than 1 cm separates opposing ossification centers
- Class 3: Less than 1 cm separates opposing ossification centers
- Class 4: Total bony ankylosis

Laboratory studies in the early stages may show an elevation of serum alkaline phosphatase and CRP/ESR. Early on, bone scan may show active ossification. Plain x-rays demonstrate positive findings about 2–3 months after the start of the process, and initially show vague densities in the soft tissues around the joint. Once the inflammatory process tapers off, alkaline phosphatase levels normalize, as do the inflammatory parameters, and bone scan findings, while plain x-rays, magnetic resonance imaging (MRI), and/or computed tomography (CT) now show mature bone.

In the early stages anti-inflammatory drugs such as indomethacin 25 mg tid for 6 weeks may alleviate the process. Similarly, treatment with didronate for 6 months can be of benefit. For established, mature heterotopic bone, surgical resection is the only treatment option. Opinion is divided on whether physical therapy is harmful or helpful. Cautious range-of-motion exercises during the early stages are probably beneficial, while aggressive manipulations should be avoided. Physical therapy probably is of no use on mature HO with impaired mobility. Surgical treatment may be contemplated in cases with significant permanent loss of passive range of joint movement. Surgery should be postponed until the inflammatory process is well-controlled. The primary goal is to allow a reasonably acceptable sitting position in the wheelchair. Such a goal does not necessarily entail total resection of all heterotopic bone; instead, the goal may be more simply met through creating a pseudarthrosis (i.e., a "false joint") by performing a *wedge osteotomy* distal to the ankylosed joint. Surgical complications include extensive bleeding, wound infection, osteomyelitis, and reactivation of the HO process. Treatment with didronate is usually continued for 3–6 months postoperatively to prevent reactivation and recurrence. Particular care must be taken when providing postoperative physical therapy, as bony structures around the previously ankylotic joint is typically highly osteoporotic, which entails risk of fracture.

OSTEOPOROSIS

Soon after injury to the spinal cord, urinary excretion of calcium and hydroxyproline increases as an early sign of bone resorption. Usually these markers revert to normal levels within 1 year post-injury. The degree of demineralization is proportional to the degree of decreased load on the skeleton. Thus, demineralization primarily affects the skeleton *below* the neurologic level of injury. In wheelchair-bound patients, osteoporosis is pronounced in the legs but not in the arms. Among persons with paraplegia, mineralization of the skeleton in the upper extremities can even increase as a consequence of the chronically increased load on the arms in conjunction with wheelchair propulsion. Within an affected extremity, demineralization is more pronounced distally than proximally. The weight load on the spinal column remains essentially normal and therefore spinal decalcification does not occur.

Plain x-rays are relatively insensitive to osteoporosis; at least a 30–40% bone loss is required to become visible. Moreover, plain films can only provide a rough qualitative assessment. A better method for assessing bone mass is *dual energy X-ray absorptiometry* (DXA). DXA enables regional quantification of bone mass.

The possibility to reverse demineralization after SCI has been studied. The most important measure is to regularly subject the skeleton to weight-bearing. However, it is difficult to achieve sufficient intensity during sessions of stand training. Functional electrical stimulation (FES) by means of cycling exercise has been shown to partially reverse demineralization, provided it is carried out regularly and with sufficient intensity. However, this method is expensive and time-consuming, something which limits its feasibility. There is no consensus on pharmacological treatment. Estrogen replacement may be given to postmenopausal women. Other treatment options that have been suggested include administration of calcium and vitamin D supplements, bisphosphonates, and even anabolic steroids. The risk–benefit analysis for long-term pharmacological treatment is complex.

Increased Risk of Fractures

Osteoporosis is associated with an increased risk of fractures. Most fractures due to osteoporosis in patients with SCI occur below the neurological level of lesion, and especially around the knee joints. Even low-energy trauma, such as falling from the wheelchair, may suffice to cause a fracture. Because of sensory loss, pain is often absent and it is therefore important to be extra vigilant for other signs of fracture, such as local swelling, increased spasticity, episodes of autonomic dysreflexia, and unexplained fever. Clinicians should use liberal indications for x-ray after even minor trauma and/or when clinical signs of fracture are present.

IMPAIRED HAND FUNCTION

Reconstructive Hand Surgery

Hand surgery for patients with SCI may in selected cases significantly improve functional outcomes. All persons with tetraplegia should thus at some time be referred to a specialist for assessment. Successful surgical outcome presumes a thorough preoperative workup and a skilled surgical specialist. Also essential is a team consisting of physiatrists, occupational therapists, and physical therapists who are able to assess the patient's hand function while considering it in relation to the total picture, and who can provide the necessary postoperative training. The patient is, of course, also key, and the individual's motivation and ability to participate are essential. The initial evaluation by a hand surgeon should be postponed until the neurological status has stabilized, which in trauma cases usually occurs about 6–12 months after the time of injury. In addition to a detailed analysis of shoulder, arm, and hand function, preoperative assessment should also include an analysis of how the patient manages daily activities such as transfers, wheelchair propulsion, and ADLs.

Reconstructive treatment began to develop in the 1940s. The therapeutic arsenal initially mainly consisted of *tenodesis*, in this case reattachment of tendons to bones, in order to achieve passive finger flexion during wrist extension and passive finger extension during wrist flexion. During the 1960s, techniques were developed for muscle–tendon transfers, initially with highly varied results. A milestone occurred with the publication of the 1975 monograph by Swedish hand surgeon Erik Moberg. The basis of Moberg's philosophy is that, after the brain, the hand is the most important remaining resource for tetraplegic patients. Persons with tetraplegia are constantly placing load on their arms and hands for transfers, and this must be taken into account when choosing a surgical procedure. Moberg also underscored the important psychosocial role of the hands as a tool for human contact. Therefore certain surgical reconstructions that resulted in stiff, clawlike hands were unacceptable. He considered the *key grip (lateral pinch)* between the thumb and the side of the index finger to be of superior value for patients with tetraplegia than the "pincer grip" between the tips of the thumb and index finger. For the large group of tetraplegic patients with a C5–C6 neurological level of injury, the goal of reconstructive surgery should be to achieve *elbow extension* and a key grip in at least one upper extremity. Most of Moberg's principles still guide hand surgery to this day.

The American Spinal Injury Association (ASIA) classification system is not sufficiently detailed to serve as the sole basis for preoperative assessment for reconstructive hand surgery. A more detailed classification is therefore used to assess residual sensorimotor function in the upper extremities. Shoulder function is often affected after a cervical SCI, which is also of significance for more distal arm and hand function. Shoulder examination is therefore included in the hand surgery assessment. A careful analysis of functional capacity in all upper extremity muscles should be carried out. Sensory function is just as important as motor function; this is because a hand devoid of sensation is hardly useful, even if motor function should be intact. Two-point discrimination is used as the main indicator of proprioceptive function. At one extreme of the classification spectrum are those patients who completely lack voluntary muscle function distal to the elbow. At the other end of the spectrum are those patients with preserved function of all muscles, with the exception of the intrinsic muscles of the hand.

Elbow extension can be achieved through a deltoid-to-triceps transfer, or a biceps-to-triceps transfer. Wrist extension can be improved in certain patients by transferring contractile function from the brachioradialis to the extensor carpi radialis brevis tendon. A *key grip* can be created in patients who have retained at least some ability for active wrist extension. An active key grip can be achieved by fusing the carpometacarpal joint of the thumb, anchoring the extensor pollicis longus tendon to the back of the wrist, and transferring the brachioradialis tendon to the flexor pollicis longus tendon. A number of alternative strategies may be used, and the more functioning muscles that remain below elbow level, the more alternatives are available.

In summary, a realistic hand surgical outcome is often said to be that the patient will be able to carry out those same activities that he could already achieve prior to surgery, only more easily and effectively. Reconstructive hand surgery thus rarely enables the patient to develop brand new skills.

Functional Neuromuscular Stimulation

Functional neuromuscular stimulation (FNS) is sometimes an alternative or complement to reconstructive hand surgery. The method, mainly developed in the United States, uses both transcutaneous nerve stimulation and implantable electrodes. For example, the *NeuroControl Freehand System*® is an implantable system that is controlled by movements of the opposite shoulder. The technique enables a patient with high SCI to activate and control a preprogrammed sequence of muscle contractions and thereby achieve a usable grasp.

23 | Compression Neuropathies

ULNAR NEUROPATHY

The ulnar nerve may be subject to repetitive trauma, especially in full elbow flexion. The course of the nerve takes it between the medial epicondyle and the olecranon, where it travels in the shallow ulnar groove, and then into the flexor muscles between the two heads of the flexor carpi ulnaris. Symptoms of neural irritation, *ulnar neuropathy*, include pain and/or paresthesias along the medial side of the hand and forearm, and sometimes also impaired fine motor hand function (Fig. 23.1). Paresthesias are triggered especially in elbow flexion, which puts tension on the nerve. Diagnosis can be confirmed through neurophysiologic testing. Treatment includes an elbow *extension splint* for use at night, and in more severe cases surgical *ulnar nerve transposition* to a more protected location anterior to the ulnar groove. In some cases this nerve may also be compressed more distally at the wrist, where it passes in the narrow Guyon canal. Compression at this site produces similar symptoms as described above, although sensation on the dorsum of the hand remains intact, since the cutaneous branches leave the nerve more proximally. Also this condition is amenable to surgical decompression.

MEDIAN NEUROPATHY (CARPAL TUNNEL SYNDROME)

Carpal tunnel syndrome is common following SCI, and subclinical (i.e., nonsymptomatic) injury to the nerve has been demonstrated through neurophysiologic testing in even more patients. Median nerve compression produces symptoms of nocturnal numbness in the three radial fingers (Fig. 23.2). The patient awakens from the discomfort, and shakes the involved hand, thereby getting some relief. More pronounced compression tends to be associated with persistent symptoms, including clumsiness, paresis, and sensory loss. Diagnosis can be confirmed through neurophysiologic testing. Treatment includes anti-inflammatory medications, a wrist *cock-up splint* to maintain wrist extension at night, steroid injection or, when other therapeutic measures fail, division of the carpal ligament (carpal tunnel release).

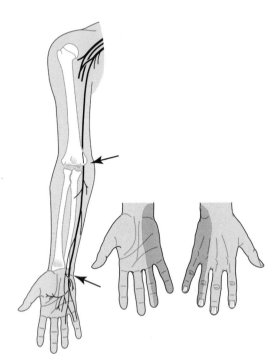

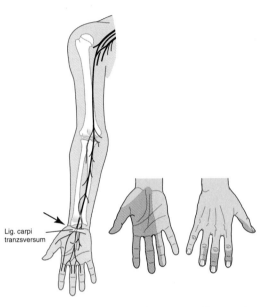

Lig. carpi
tranzsversum

Figure 23.2 Median nerve. The *arrow* indicates the site where the nerve may be subject to compression under the carpal ligament at wrist level. The *red areas* indicate the distribution of impaired sensation with compression of the nerve in the carpal tunnel.

Figure 23.1 Ulnar nerve. The *arrows* indicate sites where the ulnar nerve may be subject to compression, including the ulnar groove at the elbow level and Guyon's canal at the wrist. The *red areas* indicate the distribution of impaired sensation with compression of the nerve at the elbow level.

24 | Circulatory and Respiratory Disorders

CARDIOVASCULAR DYSFUNCTION

Cardiovascular dysfunction following SCI is due to interruption of autonomic pathways and/or, in the long term, deconditioning effects due to immobilization. In addition, general risk factors such as heredity, smoking, overweight, and poor diet also apply to individuals with SCI.

Vagotonia

One major cardiovascular complication seen during the acute stage after traumatic tetraplegia is episodes of bradycardia or even cardiac arrest caused by autonomic imbalance with relative dominance of parasympathetic activity. The precipitating factor may be vagal stimulation caused by intubation and/or suction of the airways. In high SCI, vagal impulses cannot be adequately counter-balanced due to interruption of the sympathetic innervation of the heart.

Autonomic Dysreflexia

SCI at the T6 level or rostrally (i.e., above the sympathetic splanchnic outflow) predispose to *autonomic dysreflexia* (AD). Nociceptive stimuli normally lead to sympathetic activation, but with SCI and its associated interruption of the fibers to the cerebral vasomotor centers, such activation becomes exaggerated due to loss of supraspinal inhibition. Plasma levels of norepinephrine immediately rise and correlate with symptoms and blood pressure elevation.

AD is characterized by attacks of blood pressure elevation with severe headache. Other symptoms include malaise, nausea, facial flushing, sweats, and goosebumps (Fig. 24.1). The combination of headache attacks with sweating and

facial flushing is essentially pathognomonic for AD in persons with tetraplegia or high paraplegia. Blood pressure is at least 20–30 mm Hg above the patient's baseline pressure, which is often low. Thus, to become symptomatic, the blood pressure does *not* have to be significantly elevated compared to what is normal in an individual without SCI.

Treatment

When an attack of AD is suspected, the patient should be placed in an upright position and tight clothing should be loosened. Urinary retention must be ruled out and/or treated (catheterization, irrigation of indwelling catheter). The next step is to rule out and/or treat rectal fecal impaction as the cause of elevated blood pressure (digital rectal exam and, when needed, stool removal after lubrication with local anesthetic ointment). Should a systolic blood pressure elevation above 150 mm Hg persist, the blood pressure should be lowered using a rapid-acting antihypertensive drug such as a calcium channel blocker. Other precipitating causes should then be explored, such as abdominal disorders, infection, fracture/soft-tissue injury, paronychia, thrombosed hemorrhoid, or anal fissure.

Arterial Hypotension

Systemic blood pressure is typically low in persons with SCI in the upper thoracic or cervical cord. Sitting and resting systolic blood pressure for a person with tetraplegia is typically 90–110 mm Hg. Such low blood pressure is due to decreased sympathetic activity and consequently correspondingly decreased vasomotor tone below the level of lesion. Low systemic blood pressure, assuming that it does not fall

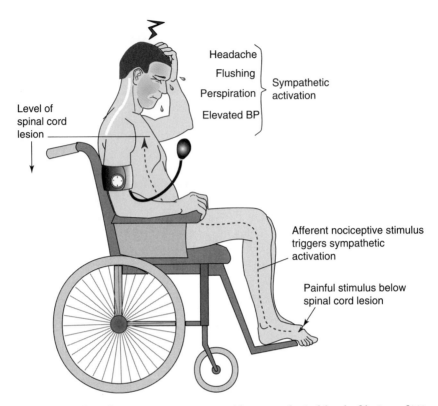

Figure 24.1 Autonomic dysreflexia (AD). In persons with a neurological level of lesion of T6 or higher, infralesional nociceptive stimuli may lead to attacks of blood pressure elevation with symptoms such as headache, sweats, and facial flushing.

below a critical level and becomes symptomatic, is not necessarily disadvantageous from a health standpoint. On the contrary, hypertension rather than hypotension is a significant pathogenic factor. It is thus postulated that low blood pressure among tetraplegic patients even might provide some protection against cardiovascular diseases.

Orthostatic Hypotension

Orthostatic hypotension is defined as a drop in systolic blood pressure of more than 20 mm Hg and/or a *symptomatic* (dizziness, faintness, etc.) drop in blood pressure when the patient sits up or stands up. Orthostatic problems are common in complete injuries at or above the T6 level, especially during the first weeks and months following SCI. The cause is impaired or absent sympathetically mediated peripheral vasoconstriction. When standing or sitting up, venous blood pools in the lower extremities and, in the absence of compensatory vasoconstriction, a fall in blood pressure occurs. Blood flow returning to the heart decreases, leading to a drop in filling pressure, end-diastolic volume, and stroke volume. This may result in cerebral hypoperfusion with symptoms such as dizziness, visual disturbances ("black-out"), weakness, faintness, and possibly loss of consciousness. Precipitating or aggravating factors include standing or sitting up too quickly, rising abruptly on waking in the morning, heavy meals (due to shunting of blood from the systemic to the splanchnic circulation), physical exertion, alcohol consumption, high ambient temperature, fever/infection, dehydration, and certain medications (e.g., tricyclic antidepressants, antihypertensives, diuretics, opioids). Neurogenic orthostatic hypotension usually resolves gradually during the rehabilitation period. Possible explanations for this physiological adaptation include compensatory changes in other vascular beds, stimulation of the renin–angiotensin–aldosterone system, compensatory receptor hypersensitivity in the vascular walls (as a consequence of sympathetic denervation), spontaneous return of the spinal postural reflexes, increasing spasticity, and/or adaptive autoregulation of blood flow to the brain.

Treatment

Treatment should focus on alleviating symptoms rather than on normalizing blood pressure. The following measures constitute first-line treatment:

- During early phases of rehabilitation, gradual mobilization on the slant board to condition postural reflexes
- Distribution of food intake into small, frequent meals
- Elevation of head at night to reduce nocturia (i.e.,. large nocturnal urine volumes) and thereby reduce hypovolemia and orthostatic hypotension in the morning
- Avoidance of rapid changes in position (sitting, standing, lying)
- Avoidance of strenuous physical activity in high ambient temperatures
- Discontinuation of antihypertensive medication
- Increased salt and fluid intake
- Use of compression hosiery and/or abdominal girdle

In addition, in rare cases, pharmacological treatment may be indicated, such as dihydroergotamine, etilefrine, or fludrocortisone. The latter medication is a mineralocorticoid, in which the mechanism of action involves some fluid retention.

Reduction in Cardiovascular Fitness

There are several causes for fitness to decline following SCI. Patients are immobilized by paresis and many become overweight. Calorie expenditure decreases and persons with SCI—especially tetraplegics—experience a decline in muscle and bone mass, while their body fat increases relatively or absolutely. Depending on level of injury, the basic energy requirement

decreases by 10–25% compared with the population at large, and the ideal weight should thus be 5–10 kg lower. In addition, these patients cannot respond with sympathetically mediated vasoconstriction (which increases venous return) or sympathetically mediated elevation of heart rate and myocardial contractility, which further limits their work capacity.

Aerobic exercise is an important component of the rehabilitation process, both initially and in the long-term. Physical activity associated with activities of daily living (ADL) is insufficient in itself to achieve an aerobic effect. The benefits of exercise include increased functional reserve capacity in daily life, as well as long-term prevention of cardiovascular disease. The more caudal the neurological level of injury and the more incomplete the injury, the greater the potential for improving aerobic fitness.

Coronary Heart Disease

Atherosclerotic coronary heart disease has in recent years become one of the leading causes of death among SCI patients. Several risk factors are overrepresented: decreased physical activity, low high-density lipoprotein (HDL) cholesterol (the "good" cholesterol), impaired glucose tolerance, increased insulin resistance, increased proportion of body fat, hypertension (in paraplegics), smoking, and psychosocial factors such as depression and social isolation. In addition, it has been proposed that recurrent chronic infections (such as urinary tract infections and infected pressure ulcers) may increase cardiovascular risk via inflammatory mediators such as C-reactive protein (CRP). Several of these factors are amenable to preventive measures. Health-promoting interventions such as smoking cessation, physical exercise, dietary modification, stress management, and regular health check-ups are obviously important for rehabilitation and long-term follow-up of persons with SCI.

From a diagnostic point of view, patients with a lesion level at or above T5–T6 pose a special problem, since the sensory loss in these cases may mask the pain of angina pectoris and myocardial infarction.

Peripheral Vascular Disease

Risk factors for atherosclerosis such as smoking, dyslipidemia, and overweight are overrepresented in persons with chronic SCI. Moreover, it has ben proposed that arterial atrophy secondary to paresis of mainly the lower extremities may be a contributing factor.

Since many persons with SCI are completely anesthetic below the level of lesion, they are unable to feel the pain of ischemia, which is otherwise a cardinal symptom that should raise a red flag. Signs of arterial insufficiency include slow-healing ulcers, trophic lesions, and weak or absent distal pulses.

Deep Vein Thrombosis and Pulmonary Embolism

Paresis of the lower extremities entails impaired muscle function and thereby decreased venous return. Furthermore, increased blood viscosity and hyperfibrinogenemia are present, especially in the acute phase. According to some studies, the incidence of deep vein thrombosis (DVT) among patients with acute SCI is 100%. With thromboprophylaxis, which is almost always given nowadays, the incidence of clinical DVT is reported to be about 2% in the first year and about 1% in the second year. The incidence of pulmonary embolism in the first year is about 0.5%, and the risk of this complication continues to be elevated throughout life.

Impaired Thermoregulation

Body heat is produced by muscle activity, digestion, and various metabolic processes. Body temperature is mainly regulated by controlled heat loss. Cutaneous receptors respond to the ambient temperature. Receptors in the preoptic region of the hypothalamus react to changes in blood temperature and activate other hypothalamic centers. These centers regulate temperature mainly via the sympathetic nervous system. When body temperature rises, sympathetic activity is inhibited, resulting in vasodilation and an increase in heat loss. Sweating increases this heat loss. When body temperature drops, the sympathetic nerves are activated, resulting in vasoconstriction and conservation of heat. Body temperature can also be increased by shivering (i.e., an involuntary muscle activity).

Fever may occur through release of endogenous pyrogens from macrophages, including interleukins and interferons. These substances are released into the bloodstream, where they lead to an upregulation of the body's thermostat. This upregulation is mediated by the hypothalamus, primarily through secretion of prostaglandins. Body temperature then increases as just described.

In the setting of complete tetraplegia, or paraplegia above T6, patients have difficulty maintaining normal body temperature at both high and low ambient temperatures. In SCI patients there is a tendency for body temperature to passively follow ambient temperature; this is known as *poikilothermia*. This is related to an interruption of the afferent temperature pathways and an inability to regulate the vascular bed and to sweat below the neurologic level of lesion. Despite such thermoregulatory disruption, most persons with SCI will react physiologically with a fever in response to conditions such as infection. In rare cases, disruption of thermoregulation in tetraplegic patients may result in chronic fever without any other explanation.

RESPIRATORY DISORDERS

Ventilatory Insufficiency

Cervical and upper thoracic SCI have a pronounced effect on respiratory function by causing complete or incomplete paralysis of the respiratory muscles. The diaphragm is the key muscle for breathing. This muscle is innervated from the C2–C4 segments of the spinal cord. The intercostal muscles are segmentally innervated from T1–12. In addition, the accessory respiratory muscles, such as the sternocleidomastoid and trapezius, which are innervated by the accessory cranial nerve and the most rostral cervical spinal cord segments, may have great significance for maintaining respiratory function among persons with high SCI. Finally, the back muscles (erector spinae) and abdominal muscles also play a role, by maintaining an erect posture and thus providing support for the diaphragm.

Respiratory function may be further compromised by SCI due to spasticity in the trunk muscles, spinal deformity such as kyphoscoliosis, chronic constipation, and side effects of various drugs that may depress respiratory function. Three major complications may result from impaired respiratory muscle function:

> - Chronic ventilatory insufficiency/hypoventilation
> - Impaired ability to cough with risk of choking, stagnation of secretions, and atelectasis
> - Lower respiratory infections and pneumonia, that may lead to an acute and serious aggravation of ventilatory insufficiency

Patients with high SCI should routinely be assessed for ventilatory function while under emergency care and during the early rehabilitation phase. These patients should be strongly advised not to smoke. In cases of esablished hypoventilation, the patient should be provided respiratory support such as continuous positive airway pressure (CPAP; see "Sleep Apnea," in Chapter 28) or should be placed on a ventilator. During long-term follow-up, and especially in the case of progressive neurologic deterioration (see Chapter 30), respiratory function should be reassessed by spirometry and similar tests.

Pneumonia

Pneumonia remains an important cause of death in tetraplegia. Patients with tetraplegia or high paraplegia are at increased risk of infection due to paresis of the diaphragm and/or intercostal muscles, which impairs the ability to dispose of secretions. Tracheostomy or endotracheal intubation further increases the risk of infection. The risk of aspiration pneumonia is also increased, especially in the acute phase, with decreased level of consciousness, gastroparesis, and paralytic ileus. Patients with high SCI should be immunized against pneumococcal infection and influenza.

The clinical picture of pneumonia may be atypical in high tetraplegia. Sensation of pain from the thorax may be absent. The ability to cough may be weak or absent due to weakened respiratory muscles. Dominant vagal tone in the acute phase leads to an increase in mucous secretions within the airways. The clinical picture is characterized by malaise, fever, tachypnea, and tachycardia, as well as elevated indicators of infection in the blood, hypoxemia, and pulmonary infiltrates on chest x-ray. Among the differential diagnoses, it is especially important to always consider pulmonary embolism.

Gastrointestinal problems following SCI fall into two main categories: (1) *direct* neurologic consequences of injury, such as changes in gastrointestinal motility and loss of sphincter control; and (2) *indirect* effects secondary to immobilization, lifestyle factors, medications, and the like. As has been pointed out repeatedly in this book, diagnosis of gastrointestinal problems may often be obscured by the absence of nociception below the neurologic level of injury. A strict bowel regimen with regular, controlled emptying while avoiding leakage is of great significance for rehabilitation outcome and quality of life. This chapter covers common consequences and complications, as well as recommendations for bowel management programs for patients with upper and lower motor neuron injuries.

ORAL HYGIENE PROBLEMS

Persons with tetraplegia find it more difficult to brush their teeth and practice good oral hygiene, something which may lead to dental plaque, caries, and periodontitis. Dryness of the mouth (*xerostomia*) is a common side effect of several drugs, such as anticholinergics, antidepressants, and certain antispasmodics. Smoking is common among SCI patients and contributes to poor oral health, with an increased risk of periodontitis in particular. Recommendations include smoking cessation, improved oral hygiene using an electric toothbrush, saliva-stimulating tablets, and sugarless chewing gum, as well as frequent checkups with the dental hygienist and dentist.

DYSPEPSIA

Gastroesophageal Reflux

Patients with tetraplegia in particular are at increased risk of *gastroesophageal reflux*. In addition to direct neurologic reasons for this, problems may arise due to frequent use of the Valsalva maneuver (bearing down) or external abdominal pressure during bowel evacuation, as well as due to a greater proportion of time spent in a reclining or semireclining position. In tetraplegia, retrosternal burning pain as a symptom of esophagitis may be absent. The sole expression of this problem may then be a recurring sour taste in the mouth due to acid reflux and/or symptoms related to complicating disorders, such as dysphagia (swallowing difficulties) or bleeding. Treatment is similar as for the population at large. It is especially important to recommend cutting back on tobacco, caffeine, and alcohol; to have patients sit up after meals; and to avoid eating right before going to bed.

Gastroparesis

Gastroparesis, i.e., the inability of the stomach to contract and thus to empty its contents, is often present during the first days to weeks following acute SCI. The ventricle is often kept empty through the use of parenteral fluids and nutrition, as well as the use of a nasogastric tube. Sluggish emptying of the ventricle and duodenum can also be present in the chronic phase. In such cases, some patients suffer from bloating and early satiety with meals. Treatment includes smaller, more frequent meals and avoidance of meals at bedtime.

Peptic Ulcer Disease

The risk of *peptic ulcer* is high during the acute phase after SCI, in part due to the acute physiological and psychological stress, and in part to the frequent use of high-dose steroid treatment.

Consequently, prophylactic treatment with proton-pump inhibitors or H_2-blockers is often recommended. During the chronic phase, long-term use of nonsteroidal anti-inflammatory drugs (NSAIDs) is the main contributing factor to the risk of gastritis and/or ulcer.

Superior Mesenteric Artery Syndrome

An uncommon but nevertheless noteworthy condition is *superior mesenteric artery* syndrome. Here, the distal duodenum is intermittently compressed between the superior mesenteric artery and the aorta. The duodenum will then be strangulated between these two arterial structures. Symptoms include epigastric fullness and sometimes pain after food intake, followed by nausea and vomiting. A sharp drop in weight, which is common in the early stages after SCI, predisposes for this syndrome.

PANCREATITIS

The risk of pancreatitis mainly increases in the early stages following SCI. Possibly, autonomic imbalance may lead to increased tone in the sphincter of Oddi, resulting in congestion and inflammatory irritation. Signs of pancreatitis include anorexia, tachycardia, fever, arterial hypotension, and/or paralytic ileus. The diagnosis is confirmed by elevated serum amylase and lipase, as well as signs of pancreatitis on abdominal computed tomography (CT).

GALL BLADDER DISEASE

The incidence of *gallstone formation* and *cholecystitis* is also increased following SCI. Diagnosis and treatment follow the usual guidelines. As with other diseases in SCI patients, the pain component will be masked when the source is located below the neurologic level of injury.

NEUROGENIC INTESTINAL PROBLEMS

Pathophysiology

For an overview of the innervation of the gastrointestinal tract, see Figure 25.1A,B. Most of the gastrointestinal problems that arise in the chronic phase following SCI involve the colon. Its principal function is to reabsorb fluid. Peristaltic contractions of the colon are coordinated with respect to both segmental and forward-propelling waves. The intestines have a highly developed "intrinsic" nervous system, known as the *enteric nervous system*, which is largely "embedded" in the intestinal wall and consists of the Meissner plexus (submucosal plexus), the Auerbach plexus (intramuscular plexus), and interneurons. Because the system is highly autonomous, colon physiology remains partially intact following SCI.

Normal defecation entails an interplay between involuntary and voluntary activities. Involuntary activities include the gastrocolic reflex, which is triggered by food intake. *Giant migratory contractions* (GMCs) arise within the colon in response to a full stomach and propel the intestinal contents through the colon toward the rectum. The stool distends the rectum and puborectalis muscle, which causes the internal sphincter to relax. This is called the *rectoanal inhibitory reflex*. Simultaneously, contraction of the external anal sphincter and the puborectalis muscle will retain the feces (known as *holding reflex*).

The activities related to defecation include voluntary relaxation of the external anal sphincter and puborectalis muscle and an increase of the intraabdominal pressure through the Valsalva maneuver, which facilitates expulsion of feces.

SCI often interfere with the normal physiological process just described. The resulting malfunction is referred to as *neurogenic bowel dysfunction*. The cardinal symptoms that characterize this condition include *constipation* and *incontinence*. From a pathophysiological standpoint, one or more of the following phenomena play a role: absent sensory function, loss of voluntary sphincter control, flaccid or spastic sphincter paresis, impaired peristaltic activity and coordination, and/or inadequate synchrony between peristalsis and sphincter activity.

Constipation

Constipation is the rule after SCI. *Paralytic ileus* is present during the acute phase and transiently leads to an inability to pass stool (this problem is addressed in Chapter 7). Constipation may be operationally defined as fewer than three bowel movements per week and/or incomplete evacuation and/or chronic abdominal distension. According to this definition, about two-thirds of all persons with SCI suffer from constipation in the chronic phase. The underlying pathophysiology differs between upper and lower motor neuron injuries.

Lower motor neuron injuries occur as a result of lesions in the conus and/or cauda equina, leading to decreased tone within the descending colon and extinction of the peristaltic reflex. The time required for the intestinal contents to pass through the gastrointestinal tract becomes prolonged, thus too much liquid is resorbed from the feces, causing the stool to become hard. The external anal

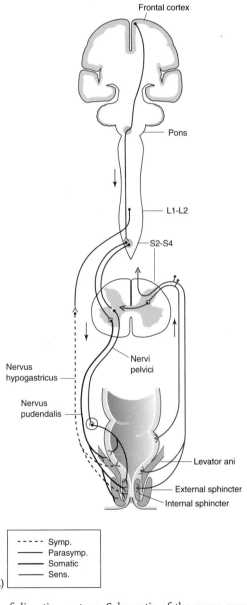

Figure 25.1 A: Nerve supply of digestive system. Schematic of the nerve supply to the distal portion of the colon. As can be seen, both voluntary (somatic) and involuntary (autonomic) neural components are present, which ensures functions such as continence.

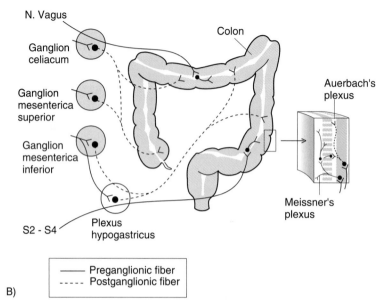

Figure 25.1 B: Nerve supply to the colon. The vagal nerve (cranial nerve X) innervates the proximal portion of the intestine. Also note the intestine's "intrinsic" nerve supply from Meissner and Auerbach plexus. Consequently, the prospects for preserved intestinal function remain despite SCI, although both incontinence and constipation are common.

sphincter becomes totally or partially denervated and thereby flaccid, preventing both reflex and voluntary contraction, thus increasing the risk of incontinence. Other factors contributing to incontinence include paresis of the pelvic floor muscles and decreased tone in the puborectalis muscle.

Spinal cord lesions above the level of the conus lead to *upper motor neuron lesions*. Such lesions will also prolong transit time through the colon, but in contrast to the situation seen in lower motor neuron lesions, spasticity increases the tone of both the colon wall and the external anal sphincter. The net effect of overactive segmental peristalsis, underactive propulsive peristalsis, overactive holding reflex, and spastic contraction of the external anal sphincter is a clear tendency toward constipation.

Diarrhea

In addition to constipation, *diarrhea* may also cause severe problems, since continence by voluntary sphincter contraction is often lost in SCI. The risk of bowel incontinence is thus very high if the stool becomes too loose for whatever reason.

Among the many possible underlying causes, diarrhea as a side effect from treatment with broad spectrum antibiotics deserves special mention. Such treatment is commonplace among SCI patients mainly due to frequent urinary tract infections. Long-term or recurrent antibiotics treatment increases the risk of *Clostridium difficile* enterocolitis. It is likewise important to consider the possibility of *stercoral diarrhea*, in which fecal impaction in the form of a solid fecaloma irritates the rectal wall, paradoxically causing diarrhea.

WORKUP

In accordance with the particulars of the case, the clinician should review diet, fluid intake, medications, and bowel regimen including bowel evacuation technique, frequency, and duration, as well as incontinence (when, how often, precipitating factors, etc.). The situation should be assessed as to gain understanding of how the current bowel regimen is working in relation to the patient's lifestyle in general. Abdominal and digital rectal exam should be included in the physical examination. Note should be taken of resting tone of the anal sphincter and puborectalis, as well as the presence or absence of the *anocutaneous reflex* (i.e., contraction of the external anal sphincter in response to stimulation of the perianal skin), voluntary sphincter contraction, and the *bulbocavernosus reflex* (i.e., reflex contraction of the anal sphincter in response to compression of the glans penis or clitoris).

Depending on symptoms and physical findings, various additional tests may be indicated, including fecal hemoglobin, stool culture, determination of *C. difficile* toxin in the stool and presence of cysts, ova, and parasites. Blood tests often include complete blood count (CBC), liver function tests, serum amylase, and electrolytes. Radiographic examinations to be considered include plain abdominal films, possibly including computed tomography (CT) and/or magnetic resonance imaging (MRI).

TREATMENT

After carrying out the relevant workup and ruling out or correcting underlying pathology, emphasis should be placed on establishing a strict bowel regimen. The purpose of this regimen is to eliminate incontinence, achieve effective bowel evacuation, and prevent secondary complications. An overarching goal is to achieve regular bowel evacuation at least three times a week. Regular, frequent, and complete evacuation of the bowel reduces the risk of bowel leakage. Implementing a good bowel regimen often requires a significant educational, multidisciplinary effort. Practical dietary counseling should be provided, with emphasis on adequate fluid intake (2–3 liters/day). Regular physical activity improves intestinal motility and should be encouraged. Microenemas are often useful, but irritant laxatives should be avoided if possible.

In lower motor neuron lesions, spinal cord-mediated reflexogenic intestinal peristalsis is reduced or absent. Therefore, bowel evacuation should be coordinated with meals in order to take advantage of the gastrocolic reflex. Since external anal sphincter tone is weak, stool should be evacuated from the rectum one or more times daily in order to prevent incontinence. The patient must be taught to insert a finger into the rectum to manually remove feces. Stool evacuation can be further facilitated through deep breathing, Valsalva maneuver, contraction of abdominal muscles, and/or clockwise abdominal massage through the abdominal wall.

In upper motor neuron lesions, the emphasis is on activating reflexes. Bowel reflexes may be stimulated through abdominal massage, suppositories, and/or enema combined with digital stretching and manipulation of the rectum. One problem that may be encountered is *anorectal dyssynergy* (i.e., paradoxical anal contraction), which means that the external anal sphincter fails to relax as the rectum contracts. However, the sphincter can be made to relax by inserting one finger into the anus to decrease resistance to evacuation. Such rectal stretching and stimulation also activates the rectoanal inhibitory reflex, which relaxes the internal sphincter, and activates the rectocolic reflex as well as the local intestinal peristalsis. Digital manipulation reportedly is most effective if stimulation occurs for about one minute and is repeated every 5–10 minutes during the evacuation process. The bowel should be emptied daily and at a minimum every 3 days.

Newer treatment options include *pulsed irrigation enhanced evacuation* (PIEE). *Functional electrical stimulation* of sacral roots (Chapter 26) can also lead to improved bowel evacuation. In recent years, surgical treatment has become more common. In addition to *colostomy*, we should also mention *appendicocecostomy* (Malone procedure) as an alternative treatment option, in which the appendix vermiformis is used to create a connection between the abdominal wall and the proximal colon. By catheterizing this stoma, 200–500 mL of isotonic saline solution can be infused to flush the colon, thereby providing an anterograde enema.

26 | Urogenital Sequelae Including Sexual Dysfunction

Up until the mid-twentieth century, renal failure was one of the main causes of death among SCI patients due to the adverse combination of recurrent urinary tract infection (UTI), urolithiasis, elevated pressure in the urinary tract, and urinary reflux. Chronically infected pressure ulcers also contributed to renal failure through the development of amyloidosis. Fortunately, antibiotics, improved bladder management programs, and regular monitoring have substantially reduced both mortality and morbidity.

In addition to the medical risks associated with urologic dysfunction following SCI, incontinence comprises an important psychosocial problem. Neurourology thus continues to play a central role in the short- and long-term management of SCI patients.

PHYSIOLOGY OF MICTURITION

The urinary bladder acts as a reservoir for urine, which is produced by the kidneys, then flows through the ureters to reach the bladder. The ureters run obliquely through the bladder wall, which reduces the risk of reflux (backflow). As the bladder empties, the urine passes through the urethra. This flow of urine is blocked by two sphincters: an internal smooth muscle and an external striated muscle sphincter. The lower urinary tract has both autonomic (involuntary) innervation from parasympathetic and sympathetic nerves, as well as somatic (voluntary) innervation.

Parasympathetic innervation is conveyed via the pelvic nerves, which originate from the S2–S4 segments of the spinal cord (Fig. 26.1). Parasympathetic activation leads to contraction of the bladder muscle (detrusor) and results in bladder emptying.

Sympathetic innervation occurs via the hypogastric nerve, which originates in the T11–L2 spinal cord segments and mainly supplies muscles in the bladder neck and proximal urethra. Sympathetic activation chiefly supports the reservoir function of the bladder by increasing the degree of contraction in the bladder neck muscles.

Somatic innervation, which comes from the pudendal nerve and originates from the S2–S4 spinal cord segments, innervates the external striated-muscle sphincter. The somatic nervous system also mainly supports the reservoir function of the bladder by increasing flow resistance through the urethra.

Sensory innervation, which is chiefly activated by stretching of the bladder wall by bladder fullness, is mediated via the pelvic nerve, while pain and temperature stimuli from the bladder mucosa are mainly conveyed through sensory fibers within the hypogastric nerve.

Voluntary control of the detrusor is initiated by impulses from the frontal cortex, which are conveyed through the pons and the reticulospinal tract. The frontal cortex is also directly connected to the pudendal nucleus by the corticospinal tract, and impulses through this system support voluntary control of the external urethral sphincter. Supraspinal control of micturition is mainly inhibitory.

When a certain threshold bladder pressure is reached, corresponding to a certain bladder volume, continence is ensured by an increase in sympathetic activation that results in contraction of the internal urethral sphincter. To further ensure continence, contraction of the external urethral sphincter increases as a result of both voluntary and reflex activity. When it is time for micturition, voluntary relaxation of the

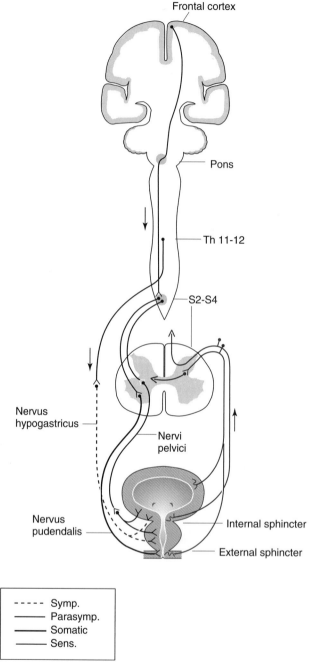

Figure 26.1 Schematic of nerve supply to the lower urinary tract. As shown, both voluntary (somatic) and involuntary (autonomic) neural components are involved.

external urethral sphincter reduces resistance to urinary flow. Sympathetic activity decreases, which results in relaxation of the bladder neck, while increased parasympathetic activity leads to bladder contraction.

A "micturition center" located in the pons is responsible for synchronizing bladder contraction and sphincter relaxation, provided that the neural pathways between this pontine center and the sacral cord are intact.

NEUROUROLOGICAL WORKUP

Neurourological workup after SCI is based on a thorough medical history, with special emphasis on the pattern of micturition. Sensory function, muscle tone, and reflexes in the perineal region need to be evaluated. The *bulbocavernosus reflex,* which is a monosynaptic reflex mediated via the sacral spinal cord, is of particular interest. This reflex is checked by squeezing the glans penis or clitoris while simultaneously inserting a finger into the rectum to detect the presence or absence of a reflexogenic anal sphincter contraction so elicited. In women, examination typically also includes assessment of potential weakness in the pelvic floor muscles and possible associated prolapse. The prostate should be checked in men.

Residual urine volume should be measured. Volumes in excess of 100 mL indicate a flow obstruction and/or ineffective detrusor activity.

A *cystometrogram* (cystometry) is a test used to assess bladder compliance, sensory function, volume, and presence of normal or disinhibited (uninhibited) bladder activity. *Pressure–flow studies* are used to assess bladder pressure at the point of maximum urinary flow. *Sphincter electromyography* can reveal either increased activity, which then usually suggests increased urethral resistance, or decreased activity, which usually indicates decreased urethral resistance.

Workup of the upper urinary tract includes *ultrasound* and/or *urography* (pyelography). Laboratory work-up includes serum urea, serum creatinine and/or serum cystatin, urine sediment, and urine culture.

MICTURITION FOLLOWING SPINAL CORD INJURY

Micturition often becomes dysfunctional after SCI. During the early stage of spinal shock a flaccid *bladder paresis* occurs, and the bladder must be emptied with a catheter (see Chapter 7). The neurourological workup is carried out after spinal shock has subsided, thus providing a baseline analysis. From this point on, neurourological monitoring becomes an integral part of long-term follow-up, mainly to prevent or diagnose any complications at an early stage.

Different pathologic voiding patterns often persist into the chronic phase, depending on the neurological level of lesion and degree of functional recovery. The most important urological problems following SCI include *incontinence, infections, urolithiasis,* and *secondary renal damage.* The most important risk factors for development of renal damage are lack of coordination between bladder wall muscles and the bladder sphincter (*detrusor–sphincter dyssynergia*), urinary tract infections (UTIs), and urolithiasis with flow obstruction. These conditions are described later in this chapter.

The optimal bladder management program should be as simple as possible for the patient to carry out, while at the same time minimizing the risk of complications. Since the number of individuals with incomplete SCI is increasing, a growing percentage of SCI patients will be able to empty their bladders in the "normal" way. In cases where normal micturition is not possible and/or accompanied by unacceptable leakage, retention, and/or infection, one of the following bladder management programs will be appropriate.

Intermittent Catheterization

Intermittent catheterization is usually the solution of choice after the immediate acute phase (Fig. 26.2). The patient should be catheterized frequently enough so that urine volumes do not exceed 400 mL when voiding. From a practical standpoint, catheterization is initially carried out every 6 hours, using a *clean technique* (i.e., with careful attention to hygiene, but without any requirement for sterility). If possible, patients should learn how to catheterize themselves, i.e., by *intermittent self-catheterization.* This assumes some residual motor function in the hands. Due to anatomical differences, this technique is usually easier for men than for women. In particular, women with adductor spasticity in the legs may have problems with self-catheterization. If the patient is unable to self-catheterize, this method of bladder emptying becomes less attractive from the standpoint of practicality, economics, and dignity, since the patient must then rely on an assistant or relative for performing the catheterization.

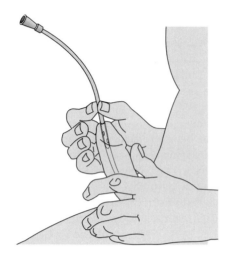

Figure 26.2 Clean intermittent catheterization (CIC). Patients with sufficiently preserved hand function are able to carry out bladder emptying by themselves, i.e., by self-catheterization. This is currently the commonest assisted method of emptying the bladder among SCI patients.

Reflex Voiding

Previously, reflex voiding or "tapping" was the commonest voiding method for persons with SCI (Fig. 26.3). By tapping and pressing over the bladder area through the abdominal wall,

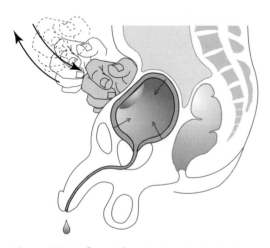

Figure 26.3 Reflex voiding (or "tapping"). Patients with upper motor neuron lesions may elicit reflex voiding by using their hands to tap on the lower abdominal wall.

patients with suprasacral spinal cord lesions may thereby typically elicit a contraction of the detrusor muscle and thus empty the bladder. The disadvantage is that bladder pressure may become high and micturition incomplete, especially in the presence of detrusor–sphincter dyssynergia. As described earlier, this approach has largely been replaced by intermittent self-catheterization.

Bladder Compression (Credé Maneuver)

The Credé maneuver comprises passive emptying of the bladder by means of external bladder compression (Fig. 26.4). This method is primarily used in conus/cauda lesions, which cause flaccid paresis of the bladder.

Suprapubic Catheter

A suprapubic catheter is an indwelling catheter introduced into the bladder through the abdominal wall by use of percutaneous technique (Fig. 26.5). This bladder management option may be appropriate in cases where intermittent self-catheterization is not possible.

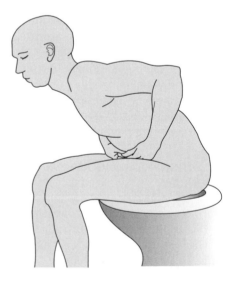

Figure 26.4 Credé maneuver. A flaccid bladder is emptied passively (i.e., in the absence of detrusor muscle contraction) by having patients press with their hands against the bladder while bearing down. This bladder emptying method is primarily used in lower motor neuron lesions.

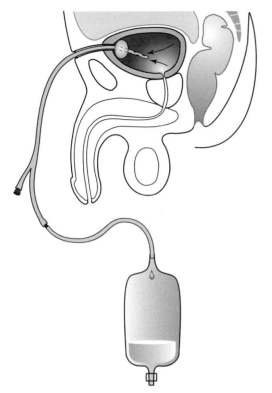

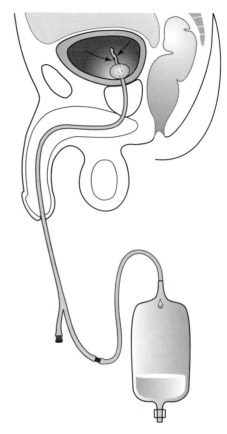

Figure 26.5 Suprapubic catheter. An indwelling catheter continuously drains urine. The catheter is introduced into the bladder through a minor surgical procedure involving the lower abdominal wall above the pubic symphysis. This method of emptying the bladder is primarily used for patients with poor hand function who thus cannot carry out clean intermittent catheterization (CIC).

Figure 26.6 Indwelling catheter. The catheter is introduced into the bladder through the urethra and secured by inflating a cuff.

Indwelling Urethral Catheter

Indwelling urethral catheters are introduced into the bladder through the urethra and then secured by inflating a cuff surrounding the tip of the catheter within the bladder (Fig. 26.6). The catheter, which may be kept open continuously or be opened intermittently, is connected to a plastic bag that collects the urine.

This bladder management option may seem appealing because it is simple and practical, but other than during the acute phase, it is contraindicated in most cases mainly because it unavoidably leads to UTI. Moreover, it is associated with a risk of urolithiasis, urethral trauma, urethral erosions and/or strictures, bladder fibrosis, epididymitis, orchitis, and bladder cancer. Therefore, in most cases, indwelling urethral catheters are inappropriate for long-term treatment; suprapubic catheters are then clearly a better option.

For those patients who nevertheless have used an indwelling urethral catheter for more than 10 years, annual cystoscopy is recommended for possible detection of early-stage bladder cancer.

Urinary Diversion Surgery

Several surgical procedures may be used to divert urine. In principle, they are based on the

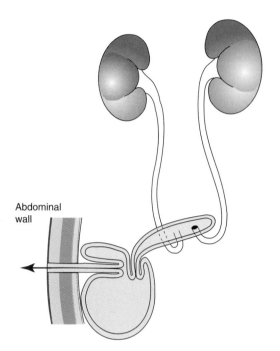

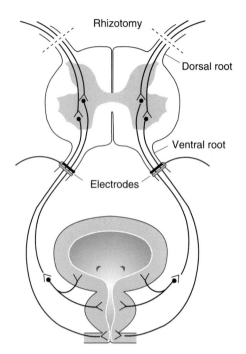

Figure 26.7 Urinary diversion. A "continent urostomy" using a Koch pouch. An artificial bladder is created from a loop of intestine into which the ureters are implanted. The bladder is connected to the abdominal wall, and by invaginating the wall of the pouch a valve effect is created that prevents leakage. The pouch is emptied intermittently by catheterizing the stoma (*arrow*).

Figure 26.8 Sacral anterior root stimulation according to Brindley. Step one of this method involves severing the segmental dorsal roots, thus converting a spastic bladder into a flaccid bladder, which increases bladder capacity and eliminates reflex contractions. Step two involves implantation of the electrodes of the stimulator on the ventral roots as to stimulate detrusor contraction and micturition.

creation of an artificial bladder, e.g., from a part of intestine, with a urostomy on the abdominal wall (Fig. 26.7). Please refer to the literature for further details.

Sacral Root Stimulation

This method is based on electrical stimulation of the ventral sacral nerve roots to empty the bladder. The electrodes are surgically placed on the ventral roots, and the dorsal sacral roots are usually severed (*rhizotomy*; Fig. 26.8). Rhizotomy, as such leads to a deafferentation of the bladder, which will abolish reflex incontinence, while increasing bladder capacity (bladder volume) and bladder compliance.

Rhizotomy unfortunately also extinguishes reflex erection and ejaculation, as well as any remaining sensation in the perineal region. A

significant part of the effect of the procedure is thus due to the conversion of a spastic bladder into a flaccid one by rhizotomy. The electrical stimulation as such causes micturition through so-called *post stimulus voiding*. The mechanism involves stimulation that initially produces concomitant contraction of the sphincter and detrusor, after which, as electrical stimulation ceases, the external sphincter relaxes earlier than the bladder, and urine is discharged.

DETRUSOR–SPHINCTER DYSSYNERGIA

Physiologically, the activity of the detrusor and the urethral sphincter is coordinated, so that micturition takes place in the presence of low intravesical pressure. Inadequate coordination results in simultaneous contraction of the detrusor and sphincter, accompanied by an increase in intravesical pressure. This condition arises in the presence of suprasacral SCI; in other words, with upper motor neuron lesions and a spastic bladder. Detrusor–sphincter dyssynergia produces high intravesical pressure during micturition, as well as increased residual urine, and therefore predisposes for infection, vesicoureteral reflux, hydronephrosis, and renal damage. Choice of method for emptying the bladder influences the consequences of the condition. For example, intermittent catheterization will eliminate the pressure consequences of detrusor–sphincter dyssynergia in conjunction with micturition, in contrast to the situation with reflex voiding/tapping.

The fact that the dyssynergia in itself is often asymptomatic, while at the same time is an important pathogenic factor for urinary tract complications is a strong argument for performing routine neurourological workup in SCI rehabilitation and follow-up.

The purpose of pharmacological treatment of detrusor–sphincter dyssynergia is to reduce detrusor pressure. This can be achieved with *anticholinergics,* such as oxybutynin (DitropanR). In addition, *α-blockers* such as prazosin (MinipressR, VasoflexR, HypoaseR) may reduce outflow resistance.

The goal of surgical treatment is to reduce outflow resistance by transurethral *sphincterotomy* or insertion of a *urethral stent.* Another treatment option is *rhizotomy of the dorsal sacral roots* (see "Sacral Root Stimulation"). Surgical treatment is rarely used today.

URINARY TRACT INFECTION

UTI is the most common type of infection among SCI patients. Inefficient emptying of the bladder, leaving residual urine, and bacteria being introduced by catheterization constitute specific risk factors. UTI symptomatology may differ in SCI patients compared with the population at large. Classic symptoms such as dysuria (i.e., painful urination), painful urgency, and suprapubic or flank pain will be absent in patients with sensory deficits. In these patients, UTI instead commonly manifests through fever, autonomic dysreflexia, increased spasticity, and/or incontinence. Adding to the diagnostic

complexity is the frequent presence of *asymptomatic bacteriuria* in patients with SCI. Presence of *pyuria* (i.e., white blood cells in the urine) indicates mucosal involvement and increases the probability that the bacteriuria reflects a clinically significant infection. However, pyuria may also occur in various noninfectious conditions such as stone formation and catheter-induced trauma of the mucous membranes.

> A common definition of "symptomatic" UTI in SCI patients is bacteriuria with $>10^5$ CFU/mL, pyuria, fever, and one or more of the following symptoms: suprapubic tenderness or flank tenderness, bladder spasm, changes in micturition pattern, increased spasticity, and/or increased dysreflexia (in the absence of other causes). The presence of high fever, chills, and pronounced malaise suggests involvement of the upper urinary tract, i.e., pyelonephritis or urosepsis.

Selection of antibiotics for treatment of symptomatic UTI should preferably be based on prior urine culture. In some cases, treatment must be initiated based on clinical experience while awaiting test results. Most UTIs in patients with SCI are caused by bacteria from the intestinal flora, primarily gram-negatives and enterococci.

Antibiotics are usually *not* indicated in case of asymptomatic bacteriuria. An exception is made for patients infected with urea-splitting organisms such as *Proteus mirabilis,* which predisposes for the formation of struvite stones (see next section). Another exception is made for pregnancy, wherein bacteriuria predisposes for prematurity.

In patients with therapy-resistant or frequently recurring UTI, the urinary tract should be worked up for anatomical abnormalities such as abscess, urolithiasis, obstruction, or strictures, as well as for occurrence of functional disorders such as vesicoureteral reflux and/or high residual post-voiding urine volumes in the bladder.

UROLITHIASIS

Urolithiasis (urinary tract stones) is significantly more common in SCI patients than in the population at large. As in the general population, the incidence of urolithiasis is higher among men. SCI is followed by two phases during which formation of stones is particularly common. The first phase occurs from about 1–2 months to about 1–2 years after injury. It is typically associated with formation of *calcium stones*. Such stone formation relates to the recent onset of paralysis and immobilization, which causes demineralization of bone and thus increased metabolism and excretion of calcium. A second phase of stone formation typically occurs about 10–15 years after injury, and relates to deterioration of bladder function with urinary obstruction, high residual volumes, high intravesical micturition pressure, vesicoureteral reflux, and/or recurrent UTI. This stage is associated with *struvite stones*. These stones are strongly correlated with UTI with urease-producing bacteria, such as *Proteus*, *Pseudomonas*, *Klebsiella*, and *E. coli*. Such bacteria cause alkalinization of the urine, usually to a pH >7.2. In this alkaline environment, in which UTI also leads to mucosal damage and inflammatory exudate, a "vicious circle" with accelerating stone formation easily arises. Moreover, *matrix stones*, consisting of mucosal debris with low crystalline content occur more often in patients with recurrent UTI caused by urease-producing microorganisms.

Stone classification can also be based on the appearance and/or location of the stones. For example, stones known as *staghorn calculi* can follow and fill up the anatomy of the renal pelvis. These are typically struvite stones. Stones in the bladder are also usually composed of struvite and may constitute a treatment-resistant haven for bacteria that may also predispose to stone formation in the upper urinary tract.

A classic symptom of urinary tract obstruction due to stones is pain, which, however, may be absent in SCI patients. Other symptoms of stones in the urinary tract include fever, nausea, vomiting, tachycardia, tachypnea, palpatory tenderness over the abdomen and flank, and/or frequent recurrent or treatment-resistant UTI.

Laboratory workup includes electrolytes, urea, creatinine, cystatin, complete blood count, urine sediment, and urine culture. Radiologic workup with plain abdominal films, pyelography, spiral computed tomography (CT),

and/or ultrasound can demonstrate stone size, location, and possible obstruction.

From a treatment standpoint, a distinction is sometimes made between "medical" and "surgical" stones. *"Medical" stones* occur without concurrent signs of infection, obstruction, or progressive renal impairment, and show no tendency for growth as demonstrated on repeated x-ray examinations.

"Surgical stones" are stones that gradually increase in size on repeated x-ray examinations, and/or result in obstruction, macroscopic hematuria, recurrent UTI, pain, and/or progressive renal failure. UTIs associated with obstructive urolithiasis are to be considered emergent and require surgical intervention, primarily to remove the obstruction. This may be accomplished through percutaneous nephrostomy. Once flow is reestablished and the infection adequately treated with antibiotics, stones may be removed by endoscopic extraction, percutaneous nephrostolithotomy, or lithotripsy (extracorporeal shock wave lithotripsy, ESWL). Open surgery is seldom needed.

RENAL FAILURE

Several factors predispose to renal failure in SCI patients. They include diminished renal perfusion, urinary flow obstruction, vesicoureteral reflux, urinary tract infections, urolithiasis, and urosepsis. In earlier times the leading cause of death, renal failure has now become a relatively rare complication thanks to improved urological management.

Acute renal failure in SCI patients mainly occurs during the acute post-injury phase, as a consequence of neurogenic, hemorrhagic, or septic shock. The toxic effects of medications or rhabdomyolysis associated with massive soft-tissue trauma may also result in renal failure. Pathophysiologically, acute renal failure is classified as prerenal, renal, or postrenal (obstructive).

In chronic SCI, acute renal failure is primarily caused by urinary tract obstruction due to stone formation.

Chronic renal failure is no longer a leading cause of death following SCI, but still poses a potential threat and is an important reason for providing lifelong medical follow-up.

Underlying factors include chronic pyelonephritis, urolithiasis with obstructive nephropathy, vesicoureteral reflux, and hypertension with nephrosclerosis. Amyloidosis (increased deposition of protein in renal tissue that impairs kidney function) secondary to chronic infections also occurs. Laboratory findings may include elevated urea and serum creatinine levels (even though serum creatinine may be unreliable due to decreased muscle mass in individuals with SCI), decreased creatinine clearance, anemia due to low erythropoietin levels, platelet dysfunction with bleeding tendency, and secondary hyperparathyroidism. Clinical symptoms of overt chronic renal insufficiency include disruption of higher cerebral functions, peripheral neuropathy, fluid retention, uremic pericarditis, and osteomalacia. For a detailed discussion please refer to specialized literature.

SEXUALITY AND FERTILITY PROBLEMS IN MEN

Very few areas in the realm of SCI care have undergone such positive developments as the opportunities for the treatment of sexual disorders and infertility. From the previous state of virtual neglect, this field is now recognized for the great importance it deserves, while at the same time therapeutic options have substantially improved.

Since 80% of traumatic SCI occurs in men, and since sexual function is also most affected in men, we will devote more space to the problems faced by men with SCI. For the equivalent discussion about SCI in women, see Chapter 29.

Sexual Physiology and Anatomy

The penis contains two dorsal tube-like chambers, the *corpora cavernosa*, and a third narrower ventral chamber, the *corpus spongiosum*. These chambers contain sinusoids capable of being filled with blood. A membrane known as the tunica albuginea surrounds the corpora cavernosa. All three chambers are also surrounded by what is known as Buck's fascia. The blood supply to the penis comes from the internal pudendal artery through the common penile artery and its branches. There are three venous systems: superficial, intermediate, and deep.

Erection arises by means of afferent input from widely differing sources such as the imagination, emotions, memories, smells, visual impressions, and somatosensory stimuli. These diverse impulses are integrated within the hypothalamus. Efferent pathways pass through the mesencephalon and brainstem down to the spinal cord level. The brainstem mainly plays an inhibitory role with respect to spinal sexual reflexes.

The penis is innervated by three systems: the sacral parasympathetic (pelvic nerve), the thoracolumbar sympathetic (hypogastric nerve and lumbar portion of the sympathetic trunk), and the somatic (pudendal nerve; Fig. 26.9). The autonomic interaction involved in the erectile process is complex. However, the dominant autonomic influence in this process is *parasympathetic*. Nitric oxide (NO) is the most important neurotransmitter for erection. The mode of actions of androgens also involves the nitric oxide system.

There are two main types of erection: *psychogenic* and *reflexogenic*. These are mediated in part through different pathways. Erection occurs through relaxation of the smooth muscles of the penile vessels, which facilitates filling the erectile tissues with blood, thereby leading to an increase in size and rigidity of the penis, which in turn increases venous occlusion that further enhances tumescence.

The male sexual climax includes two phases: *emission* and *ejaculation*. Emission is sympathetically mediated by the hypogastric nerve. In addition to the forward propulsion of sperm, this phase includes stimulation of α-adrenergic receptors to close the bladder neck and prevent retrograde ejaculation. During the ejaculation phase that follows, there is intermittent relaxation of the external urethral sphincter and spasmodic contractions of the seminal vesicles, prostate, and urethra, which discharges sperm. Propulsion is strengthened by involuntary rhythmic contractions of bulbospongiosus, ischiocavernosus, levator ani, and related muscles. Ejaculation is followed by a refractory period of varying length, during which time a second ejaculation is impossible.

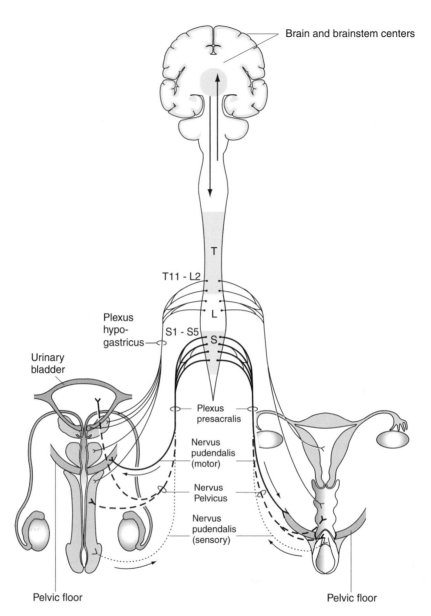

Figure 26.9 Innervation of male genitalia (left) and female genitalia (right). Note especially the thoraco-lumbar sympathetic innervation and the sacral parasympathetic innervation. In addition to this, somatic innervation occurs via the pudendal nerve. Overriding control from the brain and brainstem requires intact spinal cord connections.

Normally ejaculation and *orgasm* occur simultaneously. However, these two events are neurophysiologically separate. In addition, both ejaculation and orgasm may occur without concurrent erection, although this is less common. Orgasm is probably a conditioned reflex, which may be either *genital* or *nongenital*. Genital orgasm is experienced in the genital area and based on afferent impulses from the genitalia to the brain via the lateral spinothalamic tract. The efferent pathway for genital orgasm is probably the corticospinal tract. A nongenital orgasm can be achieved by cerebral stimuli in isolation.

Erectile Dysfunction

Men with complete SCI above the T6 level are unable to relay psychogenic sexual impulses to sacral spinal cord centers. However, the tendency for reflexogenic erection is preserved or even enhanced, although the process is "unreliable," and erection may fail during intercourse. Conversely, patients with injury to the sacral cord are unable to experience reflexogenic erections, but an intact thoracolumbar pathway can mediate a psychogenic erection. Patients whose lesion lies between these two levels will in some cases have preservation of both psychogenic and reflexogenic erection, although the interplay between these systems is lost. Patients with lower motor neuron lesions, such as those found in cauda equina injuries, have varied but often significant degrees of functional loss.

In addition to direct neurological impairment from the SCI, other contributing causes of erectile dysfunction (ED) are commonly found, such as depression, atherosclerosis, diabetes mellitus, and medication side effects.

Erectile function is often impaired following SCI and, regardless of causes, many patients will want some form of therapy to improve erectile function.

Treatment

The oral treatment with which we have the most experience as of this writing is sildenafil (Viagra). This selective inhibitor of phosphodiesterase type 5 (PDE5) regulates cyclical guanine monophospthate synthetase (GMP), an essential nucleotide for the relaxation of smooth muscle within corpus cavernosum. Sildenafil works best for men with preserved reflexogenic erection, i.e., upper motor neuron lesions. Common side effects include headache, facial flushing, nasal congestion, dyspepsia, and transient blue-tinted vision. Concomitant administration of nitrates is contraindicated, since these enhance the hypotensive effect of sildenafil. The drug should be taken 30 minutes to 1 hour before planned sexual activity at a dose of 25–100 mg. Other oral medication are available with similar mode of action.

Drugs may also be administered locally into the penis. Alprostadil or PGE1 are drugs used for local injection. The medication is injected into one corpus cavernosum using a short, thin needle. The dose of alprostadil is titrated, beginning with a maximum initial dose of 2 µg in order to avoid protracted erection and priapism (highly protracted erection posing a risk of tissue damage in the penis). This treatment is typically effective, and only persons with severe arterial disease or venous leakage have an inadequate response to this approach. Injections are given no more than once daily and not more than 3 times a week in order to minimize the risk of complications. Alprostadil or PGE1 can also be administered as small suppositories inserted in the urethra. However, efficacy in SCI patients is usually inadequate.

Mechanical treatment methods include constriction bands and vacuum pumps. The simplest is an elastic band, known as a *pubis ring,* which is placed around the base of the erect or partially erect penis. Such rings should not be left in place for more than 30 minutes. The elastic band may also be combined with a *vacuum pump.* An airtight tube is placed over the penis, after which the air in the tube is withdrawn, creating a partial vacuum that results in a "passive" erection. A constricting ring is placed around the base of the penis to maintain erection. The base of the penis is not included in this erection, which makes the erection mechanically unstable.

Finally, surgical solutions should be mentioned, such as *penile prostheses* and *sacral anterior root stimulators.* Penile prostheses should more correctly be labeled "implants," which can be soft, semirigid, or inflatable. They are implanted into the corpora cavernosa spaces. Currently, they are rarely used in men with SCI. Surgery involving sacral root stimulators includes implanting electrodes on the sacral ventral roots, as well as severing the sacral dorsal roots. This procedure leads to loss of reflexogenic erection, which makes the patient completely dependent on the stimulator or other erectile aids to achieve erection. This treatment modality is now seldom pertinent to the SCI group.

Infertility

In addition to ED, which in itself of course adversely affects fertility by preventing or complicating intercourse, SCI also often makes ejaculation impossible, a condition known as *anejaculation*. Moreover, sperm are adversely affected, both qualitatively (including impaired motility) and quantitatively. Recurrent urogenital infections may contribute to infertility in this patient group.

Although fertility is often impaired in men with SCI, contraception should not be neglected. Nor is it necessary for those who wish to have children to a priori abandon hope for achieving fertilization through intercourse. Assisted fertilization will become an option if intercourse cannot be carried out, if intercourse can be carried out but ejaculation fails, or if repeated intercourse with successful ejaculation fails to result in conception. Workup includes sperm analysis, as well as workup of the partner. Sperm may be obtained through either masturbation or through one of the methods described below.

Should masturbation fail to provide an ejaculate, *vibrostimulation* is the first-line option. This method involves applying a vibrator to the glans penis and using stimulation in repeated cycles of 1 or 2 minutes, separated by rest periods of 1 or 2 minutes. Most men achieve ejaculation within a couple of stimulation cycles. The optimal amplitude has been shown to be 2.5 mm, and the optimal frequency 100 Hz. Vibrators with these parameters, such as Ferticare R, are commercially available. This method presumes intact lumbosacral reflex arcs, and therefore is less effective or fails in the presence of conus and/or caudal lesions. About 75% of patients with the level of lesion above T10 respond to this treatment, and patients with a cervical level of lesion respond even better. Essentially the only adverse effect comprises possible autonomic dysreflexia if the level of lesion is above T6.

Electroejaculation is an option for the extraction of semen. This method triggers ejaculation via direct stimulation of peripheral nerves and even works for conus and/or cauda injuries.

Stimulation is applied with a probe inserted into the rectum. The probe is equipped with electrodes that are placed anteriorly against the prostate. Direct current stimulation with 4–15 volts generally results in ejaculation of semen, which is further manually "milked" from the penis. Patients with preserved sensory function in the perineal region are treated under spinal or general anesthesia. Stimulation should be preceded and followed up by sigmoidoscopy. The urinary bladder should be emptied with a catheter prior to stimulation, and phosphate buffer or similar solution should be instilled into the bladder in order to neutralize urine pH and thereby protect the sperm in case of retrograde ejaculation. The bladder should be emptied following the stimulation procedure, and both antegrade and any retrograde ejaculate should be preserved. As with vibrostimulation, autonomic dysreflexia is the most common adverse effect.

Yet another alternative that has become increasingly common is to surgically extract sperm directly from the vas deferens, epididymitis, or testes. These methods include *microepididymal sperm aspiration (MESA)*, *percutaneous epididymal sperm aspiration (PESA)*, or *testicular sperm extraction (TESE)*.

Fertilization can be achieved through intrauterine insemination with or without inducing ovulation, or with other assisted reproductive techniques such as *in vitro fertilization* (IVF) or *intracytoplasmic sperm injection* (ICSI), depending on practical circumstances and sperm quality.

Questions relating to sexual function and infertility should be given high priority during rehabilitation. These issues should be discussed frankly, early during the rehabilitation process. Patients are often hesitant to discuss intimate issues. The knowledge that it is possible to regain sexual function and to become a parent strengthens the patient's self-esteem, and facilitates continued rehabilitation. Patient education should be given high priority in this matter, as in many other areas.

Sexual rehabilitation builds on optimizing existing functions as well as adapting to those limitations that are unavoidable. In other words, the goal is to integrate the patient's sexual issues in the context of the total situation, which includes self-perception, bladder/bowel management, sensory function (including erogenous zones), concomitant medical problems, psychological status, relationship with partner and social network, and other issues. It is also advisable to include the patient's partner when discussing the various available treatment options, as well as ED and infertility.

27 | Pressure Ulcers

INCIDENCE AND PATHOGENESIS

Pressure ulcers has been a leading cause of death among SCI patients. Today, about 10% of deaths are related to pressure ulcers. About one-third of all newly injured patients are afflicted, and the incidence during the first and second year after the injury is about 10% annually. Once patients suffer from pressure ulcers, they are prone to recurrence. The risk is higher in complete and/or high-level injuries. Because of the lack of sensation, such individuals do not experience "warning signals" such as pain or discomfort. *Pressure ulcers are the most common "preventable" cause of hospitalization among SCI patients.*

A pressure ulcer is an area of tissue necrosis that develops when soft tissues are compressed for a period of time, usually between a bony prominence and an external surface. Typical locations in SCI patients include the sacrum, ischial tuberosities, trochanters, and malleoli. Pressure ulcers are actually areas of infarction. They arise as a result of ischemia, with an initial period of potential for reperfusion and restored tissue viability. The dead tissue in the pressure ulcer is surrounded by a penumbra zone with reversible cellular damage.

From a pathogenetic standpoint, pressure is the most important causal factor. Adverse body position due to contractures, scoliosis, and/or severe spasticity increases the risk that pressure on contact surfaces will be unevenly distributed. Both intensity and duration of pressure play a role. Transverse forces that laterally displace the dermis (shearing) increase the risk of ischemia in response to pressure. Perspiration, urine, or feces can cause the skin to become friable, thereby decreasing its tolerance to pressure. Abnormally dry skin is likewise more susceptible to damage.

Several medical factors contribute to an increased propensity for pressure ulcers. Collagen metabolism decreases below the neurological level of injury, which increases vulnerability to pressure sores and impairs the healing process. Muscle atrophy reduces pressure distribution and "padding" around bony prominences. Other risk factors include impaired venous return, anemia, fever, diabetes, and malnutrition (low serum albumin, vitamin C, and zinc deficiency). Smoking compromises peripheral circulation and is a major risk factor. Aging also increases the risk of developing pressure ulcers for various reasons. Last but not least, *psychological factors* are worthy of mention, the most important of which are depression and substance abuse.

Normal wound healing is a three-phase process. First is the *inflammatory* phase, in which bacteria and devitalized tissue are removed. Next follows the *proliferative* phase, during which granulation and scar tissues are formed. And finally, the *maturation and remodeling phase* occurs with a gradual increase in the tensile strength of the scar tissue. This healing process is strongly inhibited by concurrent wound infection.

Preventive measures are crucial. These include teaching the patient and/or assistants and family members to relieve pressure regularly every 15–30 minutes for wheelchair-bound patients, adhering to an every-other-hour turning schedule when the patient is in bed, prescribing adequate wheelchair cushions and bed mattresses, reducing sliding in bed and friction during transfers, maintaining correct body position when sitting and lying, practicing good general skin care, smoking cessation, moderating alcohol consumption, and ensuring adequate nutrition.

MANAGEMENT

Management of manifest ulcers requires a *team approach*. Treating the ulcer alone is not enough; instead, patients must be treated as a whole in which both their biological, psychological, and social situations are of great importance.

The primary purpose is to identify and address the risk factors already mentioned. The assessment also includes analysis of ergonomic factors related to sitting (especially pressure factors, presence of shearing forces, and body posture); inspection of the wheelchair, cushion, and bed; and analysis of the patient's daily routines. The available selection of cushions and mattresses offers many alternatives. Common materials include foam, air, gel, and water. Trying out appropriate assistive devices is a complex task requiring a collaborative effort involving occupational and physical therapists.

Documentation of the location, size, and depth of the ulcer should be detailed and standardized. Photos taken at regular intervals facilitate assessment of the healing process. Examination of the ulcer include an assessment of any undermining (i.e., a peripheral expansion of the ulcer under the surface of the skin). Likewise, any fistulae should be noted and documented. The appearance of the ulcer bed and wound edges, presence of exudates, and status of surrounding skin should be noted. The ulcer bed may be clean, covered by exudate, or necrotic. Underlying connective tissues, including bone, tendons, and joint capsules, may be visible or palpable in the wound bed. Wound secretion should be analyzed with respect to quantity, color, and quality. Increased exudate production is a sure sign of bacterial colonization or infection, as is the presence of purulent exudate. The ulcer may be classified according to several scales.

The most commonly used is a 4-point scale, where:

- *Grade 1* = persisting erythema in intact skin
- *Grade 2* = partial skin damage involving the epidermis, but not penetrating the dermis
- *Grade 3* = full skin thickness lesion penetrating into subcutis
- *Grade 4* = also involvement of muscles, connective tissue, joint capsules and/or underlying bone (Fig. 27.1).

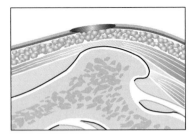

Grade 1

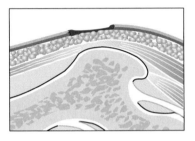

Grade 2

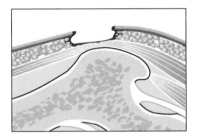

Grade 3

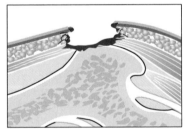

Grade 4

Figure 27.1 Pressure ulcers. The sequence of illustrations shows successively more extensive ulceration. Grade 1 is characterized by an erythema that fails to blanch. Grade 2 involves a superficial ulcer. Grade 3 entails a full skin lesion penetrating into subcutaneous tissue, and grade 4 also involves deeper tissues.

Necrotic tissue must be removed because it prevents the wound from healing, hinders assessment of the wound bed, and serves as a substrate for bacterial growth. Debridement may be sharp/surgical, mechanical (scrubbing or wound irrigation), enzymatic, or autolytic. Autolytic debridement is facilitated by occlusive bandaging, which permits endogenous body enzymes to break down necrotic tissue. However, the latter method is inappropriate during active wound infection. Once the ulcer is clean, a several treatment options are available (please refer to the literature for more detailed descriptions). A number of more or less experimental methods are also available, including electrical stimulation, growth factors, hyperbaric oxygen, electromagnetic field, therapeutic ultrasound, and vacuum treatment.

It is commonplace for pressure ulcers to become infected. Many pressure ulcers are located near the anus or urethral meatus, which greatly increases the risk of bacterial contamination. Local signs of infection include fever, erythema, edema, induration, foul odor, and increased secretion, while laboratory tests show elevated ESR, C-reactive protein, and white blood count. Common pathogens include gram-positive cocci, especially *Staphylococcus aureus* and streptococci, gram-negative bacteria such as *Pseudomonas aeruginosa*, and anaerobes, mainly *Bacteroides* species. Ulcers that on superficial inspection appear to be healed may harbor residual infectious foci deep within the tissue. In such cases diagnosis may be verified with bone scan and/or computed tomography (CT). In some cases, a deep focus of infection may manifest as a skin fistula. In such cases *fistulography* (contrast radiography) may be used to clarify the anatomy of the fistula. In other cases, the infection involves underlying bone tissue, causing osteitis and/or osteomyelitis. Bone scans are almost 100% sensitive for osteomyelitis, but unfortunately have low specificity. The purpose of a bone scan in this context is therefore mainly to rule out rather than to confirm the diagnosis.

Treatment of infected pressure ulcers includes local wound care and antibiotics. Severe cases require more extensive surgical debridement of necrotic tissue and sometimes musculocutaneous flap surgery. In cases of chronic osteomyelitis, treatment with antibiotics often must be continued for several months. Unsatisfactory therapeutic response may be due to improper selection of antibiotics, deep-seated infection, and/or fistula communicating with the urinary or gastrointestinal tract.

Typically, surgical treatment should be preceded by attempts at conservative treatment in accordance with the methods previously described. However, grade 4 ulcers rarely heal without surgical treatment. This also applies to ulcers complicated by fistulae, underlying osteomyelitis, or pyarthrosis, and to ulcers with significant undermining in the subcutaneous tissue plane. Surgical treatment includes debridement of all devitalized or necrotic tissue. Surgery for pressure ulcers is typically planned so that the skin flap will be sufficiently large to be used again, should the situation so require. If possible the surgical scar should be positioned outside the area that comes under direct pressure. Bony prominences may be reduced through partial osteotomies and through "padding" with soft tissue (usually muscle). *Musculocutaneous flaps* are usually the procedure of choice since they have a richer blood supply than other types of flaps and provide sufficient bulk to reduce "dead space" and to pad bony prominences. Postoperative care includes gradual mobilization, with careful monitoring of wound healing, as well as extensive patient education to involve the patient in actively preventing recurrence.

28 Sleep Disturbances

Insomnia is common in the general population, and even more so among SCI patients. Insomnia per se is, of course, not a diagnosis, but a symptom. There are a number of treatable causes, and insomnia in persons with SCI should therefore always be carefully assessed before prescribing symptomatic treatment with hypnotics. In this chapter we address the most important underlying conditions that cause sleep disturbances.

GENERAL CAUSES

During the early stages following SCI, patients undergo a psychological *crisis reaction,* and the anxiety component may be prominent. Depressive symptoms are equally common. Both anxiety and depression are highly likely to disrupt sleep. In addition, somatic factors may also have a negative impact. During the early phases following trauma, patients must be turned every other hour and the bladder must be catheterized every 4–6 hours. Pain and incontinence also frequently disrupt sleep.

OBSTRUCTIVE SLEEP APNEA

Sleep apnea is overrepresented in SCI, especially among persons with tetraplegia. It is also relatively common in the general population. Pathogenetically, sleep is here associated with recurring obstruction of the airways in the pharynx, which results in snoring and interrupted breathing (apnea). Apnea is defined as *suspension of breathing lasting more than 10 seconds.* Such periods result in hypoxia and carbon dioxide retention, which lead to more superficial sleep or awakening and an associated increase in the muscle tone of the pharynx, which then opens the airways. Subsequently, when deeper sleep resumes, the muscle tone of the pharynx again decreases and the process is repeated. Afflicted patients often have dozens to hundreds of such episodes of apnea each night. All this causes fragmented sleep of poor quality. This condition often results in daytime fatigue and poor performance, and may also lead to arterial hypertension and increase the risk of conditions such as stroke and myocardial infarction. The increased incidence of obstructive sleep apnea syndrome associated with SCI may be attributed to several risk factors, including obesity, high consumption of sedatives, and reduced lung capacity predisposing to collapse of the upper airways, as well as to increased neck thickness regardless of body weight.

The diagnosis should be suspected in the presence of loud snoring, frequent episodes of apnea during sleep, morning headaches, and daytime fatigue. The diagnosis is confirmed by *polysomnography*, which entails simultaneous recording of air flow through nose and mouth, oxygen saturation, snoring, thoracic, abdominal, and eye movements, electrocardiogram (EKG), and electroencephalogram (EEG). Less complex screening methods are also available.

Treatment of obstructive sleep apnea syndrome includes weight loss and avoidance of alcohol and muscle relaxants. First-line treatment is with continuous positive airway pressure (CPAP), which is administered at night using a mask to cover the nose or the nose and mouth. Pharyngeal surgery may also come under consideration.

INVOLUNTARY MOVEMENTS DURING SLEEP

Spasticity is common following SCI and frequently leads to sleep disturbances. The patient is chiefly awakened by frequent muscle spasms characterized by sudden flexion or extension of the extremities. In these cases, treatment with baclofen at night may be advantageous, especially since its side effects may include drowsiness. Clonazepam given at night is another treatment option. A relatively rare syndrome, *periodic limb movements of sleep (PLMS)*, has also been reported following SCI. It has been linked to a dopamine deficiency in the central nervous system, and is characterized by stereotypic repetitive movements during sleep.

DISRUPTION OF MELATONIN SECRETION

The sleep–wake cycle is mainly regulated by the suprachiasmatic nucleus in the hypothalamus. This structure controls functions such as melatonin secretion via an efferent neural loop that passes down through the cervical spinal cord, where it reaches the superior cervical ganglion from which it returns to the brain and innervates the pineal body. Consequently, there exists an anatomical basis for lesioning of this neural pathway in tetraplegia, and low basal melatonin levels and absence of normal physiological rhythm in melatonin secretion have in fact been demonstrated in persons with high-level SCI. Although the clinical significance has not been established, the possibility of a "SCI-specific" underlying reason for sleep disturbance has thus been suggested.

Only about 20% of patients with traumatic SCI are women. This is one of the reasons that most studies carried out to date have focused on men. Gender distribution in nontraumatic spinal cord lesions varies based on etiology, but is typically more even. This section addresses only such aspects that are either unique to women with SCI, or in which differences compared to men are significant.

FERTILITY AND SEXUALITY

Following acute SCI, women often experience a temporary loss of menstrual periods, *amenorrhea*. Transient *hyperprolactinemia* with or without *galactorrhea* (i.e., milk production in the mammary glands) may often occur. Menstruation usually resumes within 3–6 months of injury, accompanied by a return to normal fertility. This is in sharp contrast to the situation for men with SCI, where infertility remains a significant problem.

Dysmenorrhea may manifest through autonomic dysreflexia, increased spasticity, and/or urinary urgency and frequency. The symptoms may be alleviated with anti-inflammatory medications.

Sexual function may be adversely affected by impaired sensation, decreased vaginal lubrication, incontinence, autonomic dysreflexia, and positioning problems due to spasticity, heterotopic ossification, and/or contractures. In all other aspects, sexual counseling for women with SCI entails the same holistic approach as for men. Because of the increased tendency for venous thromboembolism following SCI, caution should be exercised in prescribing oral contraceptives, especially during the first year post injury, among smokers, and in persons with a history of thrombotic disease. Intrauterine devices and diaphragms also require special precaution with respect to decreased sensation in the genital area.

Pregnancy in women with SCI should be monitored by a gynecologist. Pregnancy may be associated with increased problems with urinary incontinence, urinary tract infections, impaired pulmonary function, dependent edema, constipation, pressure ulcers, and impaired mobility. The patient's current medications should be reviewed regarding potential teratogenicity, for example, benzodiazepines, carbamazepine, tetracyclines, and anti-inflammatories.

Vaginal delivery is usually the method of choice in women with SCI, except in cases in which conventional obstetrical contraindications apply. However, possible musculoskeletal obstacles such as severe spasticity, heterotopic ossification, and hip joint contractures must be ruled out. *Autonomic dysreflexia* is the most common delivery-related complication among women with a lesion level above T6. Differential diagnosis must take into account conditions such as preeclampsia. Autonomic dysreflexia in conjunction with labor can be avoided with epidural anesthesia.

INCONTINENCE

Incontinence problems are for anatomical reasons more common among women, while detrusor–sphincter dyssynergia and high intravesical pressure are less common. Urinary diversion surgery is considered more often in women, since a condom catheter of course cannot be used to provide incontinence protection.

MENOPAUSE

Menopause in women with SCI is associated with symptoms similar to those experienced by women in general. However, it should be kept in mind that menopause-related osteoporosis will compound SCI-related osteoporosis, which results in a significant increase in the risk of fracture. Changes in the skin and mucous membranes related to menopause may lead to an increased risk of pressure ulcers and urological problems. No studies are available to provide definite guidance as to whether hormone replacement therapy is more or less indicated in this patient population compared with the population at large.

Neurological deterioration following SCI may result in minor additional disability or, in worst cases, in dramatic loss of motor-, sensory-, and autonomic function above, at and below the original level of lesion. The losses of function following SCI are not static. Heterotrophic ossification, bladder and bowel disturbances, pressure ulcers, and other common causes of functional impairment have been described in previous chapters. Additionally, consequences related to the spinal cord proper have, during the latest decades, received increased attention. Deterioration of motor- and/or sensory function, increased spasticity, and pain may further reduce quality of life. Improved diagnostic tools such as magnetic resonance imaging (MRI) and surgical techniques have resulted in several new treatment options. Here, we discuss troublesome pain, spasticity, and posttraumatic myelopathy including the surgical viewpoint (Table 30.1).

POSTTRAUMATIC MYELOPATHY

Posttraumatic myelopathy (i.e., posttraumatic progressive neurological deficit related to the spinal cord itself) is reflected in the occurrence of new symptoms added to the initial neurological deficits that arose in connection with the initial trauma. A characteristic feature is the progressive nature of these symptoms over time. Thus, the condition is usually referred to as *progressive posttraumatic myelopathy* (PPM). The spinal cord is typically subject to a persistent mechanical compression following trauma. *Arachnoiditis* (i.e., scar formation of the arachnoid caused by inflammation in the acute stage of injury) is the most frequent underlying cause of PPM. MRI may or may not visualize scar tissue and/or intramedullary cyst formation (Fig. 30.1A–D; also see Fig. 30.1D in the Color

Plate section). Persistent compression of the spinal cord due to displaced bony fragments is yet another cause of PPM (Fig. 30.2). Patients with PPM either suffer from a progressive posttraumatic *noncystic* myelopathy (PPNCM) or a progressive posttraumatic *cystic* myelopathy (PPCM). The onset of symptoms related to PPM can range from months to decades post injury. However, other causes with symptoms similar to PPM (see Chapter 19) also must be excluded.

The prevalence of developing PPM is 3% and increases with severity of the initial injury.

Pathophysiology

The pathophysiological mechanisms behind PPM are not fully understood except in cases with bony compression. There is agreement about the role of scar tissue tethering the spinal cord to the surrounding tissues, such as the arachnoid (see Fig. 30.1D; also see same figure in Color Plate section). The extension of scar tissue increases with injury severity. The spinal cord is glued to the inside of the dural sac via the scar tissue, and the flow of cerebrospinal fluid (CSF) in the subarachnoid space is thus blocked. The presence of scar tissue is the crucial mechanism behind formation of both cranially and caudally located intramedullary cysts. A widening of the central canal is probably the cause of syringomyelia below the level of lesion, whereas cyst formation cranial to the level of injury probably starts as a liquefaction of contused nervous tissue in the posterior part of the gray matter (see Chapter 3).

The scar tissue causes expansion of an initial microcyst at the level of injury to an

TABLE 30.1 A brief overview of neurosurgical options comprising "Rehabilitative neurosurgery" after SCI.

Symptoms	MRI Findings	Treatment
Posttraumatic myelopathy	Tethering without cyst formation (PPNCM)	Untethering of the spinal cord
	Tethering with cyst formation (PPCM)	Untethering of the spinal cord + spinal cord cyst shunting
	Significant compression of the spinal cord caused by bony fragments	Removal of the compressive vertebra and anterior fusion
Pain problem		Intrathecal morphine therapy
		Spinal cord stimulation
		CA-DREZ lesion
		Untethering of the spinal cord
Spasticity problem		Intrathecal baclofen therapy
		Percutaneous radiofrequency thermal rhizotomy

expansile cyst ranging up to many decimeters caudally and cranially, potentially occupying a major area of the spinal cord diameter (Fig. 30.1C). It is, as mentioned earlier, assumed that posttraumatic cysts above the level of injury are not extensions of the central canal. Normal levels of proteins in cranially located cysts and lack of uptake of contrast agent following injection into the ventricular system further confirm this theory.

By contrast, it is speculated that tension in the vertebral column results in traction forces between the scar tissue and the spinal cord in patients with PPNCM (i.e., posttraumatic myelopathy without radiological signs of cyst formation). Traction results in microtrauma to the spinal cord, and ischemia gradually spreads caudally and cranially, resulting in symptoms of posttraumatic myelopathy.

Symptoms

Clinical symptoms of PPM may begin several decades following the injury. The symptoms are typically slowly increasing, although a sudden onset of symptoms is sometimes seen.

In those cases, the character of symptoms resembles those seen after spinal cord infarction. The seven cardinal symptoms of PPM are presented in Table 30.2. The frequency of symptoms listed in this table reflects those of a surgical clientele. Two to four of the seven symptoms occurred among 75% of the patients. Three symptoms were the most frequent number of manifestations, at the time of the surgical procedure.

Pain is usually presented in two forms (see Chapter 21). The first type is described as somatic pain (similar to sore muscles) localized at or above the level of injury and/or also below the injury site if the patient suffers from an incomplete lesion. The second type is a neuropathic-type pain with a similar distribution.

A progressive deterioration in motor function occurs above the level of lesion in patients with complete lesions. A loss of hand function may be the first motor sign in patients with thoracic level injuries. Patients with incomplete lesion may display a similar pattern of motor loss above the level of lesion but also additional loss of motor function in the trunk muscles (manifested as truncal instability when the person is sitting) and lower extremities. An extreme case would

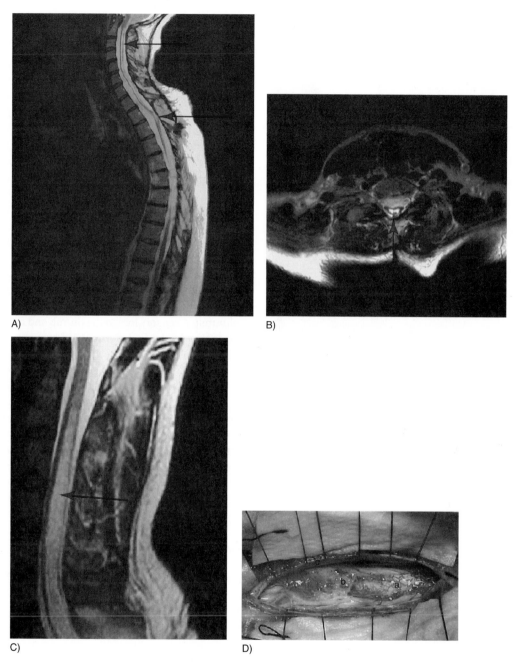

A)

B)

C)

D)

Figure 30.1 A collage showing spinal cord tethering and intramedullary cyst formation. A: Magnetic resonance image (MRI)-obtained sagittal view. The *upper arrow* shows a minor cyst located intramedullary (white structure compared to the gray color of the spinal cord). The *lower arrow* indicates posterior tethering of the spinal cord to the surrounding arachnoid tissue at disk level of T2–3. The gray colored spinal cord is retracted posteriorly in the spinal canal. B: MRI; corresponding axial view. The *arrow* marks the area of tethering. The cerebrospinal fluid is absent precisely at 6 o'clock indicating a adhesion of the spinal to the surrounding tissue. C: An intramedullary cyst (*arrow*) occupying most of the spinal cord diameter. D: Intraoperative illustration of scar formation surrounding the spinal cord. *a,* spinal cord; *b,* scar tissue; *c,* dural sac. See also Color Plate Fig. 30.1D.

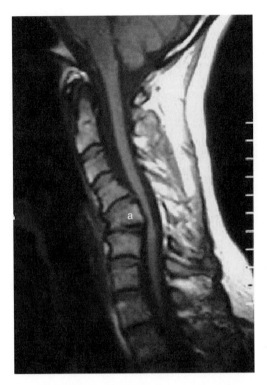

Figure 30.2 Fracture. Magnetic resonance image (MRI)-obtained sagittal view illustrating a conservatively treated fracture (*a*, damaged vertebra; C5). The spinal cord is dislocated as well as compressed at the level of injury.

TABLE 30.2 The seven cardinal symptoms (in order of appearance in the text) of PPM according to Edgar.

Symptoms	Percent
Pain problem	36
Asymmetrical motor loss	80
Increased spasticity	54
Disturbance of sensation	87
Horner syndrome	22
Autonomic dysreflexia	23
Hyperhydrosis	38

be exemplified by an initial lesion at the level of conus. An intramedullary cyst extending to the cervical region results in difficulties in writing and in transferring to and from a wheelchair,

and also reduces motor functions in the hand, such as grip and pinch strength.

Although increased spasticity is a common PPM symptom, it is highly unspecific and should thus not in its isolation be considered a sign of PPM until all other potential causes, such as pain of non–spinal cord origin and infection, have been excluded.

Disturbances in sensory function may vary in character. Deterioration in pain and temperature sensation without simultaneous loss of fine touch and proprioception (i.e., dissociated sensory loss) is the most common presentation (due to damage to the lateral spinothalamic tract). Disturbances of only fine touch and proprioception at and above the level of lesion are seen in patients with complete lesions and also below the level of lesion in patients with incomplete lesions (in both cases due to damage to the dorsal columns). A sensory loss in the thumb and index finger may be the first sign noticed by a patient using a wheelchair. A spreading of the sensory loss in this area may have a major impact on daily living because of a reduction in grip and pinch capacity, although motor strength may remain unchanged. Horner syndrome (miosis, ptosis, and enophthalmos), increased autonomic dysreflexia, and sweating are less common symptoms of PPM. The absence of these less-common symptoms does not exclude PPM but, if present, strengthens the suspicion of this diagnosis.

Investigations

The work-up and management of PPM is performed in close cooperation between the rehabilitation team and the neurosurgeon (Table 30.3). Disorders such as spondylosis of the spinal canal, persisting instability, and progressive kyphosis at the level of injury; tumors; peripheral neuropathies; and inflammatory and metabolic changes may all present with symptoms suggestive of PPM. An accurate radiological investigation, as well as a careful neurophysiologic examination including electromyelogram, sensory evoked potentials (SEP), and motor evoked potentials (MEP) are included in the preoperative work-up. The survey also includes a detailed

Table 30.3 Preoperative investigations of PPM.

Radiology
  - MRI, CT, plain X-ray
Neurophysiology
  - EMG, SEP, MEP
Functional tests
  - Spasticity
  - Neurological status
ADL and quality of life
  - FIM, COPM, SF-36

MRI, magnetic resonance imaging;
CT, computed tomography;
EMG, electromyelography;
SEP, sensory evoked potential;
MEP, motor evoked potential;
FIM, Functional Independence Measure;
COPM, Canadian Occupational Performance Measure;
SF-36, Short Form 36 Questions.

Table 30.4. Indications for surgical treatment of PPM.

Significant progressive deterioration of motor and/or sensory function
Severe nociceptive-type (muscle soreness) pain starting months to years after injury
Severe neuropathic-type pain (onset >2 years after injury)
The remaining four symptoms, if isolated manifestations of PPM, constitutes no indication for surgical treatment

neurological examination according to American Spinal Injury Association (ASIA), an evaluation of the degree of spasticity, and finally an ADL and a quality of life assessment. The final decision is mainly based on the patient's medical history and on the results of the radiological investigation. The importance of the medical history cannot be overstated, because signs of spinal cord tethering sometimes are absent on MRI. A false-negative MRI (i.e., one not showing scar formation) does not exclude the presence of PPM. On the other hand, the presence of intramedullary cysts does not, as such, indicate a need for surgical intervention.

Surgical Treatment of PPM: Indications and Goals

Indications for the surgical treatment of PPM are presented in Table 30.4. Clinical symptoms together with progressive signs of motor and sensory loss are the most common indication for surgical treatment. Presence of a progressive muscular soreness-type pain, as well as neuropathic pain with a delayed onset in relation to the trauma, may likewise both indicate a need for surgical intervention.

The choice of surgical method is based on the onset of the neuropathic pain. The computer-

assisted dorsal root entry zone (CA-DREZ) lesion procedure is preferred (as discussed in a later section), if neuropathic pain starts in connection with the primary spinal cord traumatic event. The untethering procedure will be chosen if symptoms of neuropathic pain starts 2 years or later in relation to the trauma. This depends on the type of underlying mechanism, see text ahead.

There is usually no indication for surgical treatment if increased spasticity, autonomic dysreflexia, hyperhidrosis, or Horner syndrome present as isolated symptoms of PPM.

The primary goal of surgical treatment is to halt further progression of the pathophysiological process that is based on scar formation and tethering of the spinal cord. The surgical goal is not to reverse symptoms, but rather to avoid further deterioration. A functional improvement should be considered a bonus result to the patient.

Surgical Treatment of PPM: Technical Considerations

The aim of surgical treatment is to untether the spinal cord from surrounding tissues and to create an open space for the CSF to circulate in the spinal subarachnoid space, thus also allowing the spinal cord to move without restrictions. The presence of intramedullary cysts, in addition to scar formation, will require a shunting procedure in order to reduce intrinsic compression of the spinal cord. The patient is initially placed in a prone position following the anesthetic procedure. The posterior approach is suitable since most of the scar formation will be found in the posterior aspect of the intradural space. This is probably due to a posterior accumulation of blood and inflammatory products during the initial stage of injury, during which the patient is typically lying in a supine position.

The surgical procedure starts with exposure of the dura at the level of lesion and a few segments above and below the level of lesion. This exposure enables untethering of scar tissue in both cranial and caudal directions. The presence of tethering/scar formation (see Fig. 30.1D, here and in Color Plate section and Fig. 30.3A,B), as well as intramedullary cysts (Fig. 30.4) can be verified or excluded by intraoperative ultrasonography. The dura is, after ultrasonographic investigation, opened in the midline and the spinal cord is now exposed. The scar tissue is loosened from the surrounding arachnoid/dura tissue, after which the spinal cord should regain its physiological position in the spinal canal and no restrictions to CSF flow remain at the level of lesion. Two options remain if an intramedullary cyst is present: to perform a cyst shunting procedure or to leave the cyst untouched. An additional intraoperative ultrasonography should be performed, according to Lee and coworkers, in order to visualize the cyst diameter after the untethering procedure. According to these authors, no cyst shunting is indicated if the cyst has collapsed by 50% or more compared to its preoperative size.

As the cause of cyst formation (i.e., the scar tissue) has been removed, the insertion of a shunt catheter is not considered of the essence, and could actually contribute to renewed scar formation.

Most of surgeons, however, choose to open the midline of the spinal cord (i.e., myelotomy) (Fig. 30.5; also see same figure in Color Plate section) and insert a cyst catheter, irrespective of the result of the previously performed ultrasonographic investigation. The shunt catheter is then inserted into the cyst and directed as cranially as possible, after which the caudal part is implanted into the ventrolateral subarachnoid space at least 6–8 cm below the level of tethering (Fig. 30.6; also see same figure in Color Plate section). The catheter is attached to the pia mater with unresorbable sutures to prevent shunt catheter migration. It is of extreme importance that the original dura is not closed. Instead, the original dura covering the spinal cord is replaced by an artificial dural graft (Fig. 30.7; also see same figure in Color Plate section). This prevents CSF leakage and reduces the risk for the spinal cord to reattach to the dura, a condition known as *retethering*. The aim, once the dural graft is attached to the original dura, is to achieve a watertight seal between the two. A watertight attachment prevents leakage of CSF into the blood-containing (extra dural) space and prevents blood from sleeping into the intradural space. The risk of retethering increases if blood and CSF once again mix inside of the dural graft. This may, after a period of good or excellent surgical outcome, result in a relapse of symptoms related to new scar formation and PPM. A submuscular

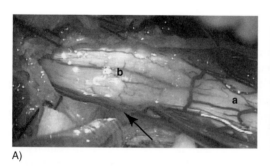 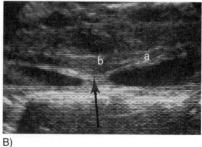

A)   B)

Figure 30.3 Scar formation. A: Intraoperative photo showing scar formation between the spinal cord and dural sac (*arrow*). *a*, uninjured spinal cord; *b*, lesion level is characterized by its grayish color. B: Intraoperative ultrasonography corresponding to the tethering (*arrow*) shown in Figure 30.3A. See also Color Plate Fig. 30.3A.

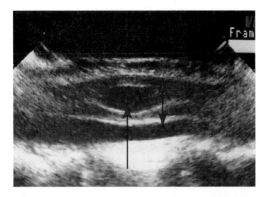

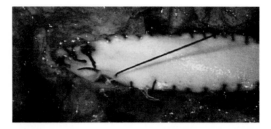

Figure 30.7 Duraplasty. See also Color Plate Fig. 30.7.

Figure 30.4 Ultrasonography obtained previous to the opening of the dura. The *single arrow* points at the intramedullary located cyst and the *double arrow* show the spinal cord diameter. The white structure at the tips of the double arrow marks the outer border of the spinal cord.

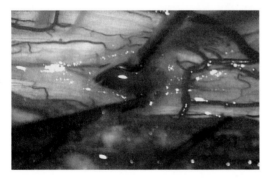

Figure 30.5 The spinal cord is exposed (midline myelotomy). See also Color Plate Fig. 30.5.

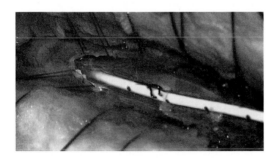

Figure 30.6 Insertion of a shunt catheter through the midline myelotomy. See also Color Plate Fig. 30.6.

drainage tube, which remains in place until the second postoperative day, is inserted, after which the fascia, subcutaneous tissue, and skin are closed. The patient is confined to bedrest until the second postoperative day.

Mobilization starts cautiously on the second postoperative day. During the entire postoperative period, it is of greatest importance that patients be turned regularly in order to avoid pressure ulcers. The risk of retethering is also at least theoretically reduced by this procedure, since regular turning counteracts new formation of scar tissue at the level of lesion. The time period of immobilization in a given position during which any blood collected between the dura and spinal cord may organize into a scar is reduced by this turning procedure. A postoperative MRI (Fig. 30.8) will show a collabated cyst and that the spinal cord has regained its normal diameter.

Surgical Treatment of PPM Caused by Persistent Spinal Cord Compression

Compression of the spinal cord can sometimes be demonstrated on MRI in patients with PPM (Fig. 30.2). Such compression may be the sole cause of PPM or may also occur in combination with other pathology, for example an intramedullary cyst. The dislocated fracture that caused the primary SCI may have been insufficiently treated in a conservative manner, a situation which was a fairly common decades in previous.

The question of how to perform the surgical procedure is complicated if both causes of PPM (i.e., tethering without/with cyst formation as well as persistent spinal cord compression) are

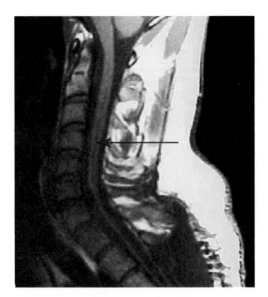

Figure 30.8 Intramedullary cyst. Postoperative magnetic resonance image (MRI) illustrating a collapsed intramedullary cyst, now seen as a thin black slit located in the middle of the gray spinal cord.

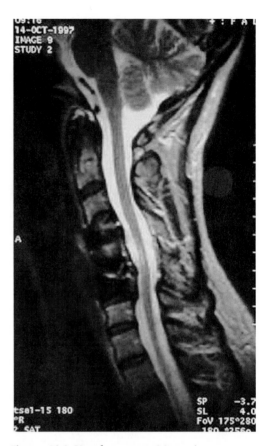

Figure 30.9 Vertebrectomy. Magnetic resonance image (MRI) following removal of fractured vertebra (compare with Figure 30.2). No sign of spinal cord compression remains.

detected by MRI. The surgeon must consider whether the first step should a decompression of the spinal cord by removing the bony fragments, or whether the focus should be directed to the tethered cord and the cyst. Although each patient with PPM and multiple changes on MRI should be assessed individually, some general principles may be applied. Removal of the compressing vertebra is, according to our view, the first step if uncertainty exists about the cause of PPM (see Chapter 12) in the case of lower cervical spine fractures and ligament injuries (C3–C7). From the patient's perspective, vertebrectomy (i.e., the surgical removal of a vertebra) is a less risky and less strenuous procedure than is the untethering operation. A postoperative MRI can further confirm the successful decompression of the spinal cord (Fig. 30.9, also see Fig. 30.2). If deterioration continues despite a successful vertebrectomy, this indicates tethering as the cause of PPM, and untethering surgery must then be considered.

The alternative surgical option is to start with the untethering procedure. If this operation results in a temporary beneficial effect and later a return of the preoperative symptoms then uncertainty will remain as to whether the symptoms now are caused either by retethering or by remaining mechanical compression. This uncertainty is avoided if the vertebrectomy is chosen as the first surgical option.

Result

Neurological deterioration ceased in 100% of the 600 patients in Edgar and colleague's study. An improvement of the preoperative motor and sensory loss, as well as a decrease in the intensity of neuropathic pain was seen in 87% if the surgical procedure was performed within 3 months of symptom onset. The success rate (here defined as some remission of previous PPM symptom) was reduced to 44% if the symptoms had been present for 6 months or more, and the success rate was further reduced to only a few percent if symptoms had been present for 12 months or more. Seventy-three percent of patients in a study by Lee and coworkers exhibited "good result", whereas 7% showed a further deterioration. Improved motor function occurred in 56% of patients in the same study, and 46% of the patients pre-operatively suffering from increased spasticity improved as regards this symptom. An improved sensory function was seen in 45%, and an improved walking ability was seen in 47% of patients with incomplete lesions. The effect on autonomic dysreflexia on the other hand, was poor.

SURGICAL (INVASIVE) TREATMENT OF PAIN

Trauma to the spinal cord results in damage to the nociceptive neurons located in the posterior horns, and ectopic stimulation may be initiated from the dorsal root ganglia (for review, see Chapter 21). Impulses from C-fibers arise and wide-dynamic-range (WDR) neurons are further activated. A condition of hyperexcitability is initiated. A connection exists between hyperexcitability in the deafferentated nervous tissue located in the dorsal horns and the occurrence of spontaneous pain. Morphological changes, such as demyelinization and biochemical alterations in the postsynaptic neurons located in the dorsal horns, may also contribute to the development of neuropathic pain. Physiotherapy and pharmacological treatment may provide insufficient pain relief. In such cases, invasive therapies should be considered. Surgical treatments of PPM have already been discussed in this chapter; now, three additional pain therapies—intrathecal administration of morphine, spinal cord stimulation, and CA-DREZ—will be presented. Unusual methods such as cordectomy, cordotomy, myelotomy, and arachnoid grafting will not be presented in this chapter.

Intrathecal Morphine Administration (Spinal Morphine Pump)

Various opioid transmitters and receptors have been localized among the presynaptic afferents

and postsynaptic neurons in the dorsal horns. Focus has been directed to two opioid transmitters, namely the dynorphines and enkephalins. The opioid receptors are designated as μ-, δ-, or κ-receptors. Morphine exerts its analgesic effect mainly through the μ-receptor, which is also the target of endogenous opioids. The analgesic effect of the opioids is achieved by the blocking of the synaptic transmission between the primary afferents and the postsynaptic neurons. The supraspinal inhibitory tracts are activated, and the transmission between the primary afferents and the postsynaptic neurons are reduced as a result of μ-receptor activation.

An implanted pump for intrathecal delivery of morphine is an option for administrating opioids in the treatment of neuropathic pain. A catheter is initially placed intradurally in the CSF space between the arachnoid and pia mater, after which the catheter is connected to an infusion pump placed in the abdominal layer of fat. The amount of drug to be delivered is defined through external presets, and drug refills are performed using an insertion needle that penetrates a central membrane in the infusion pump.

Morphine is the drug most often used in the intrathecal treatment of neuropathic pain following SCI. This treatment has previously been successful in the management of cancer-associated neuropathic pain. Its most prominent advantage lies in the possibility of avoiding most side effects associated with systematically administered morphine, since the intrathecally administered drug does not accumulate in brain tissue. The therapeutic effect of 1 mg morphine delivered intrathecally corresponds to an oral intake of 150 mg. An standard quantity of intrathecally delivered morphine varies between 1 and 20 mg during a 24-hour period, and the effect is dose-dependent. The infusion pumps used are very safe and do not restrain patients in their daily activities. The development of drug tolerance is the only real disadvantage and is reflected by the need for increasing doses of the drug. Relatively high doses may be administered, because it seems that tolerance develops more rapidly if the drug is given as a continuos infusion rather than on an as-needed basis. The development of drug tolerance may be delayed by adding other drugs such as clonidine

(Catapres®; 10 mg per 1 mg of morphine) or bupivacaine hydrochloride to the morphine solution. (It has also been reported that Catapres® may have intrinsic analgesic properties.) A pause in drug delivery, a so-called "drug holiday," may have a similar effect.

Complications such as the development of granuloma and other problems related to the catheter, as well as meningitis and myelitis have been reported. Transient side effects such as urine retention and pruritus have been reported, as well as constipation, which is considered a chronic side effect of opioid treatment. The estimated cost of an implantable spinal cord pump is about $15,000 US.

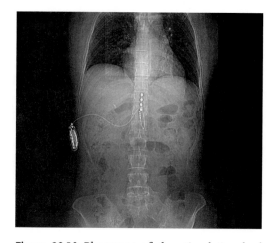

Figure 30.10 Placement of the stimulating lead during spinal cord stimulation.

The implantation of pumps for intrathecal delivery of morphine is a two-step procedure:

Step 1: A spinal catheter is inserted into the intrathecal space. This mimics the situation that will exist once the infusion pump has been implanted. The spinal catheter is connected to an external infusion pump. The analgesic effect of morphine is tested by modulating the doses of delivered morphine. Step 2 follows if delivery of the test dose results in significant pain relief.

Step 2: The implantation of a subcutaneously located pump for continuous intrathecal delivery of morphine is undertaken.

Spinal Cord Stimulation

Electrical spinal cord stimulation (SCS) has occasionally been tried to relieve central pain following SCI, although the main indication for this treatment is severe neuropathic pain of peripheral origin and conditions like failed back surgery. The effect of SCS on pain of central origin is quite discouraging. However, the method may have some therapeutic effect if given to patients with incomplete lesions suffering from a mixture of peripheral and central infralesional pain.

The implantation of an SCS device is usually carried out in a two-step procedure. In step one, a four-pole stimulator lead is introduced, usually by a percutaneous approach, into the posterior surface of the epidural space (Fig. 30.10), after which a wire harness connects the stimulator lead to an external pulse generator. The stimulator lead may be activated by either the patient and/or the doctor, and the effect of stimulation is evaluated. If this external electrical stimulation alleviates the pain, then a permanent stimulator is implanted in step two, usually in the abdominal fat. The stimulator is then regulated by a radiofrequency device. The *gate control theory of pain* states that the perception of pain is modulated by interaction of different neurons and not by activation of pain receptor neurons. This theory is one model for the explanation of the positive effect of SCS. The implanted stimulating lead activates the tracts belonging to the thicker myelinated α-fibers and peripheral receptors such as the touch and vibration receptors. The α-fibers transmit intense pain with a higher speed than do C-fibers, which are unmyelinated. The activation of the α-fiber related–tracts results in a blocking effect on C-fiber–mediated transmission. The underlying physiological and biomechanical mechanisms behind the effect of SCS are, according to Linderoth and Meyerson, only fragmentarily understood.

The level of γ-aminobutyric acid (GABA) is elevated following SCS. One theory states that GABA blocks the hyperactivity mediated by

WDR neurons, resulting in a beneficial effect of SCS. Because, as a consequence of SCI, the properties of these multireceptive neurons in the posterior horns have been changed, SCS may thus act by inhibiting the activity of these neurons.

CA-DREZ Lesioning

The technique of CA-DREZ lesioning refers to a computer-guided microcoagulation procedure at the entry zone of the dorsal roots with the purpose of ablating neurons that may demonstrate paroxysmal hyperactivity after a deafferentation injury.

During the past few decades, this method has been used to alleviate various pain conditions, and was initially used to reduce pain in patients with injuries to the brachial plexus, and with postherpetic and postamputation pain. The pain that evolves following trauma to the afferent tracts is referred to as *deafferentation pain,* and the best candidates for CA-DREZ microcoagulation are, in general, patients with this type of pain. Mechanical impact or biochemical alterations may cause the neuronal damage. CA-DREZ lesioning is a tissue destructive type of surgery, and the lesion or microcoagulation of the chosen area, usually using a radiofrequency technique, creates thermal damage to the tissue. The treatment effect is still unexplained, but three mechanisms have been suggested: interruption of ascending pain pathways within the dorsal and dorsolateral columns, destruction of pain-generating centers in the spinal cord, or a rebalancing of inhibitory and excitatory inputs within the damaged sensory network. A knife blade was used originally, but that technique has been replaced by modern lesion generators. Thermocoagulation is mainly performed using radiofrequency and specially designed electrodes (Fig. 30.11A,B). Electrical current is delivered until a predetermined temperature is reached in the tip of the lesioning electrode. It is possible to control the lesioning temperature using a heating gauge, thanks to the special design of the lesion electrode tip. It is also possible to measure the frequency of the action potentials (i.e., the electrochemical activity along the nervous tissue phospholipid membranes). Because the electrochemical degree of activity is considered an indication of the hyperexcitability in the tissue, it is possible to separate normal tissue from areas of hyperexcitability (i.e., areas of neuropathic pain origin) through a specially designed filtration technique.

The localization of areas showing hyperactivity means, theoretically, that the lesion can be directed specifically to those segments expressing hyperactivity. The distribution of the primary afferent neurons along the Lissauer tracts several segments above the level of lesion and the gate control theory of pain (convergence theory) resulted previously in a lesioning procedure involving one or a few segments above the level of injury. Now, because of the ability to identify areas of hyperexcitability, the microcoagulation procedure can be restricted to only those areas of increased excitability. The surgical procedure starts with the untethering procedure, after which a bilateral exposure of the DREZ is performed at the level of injury and sometimes up to five levels above. The reason for the extensive exposure is that a "blind thermocoagulation" (if the computer-assisted registration of hyperactivity fails) of five levels bilaterally above the level of injury will cover approximately 95% of the hyperactive areas. The lesion electrode (0.25 mm in diameter with a tip measuring 1.5 mm) is, after the identification of DREZ, inserted into the tissue, after which the registration of electrical hyperactivity begins. The lesioning electrode is then connected to the lesion generator, and microcoagulation takes place at temperatures of 75°C for 30–40 seconds. The electrical activity is again measured after thermocoagulation, and additional lesions are performed until the electrical activity is normalized. Every microcoagulation episode creates a lesion of about 1.5–2 mm in diameter. (The diameter of the lesioning tip measures only 1.5 mm in order to minimize the risk of inflicting damage to pyramidal tracts and posterior funiculi.) The lesioning is usually performed at approximately 1 mm intervals; thus, a five-level DREZ lesion includes a great number of lesions since the lesion distance is 10–15 cm on each side.

The indication for CA-DREZ lesion is severe neuropathic pain—described as pain of a sharp,

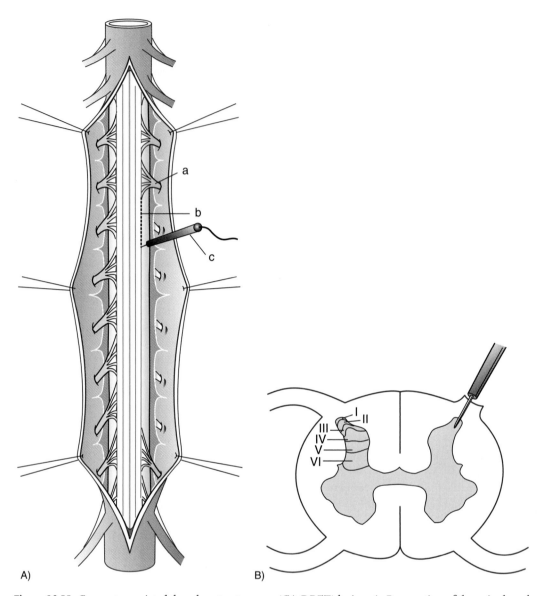

Figure 30.11 Computer-assisted dorsal root entry zone (CA-DREZ) lesion. A: Preparation of the spinal cord during the CA-DREZ lesioning procedure. *a,* dorsal root; *b,* dorsal root entry zone (DREZ); *c,* lesion electrode. B: Placement of the lesion electrode during the CA-DREZ microcoagulation process.

electrical, burning, stabbing, or "pins-and-needles" character—preferably with segmental projection at and below the level of injury. The onset of the pain should have been immediately following injury, and conservative treatment has been proved not to offer any alleviation. CA-DREZ is a method with great future potentials. Of significant interest is the result of so-called "mapping," in which efforts are being made to localize body areas affected by neuropathic pain and correlate these areas to a corresponding spinal cord segment(s). This is achieved by simultaneous stimulation of the C-fibers (light touch of the skin) and registration of the (hyper-) activity in the DREZ during surgical procedures. The future goal is to create a map portraying each spinal cord segment responsible for the neuro-pathic pain in different body areas, thus mini-mizing the lesion area to only those involved segment(s). This is of great importance, since one of the side effects, added motor loss, may occur following this type of surgery. The risk for added motor loss usually prevents lesions above the injury level of T5 since lesions five segments above T5 will potentially damage that part of the spinal cord which supplies motor impulses for hand and arm movement.

Lesioning Using Laser Technique

The laser lesioning technique is still not fully devel-oped. In this method, heat from a laser is directed to a specific area. Laser types such as carbon dioxide (CO_2), argon, and neodymium: yttrium aluminum-garnet (Nd:YAG) have been used. Side effects, such as added motor loss on the lesioned side, have been reported in a high frequency of cases, probably depending on the imprecision of the heat-generating beam. The method is therefore not used often in clinical practice.

SURGICAL (INVASIVE) TREATMENTS FOR SPASTICITY

Spasticity is, as previously mentioned, one symptom of PPM, but spasticity as an isolated symptom is not an indication for an untethering procedure. Two invasive treatments will be pre-sented in the following text that can be used in the management of spasticity if oval baclofen and other conservative treatments fail to relieve the problem: intrathecal baclofen administration (spinal baclofen pump) and percutaneous thermal rhizotomy (PTR). (We refer readers to literature of special interest for selective sensory microrootlet section [SSMS].)

Intrathecal Administration of Baclofen (Spinal Baclofen Pump)

Background and Indications

Implantation of the subcutaneously located infusion pump for intrathecal delivery of baclofen is the most frequently used invasive

method to alleviate severe spasticity. Baclofen, a derivative of GABA, acts as an inhibitor of presynaptic spinal reflexes, and monosy-naptic, as well as polysynaptic, reflexes are influenced by this drug. Baclofen has a lim-ited penetration of the blood–brain barrier, and it is postulated to exert its inhibitory effect by binding to a brain and spinal cord (central nervous system) GABA-B receptor. The effect of this is to slow down the signals sent to the muscles, thus helping to reduce stiffness and restore mobility. The possibility to achieve a high concentration of baclofen in the CSF is the main advantage of intrathecal delivery. This is of great advantage, from the anatomical point of view, since the distance to the GABA-B receptors located in Rexed lamina II is short. The baclofen concentration at the thoracic spinal cord level is reduced to approximately 50% if the drug is delivered at the lumbar level. The concentration is further reduced to 25% of original lumbar concentra-tion at the cervical and intracranial levels. The cerebral side effects associated with the oral intake of the drug are thus practically elimi-nated as a result of this reduced concentra-tion, gradients, which, of course, is a great advantage.

A spastic increase in muscular tone causes restriction of movement, pain, and/or impaired bladder function. These symptoms constitute the main indications for this type of intervention if oral intake of baclofen results in therapeutic failure and/or unacceptable side effects. The intrathecal administration of baclofen is also used to reduce spasticity among patients with multiple sclerosis.

Surgical Procedure

The placement of pumps for intrathecal admin-istration of baclofen is a two-step procedure;

In step 1, test doses of baclofen are admini-strated intrathecally either through a spinal catheter or lumbar puncture; 25 μg followed by 50 μg are delivered as test doses, after which changes in spasticity, flexor automatisms, rigidity, and bladder function are evaluated. The peak effect of the drug is reached 2–4 hours after administration, and the effect is practically gone after 6 hours. The patients are offered Step 2 if a significant beneficial response is demonstrated.

In step 2, subcutaneously located pumps are implanted for continuous intrathecal delivery of baclofen. A spinal catheter is initially inserted into the subarachnoid space at the levels of L3–L4 or L4–L5, after which it is threaded cranially up to the level of T10–T12. The caudal part of the catheter is then directed subcutaneously to the abdominal region, usually below the left or right costal arc. The catheter is then connected to the infusion pump, after which baclofen is instilled into the pump reservoir. The placement of the pump is usually in a suprafascial pocket, not more than 3 cm from the surface of the skin, as this will simplify the refilling procedure. The infusion pump is then started.

The start dose during the first 24 hours is twice as high as the lowest effective 24-hour test dose. The dose are gradually increased until spasticity and other symptoms reach an acceptable level. A 24-hour total dose of baclofen of about 200 μg is quite common. A concentration of 250 μg/L in the CSF fluid is reached after administration of 200 μg per 24 hours, compared to 24 μg/L after oral intake of 60 mg. The purpose of the intrathecal administration is to limit rather than to eliminate spasticity. A certain amount of muscular tone exerts a beneficial effect on, for instance, the ability of the trunk muscles to maintain a certain stability of the trunk.

Patients are observed in an intensive care unit following the implantation of the pump. Side effects of overdose may present with symptoms such as tiredness, indolence, confusion, bradycardia, reduced blood pressure, unconsciousness and, ultimately, respiratory arrest as the most feared condition. The complications usually occur in connection with administration of the test doses, implantation and/or starting procedure of the pump, or following changes of the delivered doses of baclofen. Patients are therefore kept under observation for 24 hours following administration of the test doses and for 5 days following the implantation procedure. Patients are also observed for 24 hours if the test dose is corrected by 5% or more.

The pump must be turned off if signs of overdose (i.e., side effects) appear. If alarming symptoms occur, this can be achieved by cutting the catheter located between the pump and its entry into the spinal canal. It is, however, more convenient to reduce or stop the infusion using the external pump-regulating device. Administration of 1–2 mg of physostigmine and 1 mg of atropine, as well as lumbar puncture to directly drain the drug from the intrathecal space, are additional measures to reverse an inadvertent intrathecal baclofen overdose. The concentration of baclofen in the CSF is reduced significantly if 30–40 mL of CSF are drained. In the long run, complications such as catheter discontinuity, orthostatic hypotension, erectile dysfunction, and tolerance adaptation is seen. A major disadvantage is the dependence on expensive equipment that requires monitoring, maintenance, and refilling three to six times per year, as the maximal shelf life of the drug is 4 months.

Percutaneous Radiofrequency Thermal Rhizotomy

Percutaneous radiofrequency thermal rhizotomy (PTR) is performed under local anaesthesia and could be summarized as a thermal lesion to peripheral nerves. The indication for this treatment is typically a severe increase of

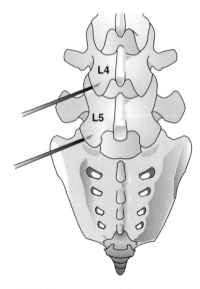

Figure 30.12 Percutaneous rhizotomy.

muscular tone in the abdominal and lower extremity musculature. A lesioning electrode is inserted 6 cm lateral to the midline and directed toward a predetermined transversal spinous process (Fig. 30.12). The needle is correctly placed in case an electrical stimulation of 0.3 V initiates muscular spasm. The peripheral nerve is then lesioned, after which a electrical stimulation is repeated. The lesioning is successful if a muscular spasm is not observed until the electrical stimulation reaches 0.5 V. PTR is usually performed bilaterally in the region between the peripheral spinal nerves of T12 and L5. Finally, the S1 root is lesioned. The effect of the procedure usually remains for up to 1 year, after which new complementary lesions can be performed.

Suggested Reading

Edgar R, Quail P. Progressive post-traumatic cystic and non-cystic myelopathy. *Br J Neurosurg* 1994;8:7–22.

El Masry WS, Biyani A. Incidence, management, and outcome of post-traumatic syringomyelia. *J Neurol Neurosurg Psychiatry* 1996;60:141–146.

Falci S, Best L, Bayles R, Lammertse D, Starnes C. Dorsal root entry zone microcoagulation for spinal cord injury-related central pain: operative intramedullary electro-physiological guidance and clinical outcome. *J Neurosurg (Spine 2)* 2002;97: 193–200.

Falci SP, Indeck C, Lammertse DP. Posttraumatic spinal cord tethering and syringomyelia: surgical treatment and long-term outcome. *J Neurosurg Spine* 2009;11 (4):445–460.

Fazl M, Houlden DA, Kiss Z. Spinal cord mapping with evoked responses for accurate localization of the dorsal root entry zone. *J Neurosurg* 1995;82: 587–591.

Hemley SJ, Biotech B, Tu J, Stoodley MA. Role of the blood-spinal cord barrier in posttraumatic syringomyelia. *J Neurosurg Spine* 2009;11(6):696–704.

Lee TT, Alameda GJ, Camilo E, Green BA. Surgical treatment of post-traumatic myelopathy associated with syringomyelia. *Spine* 2001;26:S119– S127.

Linderoth B, Meyerson B. Peripheral and central nervous stimulation in cases of chronic therapy-resistant pain. Background, hypothethical mechanisms, and clinical experiences. *Läkartidningen* 2001;98 (47):5328–5336.

Nashold BS, Pearlstein RD, eds. *The DREZ Operation.* Park Ridge, IL: The American Association of Neurological Surgeons, 1996.

Rooney GE, Endo T, Ameenuddin S, et al. Importance of the vasculature in cyst formation after spinal cord injury. *J Neurosurg Spine* 2009;11(4):432–437.

Thomas CK, Häger-Ross CK, Klein CS. Effects of baclofen on motor units paralysed by chronic cervical spinal cord injury. *Brain* 2010;133(Pt 1):117–125. Epub 2009 November 10.

31 | Paramedical Rehabilitation

WORK

An increasing proportion of persons with SCI are gainfully employed; however, according to studies from the United States, over 70% of persons with disabilities are outside the labor market, as compared with about 5% of the U.S. population as a whole. Other U.S. studies suggest that almost 60% of all persons with SCI were employed prior to the injury, compared with barely 30% post-injury (duration of injury 1–25 years). Although the situation in countries such as Sweden (i.e., our home country) is probably somewhat more favorable, the problem is indeed global.

The background to this situation is multifaceted. In a tight labor market, it is difficult for people with disabilities to find work even if they so wish. For some people, there is little financial incentive to work owing to subsidies and related factors. Individuals with a history of physically demanding work may not experience adequate motivation if "desk work" is the only realistic alternative following injury. For others, the neurological functional impairment may be so extensive and/or their overall medical status so poor that returning to work simply is unrealistic. Nevertheless, persons with SCI who do find work report a better sense of well-being, more satisfaction with life, and better overall health than those who do not work. Even if a causal relationship has not been established (since, for example, it is reasonable to assume that people who are in better health and feel healthier are also more likely to work), there is no doubt that returning to work or school is an important milestone in the rehabilitation process following SCI.

The basic should be that most persons with SCI are indeed able to carry out meaningful work, and that the objective "return to work or school" is thus desirable and realistic in most cases. The first step is to determine whether return to prior work or studies is possible. In most cases, this is a reasonable choice. However, in many cases, both physical adaptation of the workplace and changes in duties will be required. Where this is unrealistic, a variety of alternatives are available, such as looking for a radically different job with or without vocational retraining, or seeking additional education. It is regrettable if discussions of disability retirement routinely arise at an early stage. In our Western culture, work is indisputably and intimately linked to self-esteem and identity, in addition to structuring life and providing access to a social network. These factors also assume great significance also in cases where there is no clear financial advantage to returning to work. It is an essential aspect of patient education to include these considerations in the rehabilitation process from an early stage.

SCI does not necessarily entail a career disadvantage. Many examples will be found of people who became more clearly goal-oriented and achieved more successful careers after injury than before. In some cases, the SCI in itself can even become an occupational advantage, especially when working in healthcare. The individual's "injury experience" may prove invaluable for offering the best help possible to others in a similar situation.

PHYSICAL ACTIVITY

Several factors contribute to poor overall physical fitness among persons with SCI. Paralysis by itself limits mobility and therefore the potential for exercising. Psychological factors such as depression decrease motivation to exercise. These factors contribute to increase risk for cardiovascular disease, hypertension, insulin resistance, musculoskeletal complications and obesity.

As mentioned elsewhere, high-level SCI, in particular, leads to pathophysiological cardiovascular changes that further limit aerobic capacity. Moreover, paralyzed muscles atrophy to a greater or lesser extent, which contributes to an unfavorable body composition, insulin resistance, and associated adverse conditions. For many reasons, patients with SCI should become more physically active.

Arm cycling is a good exercise option for many patients, especially to achieve cardiovascular fitness. Since arm strength is also important for most patients with paraplegia and low tetraplegia, regular *strength training* should be added to the program. A modified version of *circuit training*, in which the patient goes from one strength training station to the next without pausing, has proven to be particularly effective since it combines strength and cardiovascular training. To prevent muscular imbalance, the focus is mainly on strengthening the upper back and shoulder muscles, as well as on stretching the pectorals. The strength training and cardiovascular exercise programs for SCI patients should be designed in cooperation with qualified healthcare personnel and be combined with other health-promoting initiatives, including diet modification, smoking cessation, and moderating alcohol consumption to achieve optimal results.

Functional electrical stimulation (FES) has been used mainly in the United States as a mode of exercise. Through electrical impulses, FES stimulates paralyzed muscles to contract, which exercises them. Electrically induced muscle activity leads to increased muscle mass as long as the stimulation program continues. If electrical stimulation is used for leg cycling, especially combined with "regular" arm cycling, cardiovascular benefit can also be achieved. This approach has demonstrated regression of left ventricular atrophy and, thus, improved aerobic capacity improved lower extremity circulation, improved body composition with more muscle and less fat, decreased insulin resistance and, according to some studies, some degree of anti osteoporosis effect. Naturally, such benefits presume continued, regular exercise, which is time-consuming in part due to placement of electrodes on the lower extremities. Furthermore, FES bicycles are expensive, and the exercise method has not gained a significant foothold outside the U.S.

The father of modern SCI care, Ludwig Guttmann, emphasized early on the importance of sports in the rehabilitation process because of its therapeutic value for physical, psychological, and social reasons. Many national and international centers for SCI rehabilitation have designated *recreational therapists* (RTs) and/or rehabilitation instructors. There is significant overlap and a blurred distinction between their work on the one hand and that of physical therapists, occupational therapists, and social workers. A variety of hobbies, leisure activities, sports, and athletic pursuits are available with or without major or minor adaptations. Some of the activities shown to be particularly appealing to persons with SCI include horseback riding, archery, wheelchair basketball, quad-rugby (wheelchair rugby for people with tetraplegia), wheelchair tennis, kayaking, wheelchair marathons, and sailing. In the context of sports for people with disabilities, athletes are classified according to their neurological and functional status. The purpose is to achieve the fairest grounds for competition possible by defining persons with comparable degrees of disability.

WHEELCHAIRS

The most basic type of manual wheelchair is that often seen in settings such as hospitals and airports. These wheelchairs are solely intended for short distances and must be pushed by an assistant. Such wheelchairs are not adapted uniquely to the individual, and because they are heavy and cumbersome they are only useful for very short periods of assisted use.

Modern Manual Wheelchairs

The modern wheelchair, which is intended to be an individually customized means of transport, is lightweight, with a frame constructed of materials such as aluminum or titanium (Fig. 31.1). These wheelchairs are available in a variety of designs. Many are equipped with folding

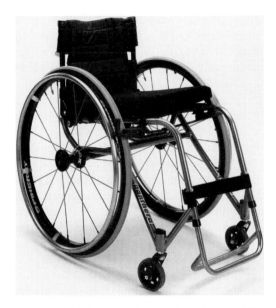

Figure 31.1 Modern wheelchair. (*Source:* Jalle Jungnell).

backrests and removable wheels. Some have the footrest built into the frame, whereas others have separate supports, which are often foldable. Regardless of design, these wheelchairs generally offer radically improved flexibility and accessibility. However, improved maneuverability also entails increased instability, with greater demands for solid training in wheelchair technique.

The most important design factor is the interface between wheelchair and user. The wheelchair may justifiably be considered an orthosis—part of the user's body—and choice of wheelchair and adaptation is thus a delicate task. The patient's body type, strength, condition, and technical skills, as well as his neurological and orthopedic status are factors to be considered when fitting wheelchair and user. This also applies to the user's situation at large, including community, occupation, and recreational and other activities.

Generally speaking, the wheelchair should be as narrow as possible, in part to improve accessibility. Backrest height is also of great importance. The better the trunk stability, the lower the height of the backrest is possible. This is desirable to achieve optimum propulsion

ergonomics. In many situations, maneuverability and stability are in opposition. For example, the longer the wheelbase, the more stable the chair, but maneuverability decreases. By angling the wheels outward in relation to the wheelchair seat, the wheelbase can be made broader. This angle is called the *camber angle*. Increasing camber angle provides greater lateral stability, facilitates quick turns, and allows the grip rings to be more ergonomically positioned in relation to the hands. Wheelchairs intended for sports usually have a high camber angle. The disadvantage to this improved maneuverability design is that the chair inevitably becomes wider.

Other important factors to consider include comfort and durability. This is certainly a consideration for the footrest, a part of the wheelchair that often bumps into external objects such as doors and walls. Footrest height will influence both the hip and knee joint angles in the seated position, and thereby also the sitting position and pressure distribution across the seat. Wheelchairs are often equipped with armrests and/or side supports to support the arms when sitting in the chair, as well as to use as a stable platform for pushing off when transferring or relieving pressure. Most modern wheelchairs are equipped with parking brakes, which are of obvious value to prevent the chair from rolling down a slanted surface, and to stabilize the chair when transferring.

Electric Wheelchairs

Electric wheelchairs may be the only realistic option for independent mobility for users with high-level SCI. However, even individuals with reasonable arm and hand function may need an electric wheelchair to cover greater distances and/or to relieve painful shoulder joints. Electric wheelchairs are available for primarily outdoor use, primarily indoors use, and in various "all-round" versions. Various assistive devices are available to help maneuver electric wheelchairs. Common examples are hand or chin-controlled joysticks, as well as sip/puff controls that can be activated by various combinations of sipping and puffing into a straw-like device.

A hybrid model combining features of both manual and electric wheelchairs is known as the *push rim activated power assist wheelchair*

(PAPAW). These wheelchairs are equipped with an electrical power assist which is activated when the patient applies torque to the wheels' grip rings.

Another recent mobility concept, similar to the wheelchair, is the *IBOT Transporter*. The IBOT is operated via a hand-controlled joystick. It has two pairs of rear drive wheels and, thanks to built-in electronic stabilizers, the IBOT can perform tasks such as climbing stairs and balancing on a single pair of wheels. Because of this latter feature, the wheelchair is able to "rise up" on its rear wheels, thereby increasing the user's reach in the vertical plane, making it possible to reach a book in a bookcase or dishes in a kitchen cabinet. However, the IBOT is heavy and expensive, and the stair-climbing feature requires either that the user has sufficient arm strength and function to "support-pull" on a railing or have an assistant.

Wheelchair Cushions

Yet another crucial part of the wheelchair is the seat cushion. The most common fillings for cushions include foam, air, or viscoelastic fluids (gel). Since users typically spend many hours a day sitting in the chair, the weight distribution and pressure-relieving properties of its cushion are of great significance in preventing pressure ulcers. However, no matter how state-of-the-art the seat cushion, it can never replace the need for meticulously fitting the wheelchair to the user's body measurements, nor can it replace the need for repeated skin inspections, pressure relief, and other prophylactic measures to prevent pressure ulcers (see Chapter 27).

DRIVING

Automotive vehicles comprise the most important assistive devices in daily life, especially following SCI. Even if public transport is a realistic option for some, and even though transportation services are often available, the possibility of driving a car should always be considered. Most SCI patients with preserved sensorimotor innervation of the rotator cuff, and even more so those with partial or completely preserved upper extremity function, may be able to drive a car,

although vehicle adaptations are often necessary. Such adaptations may involve measures to facilitate access to the vehicle and driver's seat, adjustments of controls to maneuver the vehicle, and modifications to ensure driver safety.

Choice of vehicle is important. Especially in tetraplegia, a van or minivan is preferable because it offers more space for ramps, wheelchair lifts, and special adjustable driver's seats. Vehicle doors may be electronically equipped to open and close if necessary. In regard to actual operation of the vehicle, hand controls for the accelerator, brake and automatic transmission are often necessary to compensate for absent or impaired lower extremity function. Thanks to devices such as steering knobs, power steering, and/or joysticks or other controls for single-handed operation, even persons with significant physical disabilities can become adequate drivers. With decreased truncal stability, a conventional safety belt may need to be adapted and/or expanded. A detailed description of the often sophisticated and complex vehicle adaptations is outside the scope of this book. The reader is referred to vehicle manufacturer and customizing websites for more information.

ORTHOSES

Spinal Orthoses

In the acute phase following traumatic injury to the spine, various methods can be used to fix the spinal column for purposes of transport and initial management (see Chapters 6 and 15). After the acute phase, orthoses can be used to provide additional stability and support.

Orthoses for the Upper Extremities

Orthoses for the upper extremities are mainly intended for use in tetraplegia. The purpose of orthotic support may be to prevent hyperextension of certain muscles, correct deformities, prevent joint contractures, support the wrist and hand in a functional position, support a weak wrist or hand, support weak muscles, and/or facilitate general function. Orthoses may be classified as *static* (i.e., those intended to maintain a certain position) or *dynamic* (i.e., those intended to facilitate and/or stabilize certain joint movements). The concept of orthoses may also include individually customized splints. Use of arm and hand orthoses has declined because users view many of them as frankly unesthetic, cumbersome, and generally too complicated in handling. This especially applies to technically advanced dynamic orthoses. As with other rehabilitation initiatives, fitting the orthoses must be a team effort. Hand function must be assessed in detail, especially in regard to sensorimotor function. The standard American Spinal Injury Association (ASIA) assessment is not sufficient for this purpose, and a more detailed analysis must be carried out. Such analysis should involve tests equivalent to those performed when considering hand surgery for this patient group (see Chapter 22). Successful fitting also presumes that the patient will meet both the cognitive and motivational requirements for orthosis use.

Listed here are the principles governing orthotic support in relation to level of lesion, with complete injuries as a point of departure. Naturally, with incomplete injuries, a wider array of options is available, which makes generalization difficult.

C1–C4 neurological level of injury: With this level of lesion, the arms are completely paralyzed, and orthoses are mainly used to support the arms and hands in a functional position to minimize the risk of contractures and deformities. Typically, 30 degrees of dorsal extension in the wrist and an abducted thumb position are considered desirable. For this high level of lesions "mouthsticks," which can be passive or dynamic, may be considered to be functional orthoses.

C5 neurological level of lesion: Patients with this level are also often fitted with static nighttime orthoses to prevent deformities. In addition to treating the wrists, elbow extension orthoses are sometimes used. The aim is to maintain the tenodesis grip, which positions the fingers in partial flexion. A *universal cuff* may be useful for this purpose or, alternatively, a splint or orthosis that supports the wrist in dorsal extension. The universal cuff is strapped over the hand, and

contains a sewn in pocket that can hold objects such as a fork or toothbrush.

C6-C7 neurological level of lesion: The aim for persons with these levels is to optimize biomechanics in order to achieve an effective tenodesis grip by moving the wrist. The goal is to achieve some degree of shortening in the flexor digitorum profundus and superficialis as well as flexor pollicis longus muscles, which may involve the use of an orthosis that resembles a boxing glove, such as the Moberg glove. Persons with a C6 level of lesion may benefit from using an elbow extension splint at night to preserve full extension in this joint. Such measures are unnecessary for the C7 level of lesion.

C8 functional level and lower: These patients usually do not require hand orthoses.

Orthoses for the Lower Extremities

The general purpose of lower-extremity orthoses is to provide support, substitute for lost muscle function, control severe spasticity, and/or maintain desirable skeletal position. Common lower-extremity orthoses include the foot orthosis (FO), ankle-foot orthosis (AFO), and knee-ankle-foot orthosis (KAFO). Patient assessment includes physical examination with an emphasis on range of motion, sensorimotor function, and gait. Specifically, the biomechanical dynamics during both the swing phase and the stance phase of the gait cycle are of particular interest here. The AFO may help support the sole of the foot during the swing phase and also facilitate push-off during the stance phase. The AFO may also control the position of the ankle in the sagittal plane, in order to compensate for knee joint instability due to quadriceps weakness. The KAFO is primarily used for knee instability in the sagittal plane (quadriceps weakness, genu recurvatum) or in the mediolateral direction (genu valgum, genu varum). In the United States, *reciprocating gait orthoses* (RGO) are sometimes used to stabilize the hips, knees, and ankles bilaterally. Simultaneous mechanical stability in ipsilateral hip flexion and contralateral hip extension is achieved by dynamically connecting the hip joints.

32 The Aging SCI Patient

Two main trends can be noted considering SCI in the developed world: more persons are injured at an older age, and more persons survive longer after injury. All in all, this means that problems related to the aging process have become a significant factor in the long-term management of this patient group. Obviously, the inevitable physiological aging processes also affect persons with SCI. However, changes related to aging may have disproportionately negative effects on persons with chronic SCI, since the "reserve capacity" built into various organ systems may have been depleted to a greater or lesser extent to compensate for injury-related disorders. In addition, certain sequels specifically related to SCI may lead to premature aging. This chapter briefly reviews the most important age-related problems.

URINARY TRACT

The urinary tract is subject to cumulative "wear" due to factors such as tens of thousands of intermittent catheterizations, recurrent urinary tract infections, stone formation, increased intravesical pressure, and/or vesicoureteral reflux. Long-term complications may include urethral stricture, renal impairment, even bladder cancer, all of which are more common with SCI. In men, age-related prostatic hyperplasia may create increasing flow obstruction.

GASTROINTESTINAL TRACT

Chronic constipation is common following SCI, which in turn increases the likelihood of diverticular disease and hemorrhoids. The tendency for constipation increases with increasing age and duration of disability.

SKIN

Advancing age is accompanied by cutaneous atrophy, as well as decreased skin elasticity and vascularization. Ultimately, this will compromise skin integrity, which is reflected by an increase in the annual incidence of pressure ulcers from about 15% 1 year post-injury to about 30% at 20 years post-injury.

NERVOUS SYSTEM

Both the central and peripheral nervous systems undergo degenerative changes with advancing age. This may be especially important for persons with SCI, since residual neurological function is supported by a smaller neuron population than normal. This may lead to a "post-polio like" situation, in which individual neurons, due to earlier *sprouting*, innervate a larger number of target organs (such as muscle fibers) than normal, and where the death of one such neuron therefore has disproportionately greater consequences than would normally be the case. The additional negative effects of conditions such as compression neuropathies and progressive posttraumatic myelopathy (PPM) must also be considered.

MUSCULOSKELETAL SYSTEM

In the SCI population, the musculoskeletal system is the organ system most subject to additive "wear-and-tear" trauma compared with the population at large. This especially applies, as described elsewhere in this book, to the upper extremities, where the shoulders in particular are subject to pathological changes. These problems increase over time following injury. As was also mentioned elsewhere, persons with

SCI suffer from a severe increase in osteoporosis, especially affecting the lower extremities. In addition to the osteoporosis that accompanies normal aging, SCI patients also suffer from the permanent effect of decalcification of bone that occurs shortly after injury. As a consequence, fractures of the lower extremities could be demonstrated in over 30% of patients with SCI who were followed over several decades post injury. As in the population at large, the risk of fractures is especially large among postmenopausal women.

RESPIRATORY AND CIRCULATORY SYSTEMS

Cardiovascular disease is very common in the aging general population, and now also among older individuals with SCI, especially in the presence of risk factors such as smoking, hypertension, obesity, hyperlipemia, and diabetes. Symptoms of coronary heart disease, such as chest pain, may be masked by the sensory deficit accompanying high-level injuries. Pulmonary function may gradually deteriorate, especially from smoking with chronic obstructive pulmonary disease and from spinal deformity.

MANAGEMENT

The clinical picture following SCI is not static, but changes over time. The needs of patients vary with age and over time since the injury. In rehabilitation, the desire to maximize functional ability must always be weighed against the risk of complications and problems related to wear and tear. Through health-promoting initiatives, ongoing support with personal assistance and assistive devices, regular health check-ups, and periods of "re-rehabilitation" in the outpatient or inpatient setting, the aging patient may maintain a reasonable quality of life for many years. Collaboration with the primary care network allows management of medical conditions that also occur in the population at large.

Suggested Reading

Furlan JC, Fehlings MG. The impact of age on mortality, impairment, and disability among adults with acute traumatic spinal cord injury. *J Neurotrauma* 2009;26 (10):1707–1717.

Sokolowski MJ, Jackson AP, Haak MH, et al. Acute outcomes of cervical spine injuries in the elderly: atlantaxial vs subaxial injuries. *J Spinal Cord Med* 2007;30(3):238–242.

Although successfully rehabilitated people who are left with para- or tetraplegia following SCI are not actually "ill," they do face a lifelong vulnerability to complications involving most organ systems. According to international norms, persons with SCI should be offered follow-up at least annually at a specialized center. Whether such an annual recheck focuses only on problems specific to SCI or also includes age- and gender-related screening measures may vary from one clinic to the next. Therefore it is of the essence that patients clearly understand what their annual rechecks actually cover, so that they are not lulled into a false sense of security that "everything is fine" in case the check-up is limited solely to those problems specific to SCI.

The primary purpose of regular follow-up for patients with SCI in the chronic phase is to prevent ill-health through proactive and health-promoting measures and to enable early diagnosis and treatment of complications. Annual recheck should include a structured checklist for review of common problems, as well as a general physical and neurological examination.

MEDICAL ASPECTS

Persons with tetraplegia or high paraplegia should be offered immunization against the influenza virus and pneumococci.

Skin examination should look for signs of pressure ulcers, with special attention to the sacrum, ischial tuberosities, trochanter regions, and heels. Ulcers, if present, should be analyzed in the conventional manner.

Since diabetes mellitus and low high-density lipoprotein (HDL) cholesterol levels are more common among individuals with SCI than in the general population, fasting lipids, resting blood pressure, and fasting blood sugar should be obtained, and preferably an electrocardiogram (EKG).

Two-thirds of all SCI patients have some form of significant, chronic pain problem. The approach to these problems should not be tinted by nihilism, especially not so as such problems do have a strong detrimental effect on quality of life, and many therapeutic strategies are available, as discussed elsewhere this book.

The same applies to significant spasticity. Increased spasticity during the chronic phase should always motivate a workup for underlying factors, such as posttraumatic myelopathy, infection, or pressure ulcers.

Regarding problems from muscles, joints, and bones, special mention should be given to the risk of overuse injuries in the shoulders and elsewhere in the upper extremities, as well as to osteoporosis related to paralysis and immobilization, which predisposes for fractures.

Heterotopic ossification, should it occur, typically manifests itself early during the course of rehabilitation. Diagnosis and treatment of heterotopic ossification is discussed elsewhere in this book.

Persons with tetraplegia seem to have some degree of "protection" against arterial hypertension owing to the lower level of activity within the sympathetic nervous system caused by their lesion. However, other risk factors for developing hypertension, such as physical inactivity and obesity, are present to a greater extent, which especially increases the incidence of hypertension in persons with paraplegia. When the diagnosis of hypertension is made, additional workup of underlying etiology (autonomic dysreflexia, renal artery stenosis, renal failure, hyperaldosteronism, etc.) should be carried out. Important and frequently neglected interventions include assistance with smoking cessation and moderation of alcohol consumption. Consequently, many clinicians routinely include questions on these issues in their annual rechecks. Pulmonary function may gradually decline in smokers and with increasing neurologic deficit and/or progressive spinal deformity. Arterial blood gases and pulmonary function tests (spirometry, polysomnography) should be carried out as needed.

With respect to overweight, it is well to remember that the ideal weight for a person with paraplegia is roughly 80% of the corresponding weight of a mobile person of the same height, and for tetraplegia only 60% of that weight.

Recommended laboratory tests include complete blood count, electrolytes, blood urea nitrogen, creatinine, lipid panel, liver function tests, and fasting blood sugar. In patients with diabetes, tests should also include Hgb A1c, fundus examination, and a foot check.

A screening questionnaire should be used to assess nutritional status. In the chronic phase, overweight and obesity are more common than underweight.

No increased risk of colorectal cancer has been demonstrated in relation to SCI, and the decision to include screening tests such as fecal hemoglobin and colonoscopy should be dictated by local recommendations for the population at large.

Many centers recommend that the urogenital system be checked annually, with creatinine clearance and/or renal scintigraphy and/or ultrasound of the urinary tract. Annual prostate palpation for men over the age of 40 is also often recommended.

There are no indications that diseases specific to women, such as gynecological and breast cancers, are more common in those with SCI. However, these patients are definitely at risk of not being included in the general screening system. Again, we would like to underscore that either the doctor responsible for providing spinal injury care must include these studies in their annual rechecks or else make it clear to the patient that these screening measures should be done at another healthcare facility.

The recorded history of SCI starts with the Edwin Smith Surgical Papyrus (37,71). In the well-known case 33, "Instructions concerning a crushed vertebra in his neck," the author's conclusion is that this is "an ailment not to be treated." Imhotep describes in that case symptoms associated with SCI such as loss of motion in arms and legs (tetraplegia), loss of sensation below level of injury, and loss of bladder control.

Hippocrates (circa 460–377 BC) first correlated vertebral injuries with paralysis. He introduced the "Hippocratic board" to reduce spinal deformities, and advocated, in the treatment of SCI patients, a diet consisting of four to nine pints of donkey milk combined with honey and a special mild white wine from Mendez in Egypt. Hippocrates also described the difficulties facing patients with paralysis, such as constipation, dysuria, skin problems, and edema. The Greek Galen (130–201 AD) was the first to perform animal experiments. He described that a longitudinal incision to the spinal cord did not produce loss of function, whereas a transverse incision at the cervical level resulted in loss of both motor and sensory function below level of injury. Five hundred years later, the surgeon Paulus (625–690) from the Greek island of Eagina introduced laminectomy, the removal of the vertebral arch in order to decompress the dural sac and spinal cord. In 1543, Andreas Vesalius published one of the greatest medical books ever written, *De Humani Corporis Fabrica*, in which the human nervous system was, for the first time, illustrated in detail.

The "Father of Neuroscience" Santiago Ramon y Cajal was awarded the Nobel Prize in medicine 1906 for his description of CNS structure. In 1911, Reginald Allen introduced the experimental weight-drop technique that initiated the modern era of SCI research. Both these researchers were aware of the contribution of secondary injury mechanisms to the final neurological deficit after an injury to the spinal cord. During that period, which included World War I, mortality was as high as 80% within the first 2 weeks following SCI at the cervical level. A fatalistic attitude accompanied the treatment of SCI during the period between the two world wars. However, in 1943, the modern era of rehabilitation began when Sir Ludwig Guttmann opened his Stoke-Mandeville National Spinal Centre. The creation of rehabilitation clinics that focused on the special challenges associated with SCI, together with the introduction of antibiotics, revolutionized care for this group of patients. In the decades following, improved healthcare resulted in a substantial improvement in quality of life and life expectancy. Today, for a person with SCI, life expectancy is approaching that of the general population.

Our knowledge about the pathophysiological process of SCI has increased in parallel with improved medical management. The concept of primary and secondary mechanisms of injury has been accepted both experimentally and in the acute care of these patients. All this knowledge, however, has led only to improved medical management, not to a cure. There exists no therapeutic method to restore, even partially, lost neurological function.

The prevention of secondary damage or the self-destruction of neurons following an injury and the desirable effort to rescue viable tissue is summarized as *neuroprotection*. A variety of therapeutic agents have been used, targeting one or more mechanisms of secondary injury in order to confer neuroprotection and prevent unnecessary tissue damage. The insufficient neuroprotective effects, however, have switched the focus of research to the more long-range consequences of injury to the spinal cord. Present (and future) research encompasses the field of *neural regeneration*. In 1981, breakthrough work in this field was presented by David and Aguayo (18), who concluded that, in order for axonal regeneration to occur, both intrinsic cellular and CNS environmental factors must be addressed.

The purpose of this chapter is to highlight those selected experimental and clinical studies that we believe form the basis for undertaking future challenges in the research field of SCI. We focus our discussion on methods for either preventing the consequences of secondary injury in the acute period (neuroprotection) and/or various techniques of neural regeneration in the subacute and chronic phase. Finally, we discuss possible future avenues within this research field.

NEUROPROTECTION

Neuroprotection is defined as measures to counteract secondary injury mechanisms and/or limit the extent of damage caused by self-destructive cellular and tissue processes. The hypothesis of secondary events was, during the 1970s, focused on vascular damage leading to edema, free radical formation, and norepinephrine release, whereas calcium processes, opiate receptor mechanisms, cytokine involvement, nitrous oxide formation, and lipid peroxidation were highlighted during the 1980s. Knowledge about apoptosis, energy metabolism, inflammation, and excitoxicity increased markedly during the 1990s. The coexistence of several distinct injury mechanisms post trauma has provided opportunities to explore a large number of potentially neuroprotective agents in animal experiments.

Methylprednisolone sodium succinate (MPSS) is the most extensively studied agent, Table 34.1 summarizes its reported positive effects in animal experiments.

Neuroprotection research has, in addition to characterizing injury mechanisms and testing

TABLE 34.1 Reported positive effects of MPSS in animal experimental studies.

Improves energy metabolism	Reduces edema formation by maintaining the blood–brain barrier
Reduces posttraumatic ischemia	Reduces degeneration of nervous structures
Stabilizes phospholipid membrane structures	Counteracts formation of free radicals
Reduces inflammatory response	Reduces neurological deterioration

various substances in animal experiments, been focused on a number of clinical studies aimed at minimizing neurological deficits post trauma (4). Baptiste and Fehlings published a survey of ten randomized, prospective, and controlled neuroprotective studies, considered by the authors to be most scientifically reliable (Table 34.2). Although numerous other attempts have been made to support the neuroprotective potential of the spinal cord these studies are the most quoted.

Although we concentrate our attention in this chapter on experimental studies, it should be emphasized that all types of immediate therapeutic interventions also have as their underlying objective to support the organism's intrinsic neuroprotective potential. A common and enduring problem for all treatments administered during the acute stage is knowing the length of the so-called "therapeutic window," that period of time after injury within which treatment must start to be effective. Extensive efforts have been made to translate experimental data on secondary injury mechanisms to help define therapeutic windows in clinical situations.

In a series of clinical studies (see Table 34.2) by the National Acute SCI Studies (NASCIS I-III), MPSS was given alone or in combination with either the opioid antagonist naloxone or the lipid peroxidation inhibitor, tirilazad mesylate (9,10). In addition, based on beneficial effects in animal experiments, clinical studies have been carried out with GM-1 ganglioside (25), thyrotropin-releasing hormone (TRH), the

TABLE 34.2 Summary of ten randomized, prospective and controlled neuroprotective studies (from Baptiste and Fehlings, 2006).

	Study	Animal Experimental Background	Effect on Neurological Outcome
1	NASCIS-I, 1984 MPSS in high and low doses	MPSS Antioxidative/antiinflammatory: see table 1	No difference in recovery following administration of high and low doses of MPSS
2	NASCIS-II, 1990 MPSS, naloxone or placebo	Naloxone improved impulse propagation and reduced edema formation	MPSS improved neurological recovery
3	NASCIS-III, 1997 MPSS and tirilazad mesylate	Tirilazad mesylate prevents lipid peroxidation, stabilizes phospholipid membranes, and restores the level of vitamin E in the spinal cord	MPSS improved neurological recovery
4	Japanese MPSS study, 1994 MP or placebo		MPSS improved neurological recovery
5	Maryland ganglioside study (GM-1), 1991	GM-1 stimulates axonal growth through the site of injury	GM-1 improved neurological recovery
6	Sygen® ganglioside study (GM-1), 1998		Minimal neurological recovery was seen among patients with incomplete lesions
7	Thyrotropin-releasing hormone (TRH), 1995 TRH or placebo	TRH counteracts the effect of excitatory amino acids and endogenous opioids and has antioxidant and membrane stabilizing properties	TRH improved neurological recovery among patients with incomplete lesions
8	Nimodipine, 1998 Nimodipine, MPSS, in combination or placebo	Calcium-channel blocker	No neurological improvement was observed
9	Gacyclidine study, 1999 Gacyclidine or placebo	NMDA receptor antagonist	No neurological improvement was observed
10	Decompression, 1997	Decompression performed less than 72 h, or more than 5 d, respectively, after trauma	No difference in neurological recovery between the groups

calcium channel blocker nimodipine, and the N-methyl-D-aspartic acid (NMDA) receptor antagonist gacyclidine (GK-11). Although none of these studies has shown significant beneficial clinical effects, administration of MPSS within 8 hours after injury is considered a "treatment option" (3). Despite the modest promise of MPSS, pharmacological neuroprotection for patients with SCI has fallen short of the expectations created by extensive research and encouraging observations in animal experiments.

Several nonpharmacological interventions have also been suggested to contribute to neuroprotection (70). Animal experiments have shown that early decompression reduces neurological deficits after spinal cord trauma, and a prospective, large-scale multicenter study, the Surgical Treatment for Acute Spinal Cord Injury Study group (STASCIS), has been undertaken to address this issue. A major reason for this study is the widespread reluctance refrain from operative intervention, which is commonly believed to help recovery and mobilization after acute SCI. Similarly, lowering whole body or local spine temperature has not been proven to influence outcomes after SCI.

REGENERATION

The functional consequences of SCI are determined by the level and extent of damage to pathways coursing through the white matter (Figs. 34.1 and 34.2).

With the exception of the cervical spinal cord, gray matter destruction over a few segments is usually followed by only modest functional

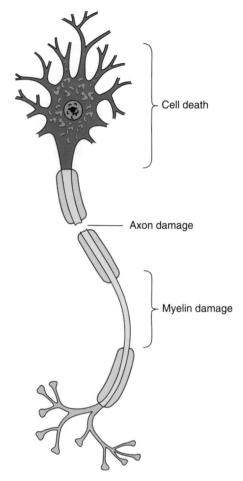

Figure 34.2 Axonal degeneration. The main degenerative events following neuronal injury are death of the neuron, interruption of its axon leading to Wallerian degeneration of the distal stump, and loss of myelin internodes (demyelination).

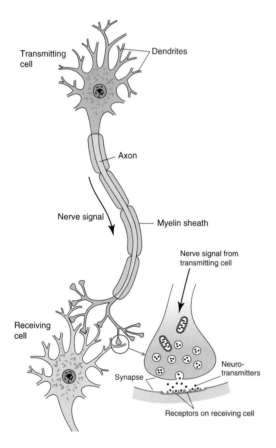

Figure 34.1 Intact nerve cell making synaptic connections with a postsynaptic neuron. The enlarged figure to the right shows the synaptic complex with the presynaptic terminal, release of its neurotransmitter and the postsynaptic site where the neurotransmitter is bound to specific postsynaptic receptors.

impairment. Interruption of descending and ascending white matter pathways (i.e., severing of axons from their nerve cell bodies) results in Wallerian degeneration of axons and myelin. Axonal injury may also cause death of the parent nerve cell body, particularly if the lesion is close to it. To restore lost functions, injured neurons must survive, and their axons must regenerate across or around the lesion site and also make functionally useful connections caudal (descending tracts) or rostral (ascending tracts) to it. As a result of mechanical compression, myelinated axons may lose their myelin (demyelination), and hence their ability to propagate nerve impulses. These axons must become remyelinated to resume impulse propagation.

The failure of injured spinal cord axons to regenerate was originally demonstrated by Ramon y Cajal in the end of the 19th century. The dogma that spinal cord neurons were unable to regenerate axons dramatically changed with the results of the experiments by David and Aguayo in the early 1980s (18). Their experiments clearly demonstrated that central nervous axons are able to regenerate, provided they are exposed to a supportive environment (peripheral nerve tissue), but that they cease to elongate when confronted with CNS tissue. During the subsequent two decades, several regeneration obstacles have been identified. Based on these findings, various regeneration strategies have been developed with the aim of modifying the growth inhibitory properties of the spinal cord environment (35,57). Here, we present some regeneration obstacles followed by a selection of interesting regeneration strategies.

REGENERATION OBSTACLES

The adult CNS environment contains a variety of mechanisms that actively inhibit axonal growth. Various processes, in the acute as well as in the chronic stage following SCI, counteract the potential of injured axons to cross the level of injury and finally to reconnect with nerve cells below the injury site. These obstacles include an insufficient growth response by the injured nerve cells (nerve cell disability) and environmental factors surrounding the nerve cell (Table 34.3).

TABLE 34.3 Regeneration obstacles.

Nerve Cell Disability	Environmental Factors
Nerve cell body response	Presence of growth inhibiting factors
	Scar tissue formation
	Formation of cavities and cysts at, below, and above the level of injury

Nerve Cell Disability

Following axonal injury, signals to the affected nerve cell body induce a shift in neuronal gene expression (62,78). In contrast to the situation in the peripheral nervous system, central neurons are able to maintain the expression of regeneration-associated genes only for a limited period, presumably due to the absence of sufficient growth-stimulating factors in their environment. As a result, the injured neurons gradually enter an atrophic state, and may eventually degenerate and die.

Environmental Factors

The injured axons are surrounded by factors that inhibit axon growth. These include NOGO-A (63) and myelin-associated glycoprotein (MAG; 76), which are both produced by oligodendroglial cells. Astrocytes, microglial cells, oligodendrocytes, and meningeal cells contribute to the formation of a scar at the injury site. The scar presents a mechanical barrier, but the main obstacle for axon growth is the presence of a chemical barrier composed of proteoglycans and collagens (21). The addition of extensive necrotic and apoptotic cell death in the injury region promotes the development of cavities and cysts in the spinal cord itself. A is fully formed, scar undoubtedly provides a mechanical obstacle to axon growth. However, this process requires many weeks to complete. The question therefore remains: Why are axons unable to grow across the injury site before the scar has formed? The most plausible explanation is that a growth-inhibitory environment is created early post injury, including the expression of myelin-associated inhibiting components, as a result of the combined activity of local glial cells and invading hematogenous cells. Finally, the emergence of mature scar tissue adds yet another obstacle to regeneration.

REGENERATION STRATEGIES

In the light of these considerations, successful regeneration in the spinal cord requires the combination of several approaches, which will be discussed in the following sections:

- Promoting intrinsic neuronal capacity for regeneration
- Counteracting early inhibitory mechanisms to axonal growth in the environment of the injured neurons
- Overcoming late inhibitory mechanisms to axonal growth in the environment of the injured neurons

Promoting Intrinsic Neuronal Capacity for Regeneration

Neurons are endowed with a normally inactive regeneration "program," which becomes activated following injury. To restore neuronal capacity following damage, injured axons need to activate their regeneration-associated genes (RAG). This activation program is markedly stimulated by appropriate growth factors (Table 34.4).

The first of these factors, named *nerve growth factor* (NGF), was identified in the 1960s. Nerve growth factors that influence the development and maintenance of neurons are often referred to as *neurotrophic factors* ("nourishing" neurons).

TABLE 34.4 Examples of growth factors (neurotrophic factors).

Neurotrophic Factors	Abbreviation
Nerve growth factor	NGF
Neurotrophin 3 or 4	NT-3/NT-4
Brain-derived neurotrophic factor	BDNF
Fibroblast growth factor	FGF
Glia cell line-derived neurotrophic factor	GDNF

Subsequent studies showed that NGF is a member of the neurotrophin family of growth factors, which also include brain-derived neurotrophic factor (BDNF) and neurotrophins (NT)-3 and -4 (NT-4). Neurotrophic growth factors are small molecules with a wide range of properties, including the promotion of neuron survival and axonal outgrowth, as well as the regulation of neuron-target interactions (Table 34.5; 26,32). The most interesting properties of these factors in the context of SCI seem to be their ability to stimulate the survival of injured neurons, as well as to regulate the expression of RAGs in a way that increases the regeneration capacity of injured axons (29,38,55,66).

Although several growth factors have well-documented effects on axonal growth, there are problems with their application in SCI. The specificities of the growth factors are incompletely known in terms of their effect on neuronal populations and peripheral tissues, such as muscle. Several growth factors stimulate axons that convey nociceptive information, which can lead to increased pain prevalence (53). Different growth factors also appear to stimulate neuronal growth at different stages in the repair process, and sometimes in an antagonistic manner (Table 34.5; 50). It is therefore a challenging task for the future to determine which growth factors are optimal for promoting survival and regeneration of different types of neuron populations, and at what time point they should be administered. Moreover, growth factors do not pass the blood–brain barrier, which raises the issue of how to deliver them in an efficient and controlled way. Intrathecal delivery via osmotic pumps containing genetically modified neurotrophin-releasing cells (e.g., fibroblasts), the implantation of slow-release cell-free systems, or gene therapy (8) are possible options. Taken together, there are

TABLE 34.5 Strategies stimulating the neuronal intrinsic regenerating capacity.

Factor	Target/Mechanism	Delivery	Effect
Growth hormones	CNS-tissue (neurons) Stimulating regeneration associated genes	Intrathecal injections Local deposition and others	Regrowth of damaged axons Functional improvement

a number of well-defined growth factors with established positive effects on axonal growth that might be used in future treatment of SCI.

Counteracting Early Inhibitory Mechanisms to Axonal Growth

Axonal regeneration is counteracted in the early period after an injury by the emergence of myelin-associated inhibitors and by factors that accelerate the formation of scar tissue in the environment surrounding the nerve cell. Here, we discuss some of the main strategies that have been adopted to counteract the effects of early inhibitory mechanisms in the nerve cell environment (Table 34.6).

Blocking Axonal Growth Inhibitory Molecules

The spinal cord of healthy uninjured adults contains powerful inhibitory substances that prevent axonal growth. These factors are vital since they stop axonal growth after the axons achieve contact to other nerve and muscle cells. Following trauma, these same factors create a major obstacle at the molecular level by delaying and/or preventing the onset of the regeneration process. Pioneering work by Schwab and collaborators led to the identification of a myelin growth-inhibiting factor, NOGO-A, a myelin protein produced by oligodendrocytes (see Table 34.6; 63). NOGO-A exerts its inhibitory effect by blocking specific NOGO-A-receptors on the surface of the axons (Fig. 34.3A–C; 24,75).

The interaction between NOGO-A and the NOGO-A receptor results in a receptor-mediated inhibition of axonal growth. This mechanism is prevented by the administration of antibodies (IN-1) that binds to NOGO-A itself (neutralizing antibodies; 17) or that act as antagonists to the NOGO-A receptor (36). Thus, intrathecal infusion of these neutralizing antibodies blocks the effect of NOGO-A, and thereby indirectly stimulates axon regeneration (Fig. 34.4).

In addition to NOGO-A, other axonal growth inhibitory proteins, such as myelin associated glycoprotein (MAG) and oligodendrocyte myelin glycoprotein (OMP) also exert their effects at the receptor level. Thus, the presence of myelin-associated inhibitors to regeneration is fully recognized. In addition to studies with IN-1 antibodies against NOGO-A, experimental studies has been performed using a passive or active immunization approach toward myelin-inhibitory molecules (Fig. 34.5, 73). Substantial anatomical regeneration and functional recovery have been reported using this approach (28). However, this approach is controversial, since other studies have reported that passive or active immunization increases structural damage and functional impairment following SCI (3,21). Recent studies have shown that the growth inhibitory influence of myelin-associated proteins can be overcome by increasing the levels of cyclic adenosine monophosphate (cAMP) in the injured axons to promote axonal elongation in the injured spinal cord (52,56).

TABLE 34.6 Strategies to counteract the early inhibitory mechanisms of the CNS environment.

Factor	Target	Delivery	Effect
Antibodies (IN-1)	NOGO-A receptors on regenerating axons	Pumps Pills?	Blocked inhibition of axonal outgrowth immunization
4-amino pyridine	Demyelinated axons	Intravenous Intrathecal	Restored signal transmission
Monoclonal antibody	ICAM	Immunization	Reduced edema Increased SCBF
Interleukins	Unknown	Systemically; IP	Switches of the inflammatory response
Chondroitinase ABC	Proteoglycans	Local infusion	Digestion of scar Functional improvement

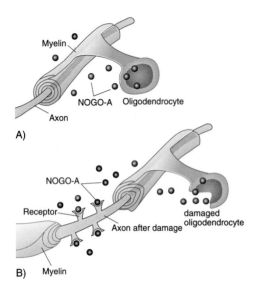

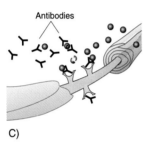

Figure 34.3 Blocking the growth inhibitory influence of NOGO-A by administration of NOGO-A antibodies. A: NOGO-A is produced and released by the uninjured oligodendrocytes. B: Binding of NOGO-A to specific receptors on injured neurons inhibits axon elongation. C: NOGO-A antibodies bind NOGO-A as well as its receptor, thereby allowing the injured axon to grow.

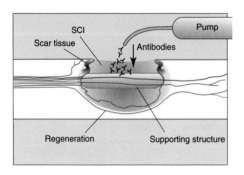

Figure 34.4 Pharmacological or bioactive agents (e.g., NOGO-A antibodies) can be infused intrathecally via a thin tube connected to an osmotic minipump.

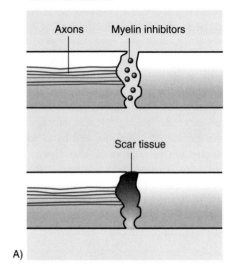

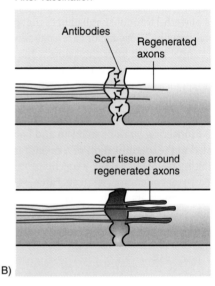

Figure 34.5 Vaccination. A: Myelin-associated growth inhibitors first prevent injured axons to cross the injury site; subsequently, the scar tissue provides additional growth inhibition. B: Circulating antibodies bind these inhibitors, thereby allowing growth of injured axons across the lesion site.

Restoration of Impulse Propagation by Modulating Axonal Membrane Properties

Contusion damage is the most frequent pathological consequence of spinal cord trauma. Transection of the spinal cord rarely occurs, and the majority of spinal cord injured patients probably have some axons that survived the acute mechanical damage as well as the effects of the secondary injury mechanisms. In both situations, degeneration of oligodendrocytes, largely by apoptosis, occurs, resulting in demyelination and thereby insecure impulse propagation or complete conduction failure. The myelin that covers the axons is partially or totally lost, resulting in impaired or completely lost impulse propagation. In addition, the propagated electrical impulses could be spread between demyelinated axons like a short-circuit in an electrical cable when the outer insulation is damaged. When an axon is demyelinated post injury, a large number of potassium channels are exposed and potassium (K^+) leaks into the extracellular space, resulting in conduction failure (Fig. 34.6).

Infusion of the fast voltage-sensitive potassium channel blocker fampridine-SR (4-aminopyridine, 4-AP) blocks the potassium channels at those gaps and makes it possible for the demyelinated axon to propagate action potentials (Table 34.6; 27). This agent has been tested in phase 2 studies, and trials are ongoing to study the effects of its administration in the early stage of the injury (15).

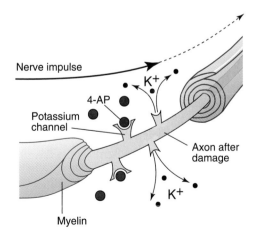

Figure 34.6 Fampridine-SR (4-AP) blocks open potassium channels and helps to maintain a resting potential.

Modulating the Immune System

Modulation of the immune system is a potentially useful strategy to reduce the inflammatory response after trauma and in this way improve the environment for neuron survival and regeneration. The inflammatory response after SCI encompasses degenerative as well as reparative processes (1,23,59). Cellular debris and breakdown products from degenerating neurons, glial cells, and hematogenous cells are eliminated through of variety of processes, thereby promoting the restoration of a beneficial environment for surviving cells. Inflammatory cells and their mediators also help to build novel structural components, including the scar, which isolates the trauma area from surrounding healthy tissues.

The inflammatory response can be divided into three overlapping phases: the phase of initiation (the phase of disintegration), the phase of maintenance (the scar-forming phase), and the phase of shutting off. All tissues harbor mononuclear cells, which together form the mononuclear phagocyte system, and have the ability to rapidly transform into macrophages in trauma and disease. Macrophages have long been known to play a key role in inflammation, including the repair of injured peripheral nerves (16). Recent studies indicate that an inadequate macrophage response in the injured CNS is an important factor behind the failure of axon regeneration in the spinal cord. In the injured spinal cord, most of the macrophages originate from microglia, the intrinsic members of the mononuclear phagocyte system. Local factors in the CNS (from, for example, astrocytes) exert a much tighter control of the activation of microglia to fully competent macrophages compared to the situation in other tissues. While this control may serve to minimize the extent of secondary damage from a fully developed inflammation, it also appears to hamper the neuroregenerative response.

To facilitate the entry of monocytes into the degenerating spinal cord white matter and their subsequent differentiation into competent macrophages may therefore promote tissue repair and axon growth.

Circulating monocytes first have to attach to endothelial cells in the capillaries to be able to

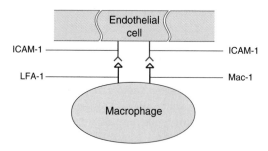

Figure 34.7 Intercellular cell adhesion molecule (ICAM)-mediated adhesion of monocytes to endothelial cells.

enter spinal cord tissue. The attachment and subsequent entry process is regulated by a set of cell adhesion molecules (CAMs (such as LTA-1 and Mac-1)) located at the cell surface (30,34) (Fig. 34.7).

Intercellular cell adhesion molecule (ICAM) is expressed on the surface of endothelial cells and is a ligand for the CAM L1, which is expressed by T cells, neutrophils, and monocytes. ICAM has also been shown to be a ligand for macrophages, and has been suggested to play a significant role in the early phase of the inflammatory response. By modulating ICAM expression, it might therefore be possible to regulate the monocyte-mediated components of inflammation following SCI. Ideally, sufficient macrophage activity should be present in the early phase to rapidly remove cell debris and breakdown products, after which the macrophage response should be attenuated to reduce their scar tissue promoting activities. This sequence of events occurs following injury to peripheral nerves, and is considered to be an important factor underlying peripheral nerve regeneration (77). An indication that such modulation is feasible and beneficial is shown by observations that administration of monoclonal anti-ICAM antibodies plays a role in regulating the presence of macrophages as well as neutrophils at the site of injury (Table 34.6; 39).

The interleukin (IL) family of cytokines play a key role in growth and function of many cell types. Some of the ILs (e.g., IL-1, IL-6, and IL-10) are important regulators of immune and inflammatory responses, and are induced or upregulated following neural trauma (13). Whereas IL-1 and IL-6 are considered

proinflammatory, IL-10 plays a role in switching off the inflammatory response, although the precise mechanism of action is incompletely known. By giving IL-10 at an early stage following SCI, the inflammatory response can be attenuated and the secondary injury process mitigated (Table 34.6). An advantage of ILs is that they can be administered systemically, even intraperitoneally, in contrast to the growth factors discussed earlier. ILs were shown to reduce edema formation and the extent of secondary damage, as well as to improve local blood flow and neurological recovery in experimental models of SCI.

In summary, ICAM and ILs are examples of molecules that participate in the inflammatory response after SCI and that are potential targets for pharmacological treatment in SCI. However, their possible use is complicated by the difficulties in determining at what time point these molecules should be administered in order to interfere in an efficient way with the inflammatory process (65).

Chondroitinase ABC: A Molecular Machete

The presence of certain molecules in the extracellular matrix is considered to counteract axonal regeneration. Proteoglycans, collagens, and adhesive proteins are the main components in the extracellular matrix (14). Chondroitin sulfate proteoglycans (CSPG) are the main contributors to scar formation following injury and therefore largely responsible for the mechanical and chemical failure of injured axons to grow beyond the level of injury. Although scar formation is hostile toward axonal regeneration, it is a natural response after injury. A bacterial enzyme was discovered 2002 with the capability of digesting chondroitin sulfate. In this pioneering work by Bradbury and colleagues, bacterial chondroitinase ABC (ChABC) was administered intrathecally following trauma to the posterior horn in adult rats (11). In this experiment, ChABC digested CSPG at the level of injury, thus reducing the scar formation (Table 34.6 and Fig. 34.8).

The enzyme acts like a molecular "machete" to reduce or eliminate the scar tissue barrier that mechanically and chemically counteracts nerve regeneration. The amount

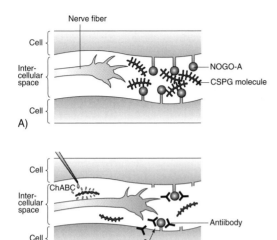

Figure 34.8 Chondroitinase ABC (ChABC) cleaves newly produced chondroitin sulfate proteoglycans, a major component in the induced scar tissue.

of regeneration-associated proteins was increased, and regeneration of afferent sensory axons as well as efferent corticospinal axons was supported. The synaptic activity was restored below the level of injury, and minor functional recovery in movement and proprioception was observed. These experiments have later been duplicated and we now await trials in a clinical setting.

Overcoming Late Inhibitory Mechanisms to Axonal Growth

The late inhibitory strategies start once scar formation has been established. In the late stage of an injury, the upper and lower stumps of the injured spinal cord are separated by a gap composed of scar tissue and/or liquid-filled cyst formation. Injured axons are unable to traverse this area and must be guided through or around it by biological or biosynthetic "bridges" or supportive structures, often used in combination with growth factors (Table 34.7). The term "filling the gap" is often used in the literature to describe different methods for bridging the mechanical obstacle created by scar formation and/or cysts.

Although supportive structures provide a permissive pathway for axonal elongation, the growing axons typically fail to reenter the spinal

cord above or below the lesion. Thus, supportive structures are only part of the solution to restore functional connections. A promising way to reach this objective is therefore to combine supportive "bridging" structures with cell replacement using transplantation from various forms of fetal tissue (Table 34.9), or more recently, stem cells (Table 34.10).

Supportive Structures

Supportive structures can promote axonal growth by serving as a scaffold for growth factors and/or as a substrate for growth-permissive interactions with regeneration axons (Tables 34.7, 34.9, 34.10). Since injured CNS axons are able to grow for extended distances in a transplanted peripheral nerve graft, peripheral nerve tissue or components of it are rational sources as growth supporting structures.

Peripheral Nerves. Of the numerous studies carried out with peripheral nerve grafts, the most remarkable results are those reported by Olson and Cheng (51). Intercostal nerve grafts were positioned to reach from gray to white matter in descending, as well as ascending directions between the stumps of a complete spinal cord transection. The graft was stabilized with fibrin glue, thus allowing the slow release of acidic fibroblast growth factor (aFGF) (Table 34.7). Axonal regrowth across the lesion site and recovery of hindlimb sensorimotor functions were demonstrated. Despite these promising results, the procedure has not been possible to implement in the clinical setting.

Schwann Cells. Since Schwann cells are the essential growth-promoting cellular element of peripheral nerve, a logical alternative to whole peripheral nerve tissue is to use isolated Schwann cells, or growth-promoting Schwann cell molecules, as guidance channels for injured spinal cord axons (Fig. 34.9).

Bunge and coworkers used "guidance channels" filled with Schwann cells and growth factors. They were able to demonstrate increased axonal growth and reduced secondary degeneration of axons, as well as functional recovery in animal models (Table 34.7; 74). The problems

TABLE 34.7 Strategies to overcome the late inhibitory mechanisms of the CNS environment –
            supportive structures.

Factor	Target	Delivery	Effect
Peripheral nerve + aFGF	Axotomized axons	Locally with glue	Structural and functional recovery
Schwann cells (SC) + Growth factors	Axotomized axons	Placement of SC transplants in guidance channels	Reduced secondary degeneration Functional improvement
Olfactory ensheathing glial cells (OEC)	Axotomized axons	Local deposition	Reduced secondary degeneration Functional improvement
Noncellular elements + stem cells	Cut axons Scar forming glia	Placement of stem cells in transplanted polymers	Improved tissue sparing Reduced scar formation Functional improvement
Erythropoietin (EPO)		Systemically	Retain neuroprotective properties
Rho	Actin cytoskeleton		Improves SCBF and locomotion
Activated macrophages		Injury epicenter	Improved motor function Reduces cyst formation

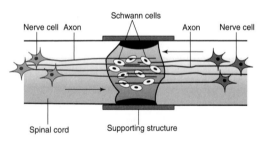

Figure 34.9 "Bridge" created by Schwann cells and extracellular matrix components provides a growth supportive substrate for injured axons.

when using Schwann cells is the hostile astrocytic reaction toward the Schwann cells in the damaged area, which decreases their ability to produce myelin.

Olfactory Ensheathing Cells. Olfactory ensheathing cells (OECs) have emerged as an attractive source for supportive structures (5). OECs envelop olfactory sensory axons along their way to the target neurons in the olfactory bulb. There is a continuous growth of axons into the olfactory bulb from newly formed olfactory sensory neurons in the olfactory mucosa. OECs are continuously

supporting this growth, and are fully integrated in the adult CNS, properties that make them interesting with regard to SCI repair (58). OECs release growth factors, as well as other growth promoting molecules, and are able to produce myelin around regenerated CNS axons (Table 34.7). Locally implanted OECs stimulate regrowth of damaged axons in the spinal cord, as well as growth of axons through areas with scar tissue formation. Furthermore, functional recovery of sensory and postural functions was observed. The mechanisms underlying functional improvement associated with transplantation of OECs are incompletely understood, but appear not only to be the result of their supportive and guiding properties, but also of their ability to promote synaptic plasticity (6). Furthermore, stem cells from the olfactory mucosa may be present in OEC transplants, and contribute to structural and functional repair (48). The capacity of OECs to fully integrate in the CNS environment and migrate through connective tissue makes them more favorable candidates than Schwann cells for supporting axonal regeneration within the injured spinal cord.

OECs can easily be harvested under local anaesthesia from the human olfactory mucosa, grown in vitro, and thereafter used for transplantation. Clinical trials with autologous transplantation of OECs into the spinal cord have been initiated in patients with chronic, complete spinal cord lesions in Brisbane, Australia. The technique and imaging results using magnetic resonance imaging (MRI) 1 year after transplantation have been reported (22).

Artificial Supportive Structures. Various artificial structures have been presented (49). As an example Schneider and colleagues (61) grafted a multicomponent polymer into the gap of the hemisected spinal cord (Fig. 34.10). The inner part of the polymer was filled with stem cells and the outer part contained a suitable substrate for axons to grow beyond the level of injury. Grafted animals showed better hindlimb functional recovery than did controls (Table 34.7).

Erythropoietin

Erythropoietin (EPO), the prime stimulator of erythroid progenitor cell proliferation, has

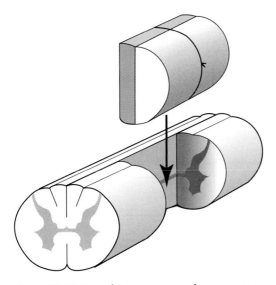

Figure 34.10 A multicomponent polymer system designed to fit into the cavity created by two spinal cord hemisections and the removal of the intercalated tissue.

been found to exert potent neuroprotective effects by diminishing lipid peroxidation and inflammation, as well as by counteracting apoptosis. The agent carbamyl erythropoietin (CEPO) retains neuroprotective properties without having hematopoietic potential. Administration of CEPO within the first 24 hours after experimental SCI reduces the neurological deficits compared to control (Table 34.7; 67).

Rho Pathway Antagonists

Rho is a GTPase-associated signalling protein that transduces extracellular signals to alterations in the actin cytoskeleton, thereby influencing cell motility (45). Injury to CNS axons induces increased Rho activity, which correlates with growth cone collapse and neurite retraction. The administration of Rho-associated kinase inhibitors such as C3 in the early period after SCI in rats promotes neurite extension, improves spinal cord blood flow, and results in improved locomotion (Table 34.7; 19). Currently, phase 1 and 2 multicenter studies are under way, using extradural administration of the Rho-associated kinase inhibitor cethrin during the first 2 weeks after injury.

Activated Autologous Macrophages

Activated macrophages are considered to play a significant role in the process of peripheral nerve regeneration, by efficient removal of myelin-associated inhibitors and the production and release of growth factors. CNS macrophages, in contrast, are significantly less activated, which may contribute to regeneration failure after SCI. Implantation of peripherally derived macrophages in the environment of the injured spinal cord has neuroprotective effects and stimulates axonal regeneration, thereby reducing spinal cord cyst formation and promoting recovery of motor function (Table 34.7; 33,64). ProCord consists of macrophages isolated from the patient's own blood and activated through a special procedure. Currently, a clinical phase 2 trial is ongoing in which ProCord is injected directly into the injury epicenter of the spinal cord within 14 days after injury.

Transplantation of Embryonic/Fetal Neural Tissue for Spinal Cord Repair

Embryonic/fetal neural tissue contains undifferentiated neurons with a potential to survive transplantation to the mature CNS, develop into mature neurons, and make functional synaptic connections in the host spinal cord. In addition, embryonic/fetal tissue contains stem cells and non-neuronal cells, which may provide trophic and substrate support for transplanted immature neurons, as well as for the injured neurons in the host spinal cord. Thus, transplantation of embryonic/fetal tissue has four prime objectives:

- To replace specific cells in order to restore lost functions
- To minimize neuronal degeneration and scar formation
- To promote regeneration and plasticity by providing a scaffold and trophic influence for axonal growth
- To serve as a "relay station" in which descending or ascending impulses can terminate and subsequently be transferred via axons from transplanted cells to neurons caudal/rostral to the lesion

Embryonic/fetal tissue has a number of properties that make it attractive in SCI treatment (Table 34.8). However, ethical aspects complicate the use of such tissue for experimental and clinical purposes. Different strategies have been used when transplanting embryonic/fetal tissue in experimental SCI studies (Table 34.9; 47).

Animal Tissue to Animal Recipients. Solid embryonic tissue transplanted to a liquid-filled cavity in the rubrospinal tract was found to counteract retrograde cell death of neurons within the red nucleus, probably due to a release of growth factors (Table 34.9). An increase in local reinnervation, as well as a functional recovery was seen after transplantation of embryonic brainstem tissue to a spinal cord segment below the level of injury.

Human Tissue to Animal Recipients. Human embryonic spinal cord tissue can survive, grow, differentiate, and become morphologically integrated

TABLE 34.8 Properties of embryonic tissue.

1	Rapid growth and cell division
2	Ability to develop to similar cells as in surrounding tissue
3	Less often rejected
4	Contain factors stimulating in-growth of vessels as well as a higher proportion of growth factors promoting survival when transplanted
5	Less sensitive to ischemia and thus able to survive in surroundings with lowered oxygen levels

TABLE 34.9 Strategies to overcome the late inhibitory mechanisms of the CNS environment – transplantation of embryonic/foetal tissue.

Factor	Target	Delivery	Effect
Solid embryonic/fetal tissue	Red nucleus axons	Transplantation to cavity	Rescue axotomized neurons
Brainstem fragments	Denervated terminal field	Injection	Local reinnervation Functional restitution
Solid embryonic/fetal tissue	Axotomized axons	Transplantation to cavity	Axonal elongation into and out of transplant
Human embryonic/ fetal tissue	Axotomized axons	Transplantation	Feasibility Cyst obliteration

following transplantation into the animal spinal cord. Human fetal tissue, including spinal cord tissue, harvested from early abortions (5–8 weeks) has been used to fill experimentally induced posttraumatic cavities, and these transplants were found to promote survival of injured neurons and axons, as well as to provide a bridge for axonal growth (Table 34.9; 79,80).

Human Tissue to Patients with SCI. Embryonic/fetal tissue has been used in humans in the treatment of Parkinson disease, diabetes, and leukemia, and in blindness due to macular degeneration. Given the observations that human embryonic/fetal tissue was able to counteract cyst expansion in experimental SCI, the question arose whether implanting such tissue into the posttraumatic cyst cavity in humans could counteract further cyst expansion in patients with posttraumatic syringomyelia. The transplant may consist of solid tissue or a suspension of cells (20,68,72). Injection of cell suspensions is associated with less injury to the surrounding tissue but solid transplants have the advantage of being harvested from older fetuses.

Experience of transplanting human embryonic/fetal tissue to patients with SCI has provided information on transplant survival, how the transplant fills the cavity, and whether rejection is provoked (Table 34.9). The final objective is that the embryonic/fetal tissue will integrate with the host spinal cord and provide structural and molecular support for cyst retraction. It is important to stress in this context that embryonic tissue transplant research today is not focused on functional recovery, but merely to study its feasibility in transplantation. This research has provoked heated ethical discussions, since the tissue is harvested from aborted foetuses.

Transplantation of Stem Cells for Spinal Cord Repair

Stem cell research has opened a new arena for regenerative science. Stem cells are the source of all cells in the organism and have the potential to differentiate to functionally competent cells of different types. They provide a repair system, and are theoretically able to divide without limitations and substitute other cells throughout an

individual's whole life. The first publication on isolation of neural stem cells was published in 1994 (46), and the first report on the use of stem cells in SCI was published in 1999 (43). In this study, embryonic stem cells from mice were injected into the damaged rat spinal cord, and the results indicated some functional recovery. The injected cells differentiated into neurons, oligodendrocytes, and astrocytes. The results proved that transplanted embryonic stem cells are able to survive and differentiate in the adult spinal cord. Stem cell research is the only field in which clear evidence has been demonstrated that cell therapy might repair damage within the CNS (40,54,69).

Embryonic Stem Cells. Embryonic stem cells are derived from in vitro fertilized eggs and thereafter donated to research with permission from the donor. Consequently, embryonic stem cells are not derived from eggs fertilized within the female body (Fig. 34.11A–C). Embryonic stem cells are obtained from the inner cells of a blastocyst, corresponding to a 4- or 5-day old fertilized egg, and thereafter transferred to a solution with special substrate. Embryonic stem cells kept in this solution without differentiation for 6 months are called pluripotent (Fig. 34.11A).

The term *pluripotent* is used to describe stem cells that are able to differentiate to cells representing all three embryonic layers: ecto-, meso- and endoderm. The neural stem cell is an example of a *multipotent* stem cell (Fig. 34.11B). When the cells in a culture are genetically identical and contain a normal set of chromosomes, they are called embryonic stem cells (Fig. 34.11A). When a cell line is established it can be stored frozen. New embryonic stem cell lines have continuously been produced. In 2001, it was reported that it was possible to control the differentiation of embryonic stem cell lines in vitro toward a certain type of cells. Thus, it is possible to isolate human embryonic stem cells from blastocysts, maintain these cells as pluripotent cells in vitro for extended periods of time, and possibly, control their differentiation to desired cell type(s). However, the risk of tumor formation by transplanted embryonic stem cells must be seriously considered (7,60).

In summary, embryonic stem cells:

- Are derived from the inner cells of the blastocyst
- Have possibilities to undergo an unlimited number of symmetrical divisions without differentiation over a long period of time
- Exhibit and keep a stable and full set of chromosomes
- Are undifferentiated and might generate differentiated types of cells to any of the three primary layers within the embryo
- Have the capacity to integrate in all kinds of fetal tissue that is under development
- Have clonogenic properties and can produce a colony of genetically identical cells

Adult Stem Cells. Adult stem cells are able to proliferate during long periods of time and generate identical copies without undergoing differentiation (Fig. 34.11C). In response to specific extrinsic factors, adult stem cells differentiate into functional cells that are appropriate for the surrounding tissue. Some adult stem cells even have the ability to differentiate into cells typical for other than the surrounding tissue although there is still no evidence that adult stem cells are pluripotent. This phenomenon—the ability to, within limits, transform into various cell types—is denoted *plasticity*.

Two fundamental strategies for the use of stem cells in the repair of nervous system diseases and trauma are used. First is the use of cells prepared in vitro with the ultimate aim of making them suitable for implantation in patients. Second is the use of growth factors and other molecules to stimulate a patient's own stem cells to repair the injury, by migrating to the injury and differentiating to the appropriate types of cells for that region. In reality, stem cell–mediated positive outcomes are likely to depend on complex mechanisms, as discussed earlier with regard to implantation of embryonic/fetal neurons. Thus, much of the morphological and functional improvements reported in experimental neural stem cell research on the injured or diseased nervous system may be the result of neuroprotective and/or neurotrophic mechanisms, rather than specific cell replacement (12).

Stem Cells for Reparation of Injured Spinal Cord. In conditions such as Parkinson disease, only one type of cell may need to be replaced, the dopamine producing cells, in order to achieve long-term alleviation of the symptoms. In a traumatically injured spinal cord, the repair procedure will be much more complex, as many different kinds of cells are affected and, hence, in need of being replaced. The primary aim of stem cell research is to restore/repair diseased white matter, often referred to as *partial repair of SCI* (Table 34.10).

The gray matter damage in SCI is of less interest since it only produces peripheral loss of function within the injured segments. The predominating functional defects following SCI are caused by interruption of axonal continuity and/or by focal demyelination as a result of oligodendrocyte degeneration (41). In both pathologies, the affected axons are unable to propagate impulses to their axon terminals. Experimentally, it has not yet been possible to achieve more than limited long-distance axonal regeneration of injured axons in the spinal cord. However, to repair a site of demyelination appears to be a more realistic goal. Therefore, the primary goal in the use of stem cells in SCI is to learn how to replace lost oligodendrocytes with cells that are able to

TABLE 34.10   Strategies to overcome the late inhibitory mechanisms of the CNS environment – transplantation of stem cells.

Factor	Target	Delivery	Effect
Neural stem cells + NT 3	Axotomized axons	Transplantation to cavity	Reconstitute cellular matrix Supporting axonal growth

make sufficient myelin for impulse propagation to resume.

McDonald and coworkers (41,42,44) used embryonic stem cells aimed at transplantation, and they initiated the cells to generate progenitor cells that differentiated to astrocytes, oligodendrocytes, and neurons. The neurons had inhibitory and excitatory properties, including the ability to form synapses. One million embryonic stem cells were injected into injured spinal cords in immunosuppressed rats. A large number of the cells died but some survived, and these cells were able to disperse in both directions within the spinal canal. Ten percent of the cells stayed in the injured area and differentiated to neurons. After transplantation, the animals showed improved motor function.

Aims of Stem Cell Research. An important goal for stem cell research is to learn how to

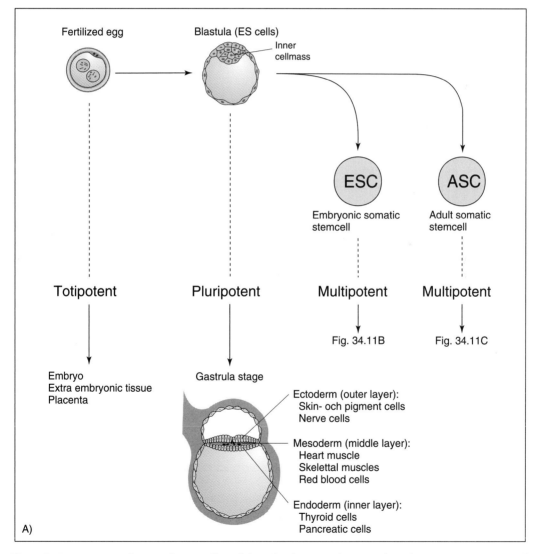

Figure 34.11 A: Principal types of stem cells and their developmental potential. With ongoing maturation of the embryo, stem cells become restricted in their developmental potential. B: Stem cells from the embryonic nervous system give rise to all intrinsic neural cells, except microglia. C: Stem cells from the adult nervous system.

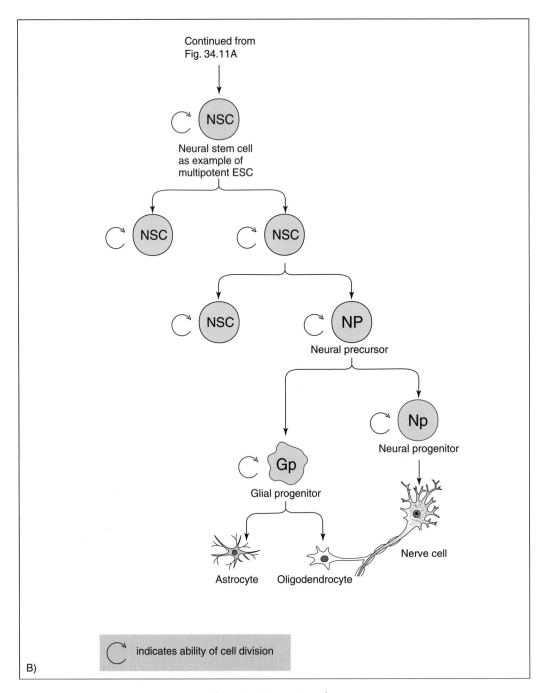

Figure 34.11 (continued).

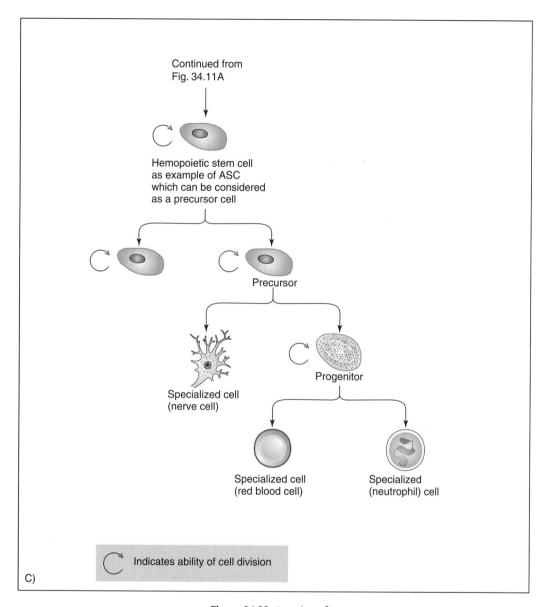

Figure 34.11 (continued).

control the differentiation of human pluripotent embryonic stem cells to a certain kind of cells, for example neurons. It is also important to learn how to identify these differentiated cells. By using growth factors or by changing the chemical composition of the surface that the cells are growing on, it is possible to stimulate stem cells to differentiate to neurons. Another method is to introduce new genes into the stem cell, so that they might differentiate into the cell type of interest.

Laboratory studies have shown that human embryonic stem cells are able to differentiate into different kinds of cells, such as cells that build vascular structures, as well as into neurons producing dopamine. However, it is still not known how stem cells are able to divide without differentiating to more specialized cell types and whether this is influenced by genetic changes. Nor is it known at which level of differentiation the human embryonic stem cells are optimal for transplantation.

Much research today is focused on the production of stem cells for use in transplantation of dopamine-producing cells in patients with Parkinson disease, β-cells in patients with diabetes mellitus, and heart muscle cells in patients with heart failure. However, in the near future embryonic stem cells will be used in SCI research, rather than in human therapy.

FUTURE CHALLENGES

In this chapter, selected examples of research on neuroprotection and neural regeneration pertinent for the search for new treatment strategies for SCI have been presented. The amount of knowledge regarding posttraumatic events following SCI has increased tremendously, particularly during the past three decades, but the challenge to cure paralysis still remains. The achievement of functional recovery in experimental models, although limited, raises hope for the future. The examples of research and development described here show very clearly that knowledge about the pathological processes is a prerequisite for future research and development, and hopefully, in a later stage, treatment options for SCI patients. No single therapy will encompass all the secondary injury mechanisms or increase the capability for regeneration of injured or transected axons. To achieve the goal of minimizing neurological deficits following SCI, several combined strategies must be used within the fields of neuroprotection and neural regeneration. The "golden" drug or treatment has not yet been developed, and new questions arise as soon as a new piece of knowledge is acquired.

Every additional increase in knowledge of SCI processes will be an important piece in the puzzle that frames the future development of new treatment strategies. Future challenges are based on further increased knowledge within every major field of SCI research, ranging from experimental basic science to pharmacological treatment and medical management. Our expectations also include improved diagnostic measures, such as MRI, that will further improve the therapeutic possibilities for patients.

There is a great need for combined treatment approaches to achieve additional functional improvement. In this chapter, strategies such as closing the gap within the injured spinal cord are discussed, but at the same time the necessity of closing the gap between researchers within various fields cannot be emphasized enough. To build bridges between scientists in the field of basic science and clinicians interested in research is a challenge in itself. The interpretation of new information of common interest demands good relations between these groups. The most important future challenge is to create a multidisciplinary approach to basic science and clinical management that enables all those who are interested in helping patients with SCI work together to test various hypothesis from a broad view.

Early treatment in the acute stage after SCI is advocated in most countries in the Western world today. Patients sustaining SCI are treated in intensive care units and submitted to early surgery in order to avoid unnecessary neurological deterioration and to establish early mobilization. This is, according to our opinion, an accepted and established treatment for the majority of these patients. But, additional questions arise, questions that must be answered through a multidisciplinary approach.

What actually is the importance of all secondary mechanisms in relation to future neurological deterioration, and could our knowledge about the secondary pathophysiological processes indicate the exact time for any eventual regeneration strategy?

Do the results of regeneration research implicate changes of the treatment protocol in the acute stage?

What is optimal tissue treatment in the acute stage, in order to facilitate regeneration? How do we optimize the chemical environment surrounding the nerve cells in order to maintain surviving nerve tissue in the acute stage in as good a condition as possible?

Is decompression of the dural sac and fixation of the spinal column in the acute stage sufficient to optimize the possibility for the spinal cord to recover? Should, if such is not the case, the dural sac be opened and the subarachnoid space be

CHAPTER 34 RESEARCH AND DEVELOPMENT **299**

exposed and flushed to eliminate blood accumulated subarachnoidally? Could such a therapeutic measure decrease or eliminate the inflammatory response and minimize the accumulation of proteoglycans and reduce the scar formation at the level of injury?

Is it meaningful to decompress and stabilize all patients, or will we, in the future, use fetal tissue, stem cells, OECs, or scaffold structures with or without neural growth factors in the acute stage as complementary treatments in some cases?

Should we delay surgical procedures until we artificially induce regeneration in a later stage and if so, when is the most appropriate time for this combined treatment?

Should a two-step surgical procedure be performed in the acute stage addressing both the compression of the spinal cord and the damage to the spinal cord itself.

Let us consider a hypothetical case of SCI at the cervical level due to a burst fracture compressing the spinal cord anteriorly. In the future, it may theoretically be possible to begin treatment with an anterior decompression of the dural sac followed by a stabilizing procedure. The patient is then rotated and placed in a prone position. The dural sac is exposed posteriorly following a laminectomy, after which it is opened through a midline incision to visualize the spinal cord. The spinal cord is probably covered with various blood products and inflammatory debris, and these products are eliminated through careful rinsing, since they are the prerequisites for scar formation (an obstacle to regeneration). Next, in our hypothetical future treated SCI patient, an artificial dura is applied in such a fashion that it counteracts the compression from posterior extradural blood. This is followed by the intradural infusion of factors that counteract scar formation and increase the speed of regeneration. This infusion cocktail includes neurotrophic growth factors, antibodies against NOGO-A receptors, 4-amino-pyridine, monoclonal antibodies against ICAM-1, and finally chondroitinase ABC. This infusion can start immediately after the application of the artificial dural sac or be administered percutaneously in conservatively treated patients. The treatment period is extended until the

estimated scar formation period, usually 2–6 weeks, ends. The inflammatory response is stopped by adding ILs, once we estimate that the injured area is cleared of damaged spinal cord tissue and debris.

Various scaffold structures are prepared during the infusion period, depending on the level and severity of injury. A second posterior approach is performed, and the artificial dural sac is opened. Scaffold structures are attached, along with Schwann cells, neurotrophic factors, stem cells, and possibly rolipram to act as a cAMP preserver. By using a special scaffold-like gel, these factors are gradually released. OECs could, in addition, be administered either through infusion or as a cell suspension (the infusion of a concentration of macrophages from the injured patient himself to counteract the inflammatory response is an exciting alternative now being tested clinically).

As our knowledge continues to increase in controversial fields such as stem cell and foetal tissue research, ethical and jurisdictional questions will have to be answered in parallel to medical questions. In the future, will it be possible to create stem cell or fetal tissue banks, or will purified adult stem cells harvested from the injured patient be used as replacement tissue for the spinal cord? Will it be possible to use such cells in the acute phase?

These speculations verge on medical science fiction; our current knowledge is not sufficient enough to give SCI patients the ultimate treatment of restoring neurological function, and the route to that goal is paved with controversy and disagreement. Our knowledge has, however, increased tremendously during the past three decades, and the hope is that continued work will eventually solve one of the most pressing of medical challenges in the treatment of SCI: the regeneration of damaged axons and the restoration of neurological function.

References

1. Andersson AJ. Mechanism and pathways of inflammatory responses in CNS trauma: spinal cord injury. *J Spinal Cord Med* 2002;25:70–79.
2. Ankeny DP, Popovich PG. Central nervous system and non-central nervous system antigen vaccines exacerbate neuropathology caused by nerve injury. *Eur J Neurosci* 2007;25:2053–2064.

3. Apuzzo ML, ed. Pharmacological therapy after spinal cord injury. *Neurosurgery* 2002;50(3 Suppl):S6–72.

4. Baptiste DC, Fehlings MG. Pharmacological approaches to repair the injured spinal cord. *Neurotrauma* 2006;23(3–4):318–324.

5. Barnett SC, Riddle JS. Olfactory ensheathing cells (OECs) and the treatment of CNS injury: advantages and possible caveats. *J Anat* 2004;204:57–67.

6. Barnett SC, Riddle JS. Olfactory ensheathing cell transplantation as a strategy for spinal cord repair–what can it achieve? *Nat Clin Pract Neurol* 2007;3:152–161.

7. Björklund LM, Sanchez-Pernaute R, Chung S, et al. Embryonic stem cells develop into functional dopaminergic neurons after transplantation in a Parkinson rat model. *Proc Natl Acad Sci USA* 2002;99:2344–2349.

8. Blits B, Bunge MB. Direct gene therapy for repair of the spinal cord. *J Neurotrauma* 2006;23:508–520.

9. Bracken MB, Shepard MJ, Collins WF, et al. Methylprednisolone or naloxone treatment after acute spinal cord injury: 1-year follow-up data. Results from the second National Acute Spinal Cord Injury Study. *J Neurosurg* 1992;76:23–31.

10. Bracken MB, Shepard MJ, Holford TR, et al. Administration of methylprednisolone for 24 or 48 hours or tirilazad mesylate for 48 hours in the treatment of acute spinal cord injury. Results of the Third National Acute Spinal Cord Injury Randomized Controlled Study. *JAMA* 1997;277:1597–1604.

11. Bradbury EB, Moon LD, Popat RJ. Chondroitinease ABC promotes functional recovery after spinal cord injury. *Nature* 2002;416:636–640.

12. Bradbury EJ, McMahon SB. Spinal cord repair strategies: why to they work? *Nature Rev Neurosci* 2006;7:644–653.

13. Brewer KL, Bethea JR, Yezierski RP. Neuroprotective effects of Interleukin-10 following excitotoxic spinal cord injury. *Exp Neurol* 1999;159:484–493.

14. Busch SA, Silver J. The role of extracellular matrix in CNS regeneration. *Curr Opin Neurobiol* 2002;17:120–127.

15. Cardenas DD, Ditunno J, Graziani V, et al. Phase 2 trial of sustained-release fampridine in chronic spinal cord injury. *Spinal Cord* 2007;45:158–168.

16. Chang HT. Subacute human spinal cord contusion: few lymphocytes and many macrophages. *Spinal Cord* 2007;45:174–182.

17. Chen MS, Huber AB, van der Haar ME, et al. Nogo-A is a myelin-associated neurite outgrowth inhibitor and an antigen for monoclonal antibody IN-1. *Nature* 2000;403:434–439.

18. David S, Aguayo AJ. Axonal elongation into peripheral nerves system "bridges" after central nervous system injury in adult rats. *Science* 1981;214:931–933.

19. Dergham P, Ellezam B, Essagian C. Rho signaling pathway targeted to promote spinal cord repair. *J Neurosci* 2002;22:6570–6577.

20. Falci S, Holtz A, Åkesson E, et al. Obliteration of posttraumatic spinal cord cyst with solid human embryonic spinal cord grafts; first clinical attempt. *J Neurotrauma* 1997;14:875–884.

21. Fawcett JW. The glial response to injury and its role in the inhibition of CNS repair. *Adv Exp Med Biol* 2006;557:11–24.

22. Feron F, Perry C, Cochrane J, et al. Autologous olfactory ensheating cell transplantation in human spinal cord injury. *Brain* 2005;128:2951–2960.

23. Flemming JC, Norenberg MD, Ramsay DA, et al. The cellular inflammatory response in human spinal cords after injury. *Brain* 2006;129:3249–3269.

24. Fournier AE, GrandPre T, Strittmatter SM. Identification of a receptor mediating Nogo-66 inhibition of axonal regeneration. *Nature* 2001;409:341–346.

25. Geisler FH, Coleman WP, Grieco G, Poonian D; Sygen Study Group. The Sygen multicenter acute spinal cord injury study. *Spine* 2001;26(24 Suppl):S87–98.

26. Gillespie LN. Regulation of axonal growth and guidance by the neurotrophin family of neurotrophic factors. *Clin Exp Pharmacol Physiol* 2003;30:724–733.

27. Hayes KC. The use of 4-aminopyridine (fampridine) in demyelinating disorders. *CNS Drug Rev* 2004;10:295–316.

28. Huang DW, McKerracher L, Braun PE, David S. A therapeutic vaccine approach to stimulate axon regeneration in the adult mammalian spinal cord. *Neuron* 1999;24:639–647.

29. Iannotti C, Ping Zhang Y, Shields CB, et al. A neuroprotective role of glial cell line-derived neurotrophic factor following moderate spinal cord contusion injury. *Exp Neurol* 2004;189:317–332.

30. Isaksson J, Farooque M, Holtz A. Expression of ICAM-1 and CD 11b after experimental spinal cord injury in rats. *J Neurotrauma* 1999;16:165–173.

31. Jones TB, Ankeny DP, Guan Z, et al. Passive or active immunization with myelin basic protein impairs neurological function and exacerbates neuropathology after spinal cord injury in rats. *J Neurosci* 2004;24:3752–3761.

32. Kirstein M, Farinas I. Sensing life: regulation of sensory neuron survival by neurotrophins. *Cell Mol Life Sci* 2002;59:1787–1802.

33. Knoller N, Auerbach G, Fulga V. Clinical experience using incubated autologous macrophages as a treatment for complete cervical spinal cord injury: phase I study results. *J Neurosurg Spine* 2005;3:173–181.

34. Kubasak MD, Hedlund E, Roy RR. L1 CAM expression is increased surrounding the lesion site in rats with complete spinal cord transection as neonates. *Exp Neurol* 2005;194:363–375.

35. Kwon BK, Tetzlaff W. Spinal cord regeneration. From gene to Transplants. *Spine* 2001; 26:13–22.

36. Li S, Liu BP, Budel S, et al. Blockade of Nogo-66, myelin-associated glycoprotein, and oligodendrocyte myelin glycoprotein by soluble Nogo-66 receptor

promotes axonal sprouting and recovery after spinal injury. *J Neurosci* 2004;24:10511–10520.

37. Lifshutz J, Colohan A. A brief history of therapy for traumatic spinal cord injury. *Neurosurg Focus* 2004;16 (1):1–8.

38. Lu P, Yang H, Jones LL, Fet al. Combinatorial therapy with neurotrophins and cAMP promotes axonal regeneration beyond sites of spinal cord injury. *J Neurosci* 2004;24:6402–6409.

39. Mabon PJ, Weaver LC, Dekaban GA. Inhibition of monocyte/macrophage migration to a spinal cord injury site by an antibody to the integrin alphaD: a potential new-anti-inflammatory treatment. *Exp Neurol* 200;166:52–64.

40. Martino G, Pluchino S. The therapeutic potential of neural stem cells. *Nature Rev Neurosci* 2006;7: 395–406.

41. McDonald JW, Liu XZ, Qu Y, et al. Transplanted embryonic stem cells survive, differentiate and promote recovery in injured rat spinal cord. *Nat Med* 1999;5:1410–1412.

42. McDonald JW, Becker D, Holekamp TF, et al. Repair of the injured spinal cord and the potential of embryonic stem cell transplantation. *J Neurotrauma* 2004; 21:383–393.

43. McDonald JW, Liu XZ, Qu Y, et al. Transplanted embryonic stem cells survive, differentiate and promote recovery in injured rat spinal cord. *Nat Med* 1999;5:1410–1412.

44. McDonald JW, Belegu V. Demyelination and remyelination after spinal cord injury. *J Neurotrauma* 2006;23:345–359.

45. McKerracher L, Higuchi H. Targeting RHO to stimulate repair after spinal cord injury. *J Neurotrauma* 2006;23:309–317.

46. Morshead CM, Reynolds BA, Craig CG, et al. Neural stem cells in the adult mammalian forebrain: a relatively quiescent subpopulation of subependymal cells. *Neuron* 1994;13:1071–1082.

47. Murray M. Cellular transplants: steps toward restoration of function in spinal injured animals. *Prog Brain Res* 2004;143:133–146.

48. Murrell W, Féron F, Wetzig A, et al. Multipotent stem cells from adult olfactory mucosa. *Dev Dyn* 2005;233:496–515.

49. Nomura H, Tator CH, Shoichet MS. Bioengineered strategies for spinal cord repair. *J Neurotrauma* 2006;23:496–507.

50. Novikova LN, Novikov LN, Kellerth JO. Differential effects of neurotrophins on neuronal survival and axonal regeneration after spinal cord injury in adult rats. *J Comp Neurol* 2002;452:255–263.

51. Olsson L, Cheng H, Zetterstrom RH, et al. On CNS repair and protection strategies: novel approaches with implications for spinal cord injury and Parkinson's disease. *Brain Res Rev* 1998;26:302–305.

52. Pearse DD, Pereira FC, Marcillo AE, et al. cAMP and Schwann cells promote axonal growth and functional recovery after spinal cord injury. *Nat Med* 2004;10:610–616.

53. Pezet S, McMahon SB. Neurotrophins: mediators and modulators of pain. *Annu Rev Neurosci* 2006;29:507–538.

54. Pfeiffer K, Vroemen M, Caioni M, et al. Autologous adult rodent neural progenitor cell transplantation represents a feasible strategy to promote structural repair in the chronically injured spinal cord. *Regen Med* 2006;1:255–266.

55. Plunet W, Kwon BK, Tetzlaff W. Promoting axonal regeneration in the central nervous system by enhancing the cell body response to axotomy. *J Neurosci Res* 2002;68:1–6.

56. Qiu J, Cai D, Dai H, et al. Spinal axon regeneration induced by elevation of cyclic AMP. *Neuron* 2002;34:895–903.

57. Raier PJ. Cellular transplantation strategies for spinal cord injury and translational neurobiology. *NeuroRx* 1(4):424–451.

58. Ramon-Cueto A, Santos-Benito FF. Cell therapy to repair injured spinal cord: olfactory ensheating glia transplantation. *Restor Neurol Neurosci* 2001;19:149–156.

59. Rice T, Larsen J, Rivest S, Yong VW. Characterisation of early inflammation after spinal cord injury in mice. *J Neuropathol Exp Neurol* 2007;66:184–195.

60. Riess P, Molcanyi M, Bentz K, et al. Embryonic stem cell transplantation after experimental traumatic brain injury dramatically improves neurological outcome, but may cause tumors. *J Neurotrauma* 2007;24:216–225.

61. Rochkind S, Shahar A, Fliss D, et al. Development of a tissue-engineered composite implant for treating traumatic paraplegia in rats. *Eur Spine J* 2006;15:234–245.

62. Schmitt AB, Breuer S, Liman J, et al. Identification of regeneration-associated genes after central and peripheral nerve injury in the adult rat. *BMC Neurosci* 2003;19:4:8.

63. Schwab ME. Nogo and axon regeneration. *Curr Opin Neurobiol* 2004;14:118–124.

64. Schwartz M, Yoles E. Immuno-based therapy for spinal cord repair: autologous macrophages and beyond. *J Neurotrauma* 2006;23:360–370.

65. Segal JL. Immunoactivation and altered intercellular communication mediate the pathophysiology of spinal cord injury. *Pharmacotherapy* 2005;25: 145–156.

66. Snider WD, Zhou FQ, Zhong J, Markus A. Signaling the pathway to regeneration. *Neuron* 2002;35:13–16.

67. Sonmez A, Kabakci B, Vardar E. Erythropoietin attenuates neuronal injury and potentiate the expression of pCREB in anterior horn after transient spinal cord ischemia in rats. *Surg Neurol* 2007;Mar 16 (Epub ahead of print).

68. Thompson FJ, Reier PJ, Uthman B, et al. Neurophysiological assessment of the feasibility and safety of neural tissue transplantation in

patients with syringomyelia. *J Neurotrauma* 2001;18:931–945.

69. Thuret S, Moon LDF, Gage FH. Therapeutic interventions after spinal cord injury. *Nature Rev Neurosci* 2006;7:628–643.

70. Vaccaro AR, Daugherty RJ, Sheehan TP, et al. Neurological outcome of early versus late surgery for cervical spinal cord injury. *Spine* 1997;Nov 22:2609–2613.

71. Wilkins RH Neurosurgical classic: XVII Edwin Smith Surgical Papyrus. *Neurosurgery* 2004;March:240–244.

72. Wirth ED 3rd, Reier PJ, Fessler RG, et al. Feasibility and safety of neural tissue transplantation in patients with syringomyelia. *J Neurotrauma* 2001;18:911–029.

73. Xu G, Nie DY, Chen JT, et al. Recombinant DNA vaccine encoding multiple domains related to inhibition of neurite outgrowth: a potential strategy for axonal regeneration. *J Neurochem* 2004;91:1018–1023.

74. Xu XM, Chen A, Guenard V, Kleitman N, Bunge MB. Bridging Schwann cell transplants promote regeneration from both the rostral and caudal stumps of transected adult spinal cord. *J Neurocytol* 1997;26:1–16.

75. Yamashita T, Fujitani M, Yamagishi S, et al. Multiple signals regulate axon regeneration through the nogo receptor complex. *Mol Neurobiol* 2005;32:105–111.

76. Yiu G, He S. Glial inhibition of CNS axon regeneration. Nature Rev Neurosci 2006;7:617–627.

77. Zhang Y, Roslan R, Lang D. Expression of CHL1 and L1 by neurons and glia following sciatic nerve and dorsal root injury. Moll Cell Neuroscience 2000;16:71–86.

78. Zhou FQ, Snider WD. Intracellular control of developmental and regenerative axon growth. *Philos Trans R Soc Lond B Biol Sci* 2006;361:1575–1592.

79. Åkesson E, Kjaeldgaard A, Seiger A. Human embryonic spinal cord graft in adult rat spinal cord cavities; survival, growth, and interactions with the host. *Exp Neurol* 1998;149:262–276.

80. Åkesson E, Holmberg L, Jonhagen ME, et al. Solid human embryonic spinal cord xenografts in acute and chronic spinal cord cavities: a morphological and functional study. *Exp Neurol* 2001;170:305–16.

Index

Note: Page numbers followed by f and t denote figures and tables, respectively.